Madness and the Demand for Recognition

International Perspectives in Philosophy and Psychiatry

Series editors: Bill (K.W.M.) Fulford, Lisa Bortolotti, Matthew Broome, Katherine Morris, John Z. Sadler, and Giovanni Stanghellini

Madness and the Demand for Recognition

A philosophical inquiry into identity and mental health activism

Mohammed Abouelleil Rashed

Wellcome Trust ISSF Research Fellow,
Department of Philosophy,
Birkbeck College, University of London,
United Kingdom;
Visiting Lecturer,
Department of Philosophy,
King's College London,
United Kingdom

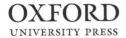

OXFORD
UNIVERSITY PRESS

OXFORD
UNIVERSITY PRESS

Great Clarendon Street, Oxford, OX2 6DP,
United Kingdom

Oxford University Press is a department of the University of Oxford.
It furthers the University's objective of excellence in research, scholarship,
and education by publishing worldwide. Oxford is a registered trade mark of
Oxford University Press in the UK and in certain other countries

© Oxford University Press 2019

The moral rights of the author have been asserted

First Edition published in 2019

Impression: 1

Published in the United States of America by Oxford University Press
198 Madison Avenue, New York, NY 10016, United States of America

British Library Cataloguing in Publication Data

Data available

Library of Congress Control Number: 2018949669

ISBN 978–0–19–878686–3

Printed in Great Britain by
Ashford Colour Press Ltd, Gosport, Hampshire

For Rachel

And the moments when I'd been soaring with eyes full of horizon and a heart branded like a contour map with the outlines of rocky sunrises and the fractal branching of so many threads of understanding . . . these seemed like the most important moments of my life. I didn't want to chalk them up to pathology, give them ugly labels like mania and delusion that seemed to invalidate them, make them less real. I didn't want to eradicate them all for the sake of "stability" . . . Yet as much as I resisted their words, they were all I could find, and over and over again these incredibly limited, awkward words seemed like the barest blueprints to my soul.

Jacks Ashley McNamara,
artist and activist

Thou only hast taught me that I have a heart—thou only hast thrown a light deep downward, and upward, into my soul. Thou only hast revealed me to myself; for without thy aid, my best knowledge of myself would have been merely to know my own shadow—to watch it flickering on the wall, and mistake its fantasies for my own real actions.

Nathaniel Hawthorne, a letter to Sophia Peabody
October 4, 1840, ½ past 10 A.M.

Foreword

Honored with the task of introducing this exemplary volume—an important book, at a critical time—I want to begin by placing Mohammed Rashed's project within its historical and disciplinary context, before drawing attention to some of its most notable, and admirable, qualities.

Mental health and ill health intersect with a host of traditional philosophical concerns—reductionism, agency, responsibility, knowledge, belief, rationality, and self-identity, to name a few—and since the last quarter of the twentieth century, philosophical attention has been drawn to the ways mental disorder confounds, and illuminates, these and allied concepts. By the 1980s and 1990s, philosophy and mental health, or as it was more often known in the United States, the philosophy of psychiatry, emerged as a distinguishable research area within academic philosophy, affording focused conferences and associations, specialized monographs and collections in scholarly presses, and a widely respected scholarly journal.

From the start, the new research field was eclectic, notably broad in its interests and methods, and contentious. Unlike many medical conditions, mental disorders are rarely (or arguably, never) a-symptomatic. Nor, thus far, can they be verified independently of first person symptom-descriptions. And this distinctive epistemic feature has fostered involvement with phenomenological ideas inherited from thinkers such as Husserl, Heidegger, Jaspers, and Merleau-Ponty. Within psychology during these decades, in addition, a functionalist cognitivism and neuroscience, agreeable to philosophical language and presuppositions, came to replace behaviorism. Beyond these very general trends, the subareas of philosophy registered particular challenges posed by psychopathology. Philosophers of science have refined their conceptions of kinds through a consideration of mental diseases, for example. The treatment and care of the mentally ill have attracted the attention of bioethics. Those analyzing agency recognized the puzzles raised by addiction. And traditional analyses were required to acknowledge the anomalous epistemology of delusions. Disagreement here has always been wide, and deep. Undertaken alongside an increasingly biological and reductionist medical psychiatry and neuroscience, much of this work accepts, or makes peace with, the diagnostic categories and methodological presuppositions of models employed by medicine, where those with mental disorder are construed as blameless victims of misfortune, indistinguishable from people disabled by other forms of ill health, and as dependent on their medicines as the diabetic on her insulin. Irreconcilably contrary, meanwhile, were the antipsychiatry claims of Szasz, Laing, Foucault, and the feminists. Mental illness was not an illness at all; medical psychiatry was an organized, predatory force, to be resisted.

Concurrent with such theoretical inquietude during those decades, radical, real-world changes were taking place. The effects of the 1970s mental patients' rights movement (along with other factors) had emptied the asylums. Psychopharmacology increasingly rendered physical restraints unnecessary and, at least in the eyes of many, left long-term psychotherapy otiose. In the clinic, appeal to psychoanalytic and psychodynamic ideas was being replaced by evidence-based psychiatry. And, as Mohammed Rashed documents in his opening chapter, the power of collective political action was making itself felt by those sharing what is today politely termed a "mental health history."

In all the otherwise eclectic, wide-reaching, and take-no-prisoners theoretical discussion, little philosophical attention was given to the words of consumers, survivors, and users, or to the rhetoric emerging from political interest groups formed by those subject to psychiatric diagnoses and treatment. Following Descartes' infamous remarks in the First Meditation, these voices were assigned the epistemic role of incomprehensible ravings, when not entirely ignored. Even as first person accounts of the experience of disorder were increasingly acknowledged to be an indispensable resource, and long after mental health services had begun to include consumers and service users in advisory roles, this more politically toned rhetoric was side-lined, and largely neglected in academic and theoretical research—within psychiatry, as we can perhaps more readily expect and understand, but also within the Philosophy of Psychiatry and of Mental Health.

In light of such neglect by others theorizing about mental disorder, that Mohammed Rashed has chosen to consider the claims arising from these consumer and user movements, is itself noteworthy. Equally noteworthy is that among the diverse range of claims arising from these movements, he has chosen to focus on the most radical version: not the request for less stigmatizing language; not the polite call for a seat at the table ("nothing about us without us"), or claims of authority derived from first-hand experience of symptoms; not the indignant complaint expressed by "survivors" of the mental health treatment that injustice has been done, and their semantic authority nullified; not the request for equality of mental with other disabilities, or the call for even-handed consideration of neuro-atypical and neuro-typical traits. Rashed's particular, and particularly confronting focus is on the credo that madness is an identity, arising from its own distinctive culture, and worthy of full political and interpersonal recognition. In the "mad and proud" attitude of what is here named mad-positive activism, madness is an attribution from which to draw strength, comfort, and self-definition.

This decision is part philosophical and part historical: Mad Pride is both the latest wave of activism, as Rashed points out, but also the one that makes the most serious demand on social norms and understandings. In addition, I would add, it evokes a Western cultural preoccupation. That amidst all the suffering, compromised practical and emotional functioning, and cruelly discriminatory treatment, madness has a compensating, glamorous aspect, is a long-recognized link, and one not lost on mad-positive activists, with their talk of "dangerous gifts." The haunting question from the pseudo-Aristotelian Problems (Why is it that all brilliant men suffer from melancholia?) reoccurs through the ages: through Galen, Ficino, Shakespeare, Burton, and the Romantics, to the early twentieth century. (Even Freud, the aspiring scientist, assigns to the melancholic "a keener eye for the truth.") Bespeaking the spare normative economy of the eighteenth century, these once-valued compensations have today been demoted—what is glamor, compared to pain and uselessness? Art and culture may be served by rare cases of manic inspiration; but overall, mental disorder must be judged to possess unmitigated disutility, both in the suffering it brings (or portends), and in its aggregative effects on productivity. The link to creative energy, exuberance, and profundity of thought and feeling, has been largely severed. (In a cynical exception, drug companies list the mad geniuses of the past to enhance sales of antidepressants.) As well as taking on the most philosophically challenging and current of these activist viewpoints, then, the following work serves to remind us of themes from our cultural past that have been all but eclipsed by modernity.

Approaching this set of ideas with meticulous care, Rashed explores, dissects, explicates, and interpolates the claims of mad activism, exposing their theoretical implications, and allowing us to see their philosophical force. As well as situating them within mainstream philosophical research on mental disorder, he relates them to a body of theory that had not previously thought to examine them, Hegelian descendants from the social theory of thinkers like Honneth, and Taylor. And he subjects the whole to a thorough and respectful critique that is an exemplary model for how theorizing about mental disorder ought to be undertaken. *Madness and the Demand for Recognition* is, I believe, of the utmost importance to research developments in the philosophy of mental health and psychiatry. In the current era of identity politics, it shows the way through to a more complete and comprehensive application of philosophy to both medical science and real-world political culture.

Defining, understanding, and critically assessing Mad Pride, the following pages show, is a complex endeavor. The nature of recognition; the casual equation of identity with culture; the claimed analogies linking contemporary pride, and disabilities rights movements; the interlocking aspects of identity formation and capacity, and the place of self constructs in relation to these; and the value and scope of the "cultural adjustments" that go beyond prevailing medical conceptions of disorder each demand patient, nuanced analysis, and theory-informed interpretation. There are no easy answers here, and Rashed offers none. Yet he has given us a discussion that is fair, compelling, intelligent, and sympathetic. He also provides a detailed way forward, identifying what could work, and what can and should be done—a burden, he shows, that falls as much, or more, on the broader society, as on those who would forge mad identities for themselves. Those identifying as mad could not hope for better philosophical treatment, nor for a fairer and more useful analysis of, in his words, how to reconcile madness and society, in light of the polarities that have made Mad Pride a fiercely contested idea.

Jennifer Radden
Emerita Professor of Philosophy,
University of Massachusetts, Boston

Preface

I find it telling that the concept of mental illness tends to be applied to individuals and not communities. We have seen attempts to apply it to groups of people, to character-ize some societies as "sick" or "deluded" by virtue of their barbaric practices and ideo-logical commitments. But such claims can only be taken metaphorically, the power of the metaphor deriving from the meaning of these terms in the individual case. In psychiatric practice, one person can be deluded, two persons can be deluded—perhaps even three—but at a certain increment of numbers we no longer find it appropriate to continue using these concepts: we talk, instead, of cultural and ideological differences. Why is this so? There is no doubt that being part of a group protects, and doubly so. It offers a context of mutual affirmation of one's experiences and convictions. And, from the outside, it proves that the persons involved in this group, irrespective of what we think of their beliefs and practices, are capable of forming a community; they possess the capacity for sociality, a capacity whose absence is often considered the hallmark of certain mental health conditions. If the group protects, how is society to respond to attempts within mental health activism to form communities, to transform the mean-ing of conditions typically considered to be mental disorders, to present madness as grounds for culture and identity, and to demand recognition of the validity and value of Mad culture and Mad identity: How is society to respond to Mad Pride and mad-positive activism? I wrote this book to attempt to address this question.

When I began to consider an answer to this question, I was struck by the complex-ity and range of the issues that I had to engage with in order to be able to address it satisfactorily. To begin with, there is the need to come to an understanding of the claims and demands of Mad Pride and mad-positive activism (Mad activism), and to place them in relation to past and current approaches in mental health advocacy and activism. Then there is the problem of how to reconcile the view of madness as a disorder (or a dysfunction or an illness) of the mind—as a set of phenomena that cause significant distress and disability—with the view that madness can be grounds for culture and identity. Then there is the presentation of the demand as a demand for *recognition*, which immediately raises thorny philosophical issues concerning the meaning of recognition, why recognition matters, the justification and adjudication of demands for recognition, and the various ways in which society can respond to them. Beyond all this, there is the challenge of reconciling madness—often assumed to mani-fest in various impairments in identity formation—with the understanding of identity presupposed by the theory of recognition. And, finally, there remains the question that began this cascade of concerns: How should society respond to Mad activism's demand for recognition?

The range of issues just outlined meant that I had to venture into academic dis-ciplines and philosophical traditions and concerns that have not been sufficiently recognized in the philosophy and psychiatry literature. The resurgence of philosophical interest in psychiatry and mental health since the mid-1980s has been associated with a distinctive set of important concerns that include: the definition of the concept of mental disorder; the boundaries of illness; the philosophical phenomenology of the various mental health conditions; issues in philosophy of science such as causality, explanation, and classification; ethical issues in psychiatric practice; intersubjectivity and empathy in the clinical encounter and in specific mental health conditions. This book draws upon these research fields as required and, in addition, upon the following literatures: the activist literature, Mad studies and Disability studies literatures, and philosophical literature on the concepts, theories, and politics of identity and recognition. The latter, in particular, is notable by its relative absence in philosophy and psychiatry. I am referring here to a tradition of philosophical thought on recognition, freedom, and identity that finds its roots in the work of Georg Hegel and Immanuel Kant, and continues in the present day through the work of Charles Taylor and Axel Honneth, with alternative perspectives by Nancy Fraser, Kwame Appiah, and Richard Rorty, among others. By engaging with this literature, I developed in Part II a theoretical framework for thinking through the complex issues noted earlier and addressed in Parts III and IV of the book. In addition, I hope to have provided a formulation of identity and recognition that can be helpful for philosophers and social theorists grappling with other problems in mental health and psychiatry and with social movements in general.

It is common to refer to every current wave of activism as the final frontier in social change. I would not use that phrase, not only because it has so often been misused, but because there is no telling how far society can and will change, or what the next set of social shortcomings and accompanying demands for redress are going to be. But one thing I have no illusions about in writing this book is that the topic it deals with is controversial. Constructions such as Mad Pride and Mad identity tend to evoke passionate reactions, ranging from unconditional acceptance of such constructions to accusations that they are oxymoronic and incoherent. Partisan responses of this kind tend to characterize controversial issues in general; we have seen them and continue to do so in many of the pressing social issues of our time such as climate change and gay marriage. People tend to fall on one side or other of the issue, which limits the possibility of rational assessment and debate. In the domain of mental health, we see this today in the so-called diagnosis wars carried out on social media, and most clearly illustrated on Twitter. Psychiatrists and critical psychologists are pitted against each other, constantly arguing past each other, with one side seeing psychiatric diagnosis as a helpful or indispensable tool for providing mental healthcare, and the other side seeing it as an artificial construction that prevents mental health practitioners from understanding the social and political origins of mental distress. Mad activism is too important and far-reaching to be stuck in a similar closed circle of partisan commitments. It would be foolish to suggest that a book can provide a solution for this problem, but I hope that it manages to provide a philosophical framework for reconciling skeptics and supporters of Mad activism or, at least, to clarify their genuine loci of disagreement.

Accordingly, in some respects, I see my role as one of mediator, and I bring to this role various aspects of my experience and learning. In my philosophical training I spent much time thinking about the concept of mental disorder, the boundaries of illness, and the phenomenology of the conditions referred to in psychiatry as schizophrenia and bipolar disorder. Before moving on to fulltime research, I trained in psychiatry in London on the Guy's, King's College, and St. Thomas' hospitals training scheme. I worked for a few years on acute inpatient units, rehabilitation units, and outpatient clinics. I witnessed the immense suffering and the cognitive and emotional challenges associated with the various conditions that doctors treat. On the other hand, I was aware that there was something fundamentally lacking in the rather austere, limited language of clinical psychiatry, and its one-size-fits-all approach. It did not describe my experience of the world, or that of many others. In my research I began thinking about alternative approaches to psychiatry, and I conducted an ethnographic study of a community in the Dakhla Oasis of Egypt where there was no mental health provision. I experienced an alternative cultural system where people understood and managed the range of mental health phenomena through entirely different narratives and social structures of healing and support. I was able to see the benefits and drawbacks of such systems. My experience as an ethnographer is key to how I view the endeavors of Mad activism, which I regard as attempts to broaden the cultural repertoire as it pertains to madness beyond medical and psychological models of illness, an issue that I address in Part IV. My intention throughout this book has been to engage fairly and respectfully with the claims and demands of Mad activism. Mental health is something that concerns all of us, and creating a society where there is a diversity of narratives in which people can find themselves is an important aim. In this respect, reconciling madness and society is a worthwhile goal, and I hope this book contributes toward that goal.

Mohammed Abouelleil Rashed
London, January 2018

Acknowledgments

I began working on this book in 2013, but the ideas and experiences that led me to think about the issues in its pages go further back. In those years I have been influenced and inspired by far too many people to be able to mention them all here. I must begin by thanking the generous people who had shared their stories with me during my time as a clinician in London and as an ethnographer in the Dakhla Oasis of Egypt.

Special thanks to Derek Bolton and Werdie van Staden for their mentorship and friendship. I have learnt a lot from their knowledge of philosophy and psychiatry and from their wisdom—their keen sense of what is distinctive about our field and why it matters. Our discussions and collaborations along the years have certainly shaped my intellectual views and commitments.

Parts of this research were carried out while I was a research fellow at three institutions: the Institute of Advanced Studies (IAS) at University College London; the Division of Philosophy and Ethics of Mental Health at the University of Pretoria; the Department of Philosophy at Birkbeck College, University of London. I am grateful to my colleagues at these institutions for their engagement with, and feedback on, various presentations of my work. In particular, I would like to thank Tamar Garb, director of the IAS, for the stimulating research environment she had created at the Institute and for the opportunity to be part of it. I am also grateful to James Wilson for his guidance and support during my time at the IAS. Since 2008 I have been a member of a philosophy of psychiatry group composed of King's College London alumni. On many occasions, I have had the opportunity to present my research and to discuss ideas with the group. Thank you for your valuable feedback. I would like to thank Werdie van Staden, Derek Bolton, and Rachel Bingham for reading and commenting upon parts of the manuscript. Special thanks to Chetan Kuloor and Amr Shalaby—they know why.

As the coming pages attest, I have been hugely influenced by the rigorous and subtle philosophical work of Jennifer Radden. Her writings on identity and mental health have been key to my understanding of these issues. I am greatly honored to have her introduce my book. Another obvious debt is to Charles Taylor, for it was on reading his essay "The Politics of Recognition" several years ago, that I acquired an entirely new perspective for thinking about mental health, madness, and society.

Thank you to Charlotte Holloway of Oxford University Press for her impeccable editorial assistance, and for remaining supportive throughout the whole process.

I have worked on this book at various locations. The bulk of the research and the writing were accomplished mostly in London but also in Pretoria and Cairo. In July 2017 I spent two weeks in Alexandria that saw me through a particularly challenging stage in the book; I found patience and, ultimately, inspiration in the city's coffeehouses by the Mediterranean. In December 2014 I spent one week in Coffee Bay during South Africa's bright summer. It was during my morning walks by the Indian ocean of the Wild Coast that the concept of the book as a whole finally came together.

I am grateful to my parents Nadia Abdelaziz and Mahmoud Abouelleil, and to my daughter Adele, for their encouragement and support. Finally, this book would not have happened without the philosophical acuity and moral support of my partner Rachel Bingham. Her influence on my thinking and my work has been profound.

Source Acknowledgments

Grateful acknowledgment is made to the authors and publishers of copyright material which appears in this book, and in particular to the following for permission to reprint material from the sources indicated:

The Guardian: extracts from Rachel Dolezal: "I wasn't identifying as black to upset people. I was being me," December 13, 2015, Copyright Guardian News & Media Ltd 2018.

Jacks McNamara: extract from *Navigating the Space between Brilliance and Madness: a Reader and Roadmap of Bipolar Worlds*, The Icarus Project, www.theicarusproject.net.

Ohio State University Press: extract from Joel Myerson: *Selected Letters of Nathaniel Hawthorne* (OSU Press 2002).

Ken Paul Rosenthal: quotations from the documentary *Crooked Beauty* (2010), the first movie in the *Mad Dance Mental Health Film Trilogy*, www.kenpaulrosenthal.com.

Contents

Introduction

Madness is a complex and contested term. Through time and across cultures it has acquired many formulations: for some people madness is synonymous with unreason and violence, for others with creativity and subversion, for others it is associated with spirits and spirituality. Among the different formulations, there is one in particular that has taken hold so deeply and systematically that it has become the default view in many communities around the world: the idea that madness is a disorder (or a dysfunction or an illness) of the mind. Medical interest in madness is not new—it stretches back, at least, to Ancient Greece—but medical dominance over madness can be traced back to the late nineteenth century. We encounter madness after more than a century and a half of sustained medicalization; the subsuming of madness under scientific (medical and psychological) idioms and their associated practices. According to the dominant view today, madness—or as it would be classified in terms of the various subtypes of schizophrenia, bipolar disorder, and psychosis—is a disorder of the mind caused by the interaction of multiple factors that include the biological, psychological, and social. It is a view that has taken significant hold on the cultural imagination, supplanting alternative views. It has become fundamental to healthcare planning and funding at the governmental level. It delineates the aims of local and global research programs concerning the causes of mental disorders and the interventions that can alleviate disorder. Yet the dominance of this view is being challenged within certain strands of mental health activism.

Dissatisfaction with the treatment of individuals considered to be "mad," "insane," or "mentally ill" goes back a long way, but the 1970s are generally regarded as the starting point of a distinctive wave of activism that persists to this day.[1] In the wake of the efforts of black, gay, and women's civil rights movements, a number of broadly connected mental health ex-patients movements began organizing for the civil rights of users and survivors of psychiatric treatment and for reform of mental health institutions. In time, the mental health consumer/survivor/ex-patient (c/s/x) movements grew and diversified and today various discourses and initiatives can be identified: in addition to long-standing concerns with coercive interventions, lack of involvement in recovery, limited access to treatment, and social stigma and discrimination, some activists have resisted the medicalization of madness. Mad Pride and mad-positive

---

[1] A note on the use of scare quotes, which are quotation marks placed around terms whose meaning or legitimacy are contested. Many of the key terms used in this book are contested, for example: madness, mad, schizophrenia, bipolar disorder, mental disorder, and mental illness. To use scare quotes every time one of these terms is mentioned would result in numerous instances on every page; it would be unwieldy and distracting. Accordingly, I only use scare quotes in two situations: where the emphasis in the usage of a term is the fact that it is contested, and to indicate that I am referring to a concept.

activism (henceforth Mad activism) seeks to counteract discrimination by rejecting the language of "mental illness," "disease," and "disorder." Activists reclaim the term "mad," reverse its negative connotations, and present madness as grounds for culture and identity.

A key difference between Mad activism and treatment-focused/service-improvement endeavors is the former's formulation of the problem as one to do with respect and recognition. What is at stake is the entire way in which people's identities are publicly represented and valued, with the dominant, reductive view of madness as a disorder of the mind being seen as an affront to a positive identity. The goal is not so much to reform psychiatry (though that also is on the agenda) but to effect cultural change in the way madness is viewed. In this respect, the aims of Mad activism overlap with those of other movements that organize around issues of identity and recognition. In the domain of sexual orientation and gender, for example, Gay rights and Trans rights are not only concerned with countering discrimination in employment opportunities, for instance, but with achieving symbolic and cultural reparation in the wider society. A key aim is for being gay or being transgender to be viewed as a valid way-of-life, and for individuals to develop positive identities that society would recognize and reflect back to them as such. In those terms, gay individuals in some parts of the world have been able to achieve some redress, while recognition of transgender identities is being worked-out at present. In contrast, madness and Mad individuals lag behind, with professional and social views dominated by a cluster of terms emphasizing deficit and disorder. Mad activism is trying to change this, and it is this radical and, potentially, far-reaching activism that is the focus of this book. What are the claims and demands of Mad activism?

A review of Mad activism (Chapter 1) shows that dissatisfaction with the dominant view of madness can be formulated into a claim and a demand:

- The claim: Madness is grounds for culture and identity
- The demand: Society should recognize the validity and worth of Mad culture and Mad identity

This book is an examination of this claim and of the demand for recognition. Before I can present an outline of the overall methodology and argument, we must contend at this early point in the exposition with two kinds of response that we may encounter: skeptical and supportive. Both responses do not see the point of conducting the examination attempted in this book. Skeptics unconditionally reject the claims and demands of Mad activism, while supporters unconditionally accept them. Skeptics can make several arguments, all of which rely upon a version of the view that madness is a disorder (or a dysfunction or an illness) of the mind, along with the idea that this view implies falsity of the claim that madness can be grounds for culture and identity—skeptics essentially respond to Mad activism's objections to this view by insisting on that view. That, of course, is not a reasonable way to address a political demand. Skeptics who are mental health clinicians may respond in this way because they do not consider the claims of Mad activism to be about the individuals they see in the clinic and on acute wards, rehabilitation units, and psychiatric intensive care units. These individuals, the skeptics can point out, are too unwell for the claims of this movement to apply to them: they are unable to function in the most basic of ways let alone make political demands and construct culture and identity. Other skeptics can be patients/clients who understand their experiences and situation in terms of medical concepts; Mad activism does not speak to them for they consider themselves to be ill. Aside from the clinic, skeptics among the academic and the nonacademic public may view Mad activism with interest yet suspicion that there is something oxymoronic, if not dishonest, about constructions such as Mad Pride or Mad identity: madness, they could point out, is essentially negative and associated with illness and irrationality; whence the positive conceptions?

Underlying the skeptic's unconditional rejection of Mad activism is an unjustified generalization. Skeptics take the view of madness that fits their experiences (and, in some cases, their prejudices) to be the paradigm case. They then generalize from this to all of madness. But we must not take one view as constituting all we can think and know about madness: such a move, as we know all too well, is at the heart of various forms of discrimination in society such as those based on race or gender. Madness is not one thing, and neither are people's hopes about what they want to achieve through activism, or even if they can or want to take part in activism. Throughout the history of the Gay rights movement, there were individuals in society who wanted to be "cured" of homosexuality; it was and remains wrong to take such individuals as evidence that Gay activism was/is misguided. Similarly, the fact that some individuals wish to medically frame and treat their experiences, or may appear to lack capacity for certain decisions, should not be taken as evidence that Mad activism is oxymoronic. Does that mean that Mad activism can only speak for a limited number of individuals, those who are already making the demand for recognition? As a starting point, yes. But what the activists are trying to achieve can have repercussions that go far beyond the activism itself: through their efforts to render intelligible and to popularize a number of alternative narratives of psychological, experiential, and emotional diversity, Mad activists are playing a key role in broadening our cultural repertoire as it pertains to madness. In these efforts, many stand to benefit, as I argue in Chapters 9 and 10.

In contrast to skeptics, supporters unconditionally accept the claims and demands of Mad activism. For them, there is nothing to examine, just a lot of work to do to question the dominant view of madness and to achieve symbolic and cultural change in society. That, indeed, may be the position we arrive to at the end, but we have to *arrive* there: we cannot assume it at the outset and this is for a number of reasons. We owe it to Mad activists to take their claims and demands seriously, which requires engagement with these views in a process whose outcome cannot be prejudged; anything less would undermine the value and sincerity of the position we hold. We owe it to the skeptics to demonstrate to them the validity of the claims and demands, the importance of what Mad activism is trying to achieve, and how these achievements can be relevant to the skeptics themselves. We owe it to society in general to get right our recommendations on the direction of moral and social change. If the claims of Mad activism lack coherence, and if the demands lack normative force, then they should not command our sense of obligation. Yet to establish this we need to examine those claims and demands: we need to get it right.

Neither unconditional acceptance (the supporter's position) nor unconditional rejection (the skeptic's position) will do. But it will not do either to ignore Mad activism—to make no effort to take a considered position toward it—and this is for two reasons. First, if the claims put forward are coherent and the demands for recognition justified, then society has a problem at its hands evident in the dominance of reductive and pathologizing language about madness that would not be accepted today as a way of talking about other social identities. Second, Mad activism presents us with a valuable opportunity to question our ideas about identity, self, agency, and rationality to name some key concepts. It is a chance to ask if positive definitions and uses of these concepts exclude many individuals, perhaps unjustifiably so. For these reasons, we must not ignore Mad activism. In the spirit of respect for a particular viewpoint, this book sets out to examine and respond to the claims and demands of Mad activism.

Synopsis

This book is an extended philosophical argument that addresses the following questions derived from the claims and demands of Mad activism:

- Can madness be grounds for culture or identity?
- Does the demand for recognition possess normative force and, if it does, how should society respond to it?

These questions are addressed, respectively, in Part III and Part IV of the book. Part I offers an overview of activism in mental health and responds to key objections to Mad activism. And Part II presents background arguments in the philosophy and politics of identity and recognition. The nature of the questions and the overall subject matter require that we engage with a range of literatures: mental health activism literature; philosophical literature on the concepts and politics of identity and recognition; philosophy of psychiatry literature on the concept of mental disorder, delusions, unity and continuity of self, and specific mental health conditions; Mad studies and Disability studies literatures. In what follows I present an outline of the approach and content of each part, indicating how the argument of the book as a whole hangs together.

Part I: Madness

Chapter 1 begins with an overview of developments in mental health activism in the United Kingdom and the United States from the late nineteenth century to the present day. It outlines the discourse of "mental hygiene," the "antipsychiatry" of the 1960s, the 1970s civil rights movements, and the consumer/service-user/survivor movements. A historical overview allows us to appreciate the distinctiveness and, in some ways, the radical nature of Mad Pride activism relative to older and other contemporary endeavors. The rest of the chapter is devoted to describing the activities, claims, and demands of Mad Pride activism as they emerge through key writings, publications, and manifestos by activists. Chapter 2 responds to objections that have been put forward to Mad activism to the effect that madness is inherently disabling and distressing. For the objectors, these problems undermine positive constructions such as Mad Pride and Mad identity. I respond to these objections as follows: on the question of disability, I develop two bulwarks against the tendency to assume too readily the view that madness is inherently disabling: the first arises from the normative nature of disability judgments, and the second from the implications of political activism in terms of being a social subject. In the process of making these arguments, I explore the social model of disability in light of debates on naturalism and normativism, the applicability of the social model to madness, and the differences between physical and mental disabilities in terms of the unintelligibility often attributed to the latter. On the question of distress, I demonstrate that a phenomenon can be distressing and valuable, and this despite distress or, sometimes, because of it. With the subject matter in place, I now move on to Part II where I lay down the philosophical foundations for this book.

Part II: Recognition

Part II presents a philosophical account of identity and recognition, an account that is essential to addressing the questions in Parts III and IV (Can madness be grounds for culture or identity? Does the demand for recognition possess normative force and, if it does, how should society respond to it?). The philosophical literature on the concepts, theories, and politics of identity and recognition is huge and criss-crosses several philosophical schools and styles of argument. Further, it is a literature that has many unresolved issues and taps into long-standing problems in epistemology, ontology, moral philosophy, and political philosophy. In order to be able to address the questions just noted, I develop a formulation of identity and recognition that we can work with and that can allow us to make progress. My account seeks to achieve four aims: an understanding of the concept of recognition; an understanding of the concepts of individual and social identity; an argument for the normative force of demands for recognition (in general); a view on possible social and political responses to demands for recognition. In so far as possible, I ground my account in primary sources; for the concept of recognition I work with Hegel's exposition in the *Phenomenology of Spirit* (while siding with Robert Pippin's and Terry Pinkard's interpretations of Hegel's work); for the concept of identity I work, primarily, with the account developed by Charles Taylor; for the politics of recognition I work with key arguments by, among others, Axel Honneth, Nancy Fraser, Richard Rorty, and Kwame Appiah. Part II is essential to the argument of the book as a whole but can also be read independently as a perspective on the theory and politics of recognition.

Part III: Routes to recognition

With the background prepared, Part III examines whether madness can be grounds for culture or identity. Culture and identity are two routes by which social groups make the case for the validity and value of their way-of-life or shared self-understandings. Mad culture is examined in Chapter 6 and Mad identity in Chapters 7 and 8. In Chapter 6 I begin by outlining several concepts of culture followed by an assessment of whether Mad culture satisfies the relevant concept. As will be seen, Mad culture does not fit neatly with typical understandings of a societal culture. However, even if it does, a consideration of the moral basis for cultural rights leads us to identity and not to culture as the primary issue at stake.

Chapters 7 and 8 examine the viability of Mad identity as a route to recognition. The key problem that confronts us here is, in effect, a paradox: how can madness be grounds for identity given that phenomena such as delusions, passivity experiences, hallucinations, and extremes of mood, as commonly assumed, *undermine* the requirements for identity formation? Madness, it seems, cannot be grounds for identity: it lies outside the scope of recognition. I explore and respond to this objection in two stages. First, I outline three requirements for identity formation that need to be satisfied by any potential demand for recognition: this is for the identity claim to be of a certain epistemic status; to be an expression of a unified mental life; and to persist over a sufficient period of time. Second, I examine key phenomena of madness in light of these requirements. In each case I begin by interrogating the ways in which the phenomenon in question is judged to impair the relevant requirement, and I continue by demonstrating the complexity inherent in such judgments. For example, thought insertion is typically considered to indicate disunity of self, evident in the subject's inability to identify with its own mental states (in this sense thought insertion undermines the second requirement for identity formation noted here). By identifying the premises implicit in such a judgment, I demonstrate its reliance on a range of distinctive cultural psychological assumptions pertaining to self and authorship of mental states. In a different cultural context, thought insertion (passivity phenomena more generally), rather than constituting disunity of self, can actually be the basis for a potentially enriching self-understanding. A similar procedure of analysis and unpacking is performed for delusions and for the discontinuities of self often seen in schizophrenia and bipolar disorder. The aim of Chapters 7 and 8 is to establish, as a possibility, that these phenomena can be brought within the scope of recognition.

With this possibility established, Chapter 9 examines how it can be achieved. I explore this through the notion of "ordering madness," an endeavor that requires the fulfillment of two conditions: (1) preserve something of the phenomenology of madness, and (2) resolve impairments to identity formation. Only if these two conditions are satisfied can madness be brought within the scope of recognition, not as a psychiatric condition or a psychological construct, but as itself. I argue that only Mad narratives—the narratives of psychological, emotional, and experiential diversity advanced by activists—can satisfy these two requirements, whereas subjective narratives and professional narratives fail in this respect. In conclusion, madness can be brought within the scope of recognition: the notion of Mad identity is not incoherent.

Part IV: Approaches to Mad activism

Having defended the notion of Mad identity and demonstrated in what way madness can be brought within the scope of recognition, the final question can now be addressed: Does the demand for recognition of Mad identity possess normative force and, if it does, how should society respond to it? Building on the account of identity and recognition developed in Part II, Chapter 10 argues that the demand for recognition of Mad identity possesses normative force if the demand passes adjudication. In general terms, this requires that the identity in question is not trivial, morally objectionable, or irrational. I examine Mad identity in light of these three require- ments: Mad identity is neither trivial nor morally objectionable, but the question of irrationality is more complex. An identity is irrational if it is constituted by claims whose truth can, in principle, be determined (and where such claims are false). Determining the epistemic or logical status of a claim presupposes a standpoint of assessment; if we adopt the stance of scientific rationality we are in a position to make such assessments. However, such a stance is not always an appropriate one to adopt. For some identities, it would be inappropriate to assess their constituting claims in terms of their epistemic or logical status; their claims are better apprehended in their performative and expressive aspects. In other cases, there might be experiences that overdetermine the framework that can adequately express them, hence that frame- work cannot be summarily rejected; it calls for examination and understanding. The Mad narratives discussed in this book, I argue, involve claims that can be appre- hended in these different ways, and hence cannot simply be dismissed as irrational.

How should society respond to these valid demands? Drawing on the account devel- oped in Chapter 5, Chapter 10 outlines a response to misrecognition where both polit- ical activities and interpersonal reconciliation play a key role: I discuss four aspects of this response: the intended outcome—the final aim—of responding to misrecognition; the vehicle through which this outcome can be realized, which is "conversation"; the attitude that should inform these conversations (an attitude of reconciliation); and the activities that can facilitate reconciliation. Chapter 10 then concludes by consider- ing (hypothetically) the fruits of a successful process of reconciliation. These consist in the broadening of our cultural repertoire as it pertains to madness beyond medi- cal and psychological constructs and frameworks, to include in addition a range of Mad narratives. In this sense, Mad narratives can be understood as a cultural form of societal adjustment; a "cultural adjustment" that can bring benefits to many people in society, and not just to the activists demanding recognition. Finally, Chapter 11, the Conclusion, ties together several arguments in the book and charts two pathways to reconciliation: reconciling skeptics and supporters of Mad activism, and reconciling madness and society.

Part I

Madness

Chapter 1

Mental health activism and the demand for recognition

1.1 **Introduction**

There is no doubt that current developments in mental health activism—if not the phrase itself—would have been incomprehensible to the founders of modern psychiatry. For Emil Kraepelin (b. 1856), the famous German psychiatrist who coined the term Dementia Praecox (the precursor to the term *Schizophrenia*), madness was a chronic, degenerative, incurable affliction characterized by disorders of thinking, feeling, acting, and willing (Kraepelin 1909). The "mad" had nothing to say that would amount to more than elucidation and confirmation of their madness, let alone make political demands. The silencing of madness is a key theme in Foucault's (2001) revisionist history, originally published in 1961. For Foucault (2001, p. xii), once madness is delegated to physicians and conceived of as mental illness, no further dialogue is possible: the language of psychiatry becomes "a monologue of reason about madness," a mechanism by which mad people are silenced. The history of mental health activism can be viewed as an ongoing attempt by various groups to break this silence, to find a voice that would push back against the medical monologue about madness, and against disqualification and discrimination in society.

In presenting an account of mental health activism, it is necessary to emphasize from the start that this is not an uncomplicated narrative with a single dominant voice or an agreed upon set of strategies. The maltreatments and injustices experienced by users and survivors of mental health services are well known and include: excessive violation of their autonomy through coercive legislation and treatment; lack of inclusion of their voice in decisions pertaining to their care and recovery; reduction of their experiences to narrow biomedical and cognitive models of illness; stigma and disrespect in society ranging from unjustified perceptions of dangerousness and deficit to actual discrimination in employment possibilities. Attempts to address these problems have generated many different responses. There are those who campaign for reform of mental health services without rejecting medical understandings of madness and psychological distress; those who seek to depathologize a certain phenomenon—voices for example—by normalizing it and demonstrating its commonality in the population, while others seek to do the same while presenting voice-hearing as a special and unique experience; others still who draw affinities between the Mad and Disability movements, aiming to emulate the success of the latter in promoting favorable social change.

But it is a particular recent approach to mental health activism that has taken the challenge right to the heart of social views on mental health and mental disorder: this is Mad Pride and mad-positive activism. These activists, as Schrader, Jones, and Shattell (2013, p. 62) wrote, "have moved beyond treatment-centred activism to articulate a broader culture of madness." A key aspect of their endeavors is the rejection of the language of "mental illness," "disease," "disorder," the reclamation of the term mad and its redefinition in a variety of ways. In this respect activists have highlighted the "connections between madness and art, theatre, spirituality, and a valuable sensitivity to individual and collective pain" (Schrader et al. 2013). They have challenged the view of madness as illness in favor of the view that madness can be grounds for identity and culture. They have drawn explicit analogies with the black and gay civil rights movements and their fight for equality and recognition. And they have demanded social change to affirm the validity and worth of Mad identity. By doing so, activists have brought mental health activism squarely within the ambit of moral and political discussions on identity and recognition, and have made it clear that what needs to change is far bigger than the profession of psychiatry, it is society itself. This book is concerned with this kind of far-reaching activism.

As a prelude to an account of Mad Pride activism, I begin with a historical overview of mental health activism in general. This is important for two reasons: first, in order to fully appreciate the distinctiveness of Mad Pride discourse it is helpful to see it in light of past and present activist discourses; second, some concepts and ideas that recur at certain points in the book—such as the move from illness to identity and the concept of consciousness-raising—were initially raised in earlier periods of activism. Accordingly, this chapter begins with a brief historical account up to the emergence of Mad Pride, followed by a discussion of the meaning of madness in this context. It continues with an account of Mad Pride that focuses on the discourses involved and the demands made, and concludes with an overview of philosophical engagement with this activism.[1]

1.2 A brief historical account of activism in mental health

1.2.1 Early advocacy and activism

The modern consumer/service-user/survivor movement is generally considered to have begun in the 1970s in the wake of the many civil rights movements that emerged

---

[1] The majority of groups and networks in mental health advocacy and activism run websites and blogs in which they describe their history, activities, campaigns, and events. In this chapter, links to such sites are frequently cited. Unless otherwise indicated, as of September 2018 all links are in working order. However, groups can cease to campaign, websites change domains, are sometimes not maintained, and may run out of funding. Accordingly some links may, in time, cease to work.

at the time.[2] The Survivors' History Group—a group founded in April 2005 and concerned with documenting the history of the movement—traces an earlier starting point.[3] The group sees affinity between contemporary activism and earlier attempts to fight stigma, discrimination, and the poor treatment of individuals variously considered to be mad, insane and, since the dominance of the medical idiom, to suffer with mental illness.[4] In their website which documents Survivor history, the timeline begins with 1373, the year the Christian mystic Margery Kempe was born. Throughout her life, Margery experienced intense voices and visions of prophets, devils, and demons. Her unorthodox behavior and beliefs upset the Church, the public, and her husband, and resulted in her restraint and imprisonment on several occasions. Margery wrote about her life in a book in which she recounted her spiritual experiences and the difficulties she had faced.[5]

The Survivors' history website continues with several recorded instances of individual mistreatment on the grounds of insanity. But the first explicit evidence of collective action and advocacy in the United Kingdom appears in 1845 in the form of the *Alleged Lunatics' Friend Society*: an organization composed of individuals most of whom had been incarcerated in madhouses and subjected to degrading treatment (Hervey 1986). For around twenty years, the *Society* campaigned for the rights of patients, including the right to be involved in decisions pertaining to their care and confinement. In the United States, around the same time, patients committed to a New York Lunatic Asylum produced a literary magazine—*The Opal*—published in ten volumes between 1851 and 1860. Although this production is now seen to have painted a rather benign picture of asylum life, and to have allowed voice only to those patients who were deemed appropriate and self-censorial (Reiss 2004), glimpses of dissatisfaction and even of liberatory rhetoric emerge from some of the writing (Tenney 2006).

An important name in what can be considered early activism and advocacy is Elizabeth Packard. In 1860, Packard was committed to an insane asylum in Illinois by her husband, a strict Calvinist who could not tolerate Packard's newly expressed liberal beliefs and her rejection of his religious views. At the time, state law gave husbands this power without the need for a public hearing. Upon her release, Packard campaigned successfully for a change in the law henceforth requiring a jury trial for decisions to commit an individual to an asylum (Dain 1989, p. 9). Another important campaigner is Clifford Beers, an American ex-patient who in 1908 published his autobiography *A Mind That Found Itself*. Beer's biography documented the mistreatment he experienced at several institutions. The following year he founded the National Committee

---

[2] The following account outlines key moments, figures, groups, and strategies in mental health advocacy and activism; it is not intended to be exhaustive but rather to illustrate the background to the Mad Pride movement and discourse.

[3] The timeline can be found at: http://studymore.org.uk/mpu.htm. (The website states that Survivor history is being compiled into a book.) See also Campbell and Roberts (2009).

[4] In contrast to Survivor history, there is a tradition of historical and critical writing on the history of "psychiatry" and "madness," and on the development of lunacy reform and mental health law. Notable names in this tradition are Roy Porter, Andrew Scull, and Michel Foucault.

[5] See Peterson (1982, pp. 3–18).

for Mental Hygiene (NCMH), an organization that sought to improve conditions in asylums and the treatment of patients by working with reform-minded psychiatrists. The NCMH achieved limited success in this respect, and its subsequent efforts focused on mental health education, training, and public awareness campaigns in accordance with the then dominant concept of mental hygiene (Dain 1989, p. 6).

1.2.2 **1900s–1950s: "Mental hygiene"**

On both sides of the Atlantic, mental health advocacy in the first few decades of the twentieth century promoted a mental hygiene agenda.[6] Mental hygiene is an American concept and was understood as "the art of preserving the mind against all incidents and influences calculated to deteriorate its qualities, impair its energies, or derange its movements" (Rossi 1962). These "incidents and influences" were conceived broadly and included "exercise, rest, food, clothing and climate, the laws of breeding, the government of the passions, the sympathy with current emotions and opinions, the discipline of the intellect," all of which had to be governed adequately to promote a healthy mind (Rossi 1962). With such a broad list of human affairs under their purview, the mental hygienists had to fall back on a set of values by which the "healthy" lifestyle was to be determined. These values, as argued by Davis (1938) and more recently by Crossley (2006), were those of the educated middle classes who promoted mental hygiene in accordance with a deeply ingrained ethic. For example, extramarital sex was seen as a deviation and therefore a potential source of mental illness. Despite this conservative element, the discourse of mental hygiene was progressive, for its time, in several ways: first, it considered mental illness to arise from interactions among many factors, including the biological and the social, and hence to be responsive to improvements in the person's environment; second, it fought stigma by arguing that mental illness is similar to physical illness and can be treated; third, it promoted the prevention of mental illness, in particular through paying attention to childhood development; and fourth, it argued for the importance of early detection and treatment (Crossley 2006, pp. 71–5).

In the United States, Clifford Beer's own group, the NCMH, continued to advance a mental hygiene agenda. The NCMH eventually became the National Mental Health Association, a nonprofit organization that exists since 2006 as Mental Health America.[7] In the United Kingdom, mental hygiene was promoted by three interwar groups that campaigned for patient well-being and education of the public. These groups merged, in 1946, to form the National Association for Mental Health (NAMH), which changed its name, in 1972, to Mind, the name under which it remains to this day as a well-known and influential charity.[8] In the late 1950s, these two groups continued to educate the public through various campaigns and publications, and were involved in training mental health professionals in accordance with hygienist principles. In addition, they were advocates for mental patients, campaigning for the government

---

[6] This section benefits, in part, from Crossley's (2006, chapter 4) account of mental hygiene.

[7] Mental Health America. Online: http://www.mentalhealthamerica.net/

[8] Mind. Online: http://www.mind.org.uk/

to improve commitment laws, and, in the United Kingdom, working with the government to instate the move from asylums to "care in the community."

Even though the discourse of mental hygiene was dominant during these decades, the developments that were to come in the early 1970s were already taking shape in the emerging discourse of civil rights. A good example of these developments in the United Kingdom is the National Council for Civil Liberties (NCCL), better known today as Liberty. Founded in 1934 in response to an aggressive police reaction to protestors during the hunger marches, it became involved in 1947 in its first "mental health case": a woman wrongly detained in a mental health institution for what appeared to be "moral" rather than "medical" reasons.[9] During the 1950s, the NCCL campaigned vigorously for reform of mental health law to address this issue, and was able to see some positive developments in 1959 with the abolition of the problematic 1913 Mental Deficiency Act and the introduction of tribunals in which patients' interests were represented.

1.2.3 1960s: The "antipsychiatrists"

During the 1960s criticisms of mental health practices and theories were carried through by several psychiatrists who came to be referred to as the "antipsychiatrists." Notable figures included Thomas Szasz, R. D. Laing, and David Cooper. Szasz (1960) famously argued that mental illness is a myth that legitimizes state oppression (via the psychiatric enterprise) on those judged as socially deviant and perceived to be a danger to themselves or others. Mental illnesses for Szasz are *problems in living*: morally and existentially significant problems relating to social interaction and to finding meaning and purpose in life. Laing (1965, 1967) considered the medical concept of schizophrenia to be a label applied to those whose behavior seems incomprehensible, thereby permitting exercises of power. For Laing (1967, p. 106) the people so labeled are not so much experiencing a breakdown but a breakthrough: a state of ego loss that permits a wider range of experiences and may culminate in a "new-ego" and an "existential rebirth." These individuals require guidance and encouragement, and not the application of a psychiatric label that distorts and arrests this process. David Cooper (1967, 1978) considered schizophrenia a revolt against alienating familial and social structures with the hope of finding a less-alienating, autonomous, yet recognized existence. In Cooper's (1978, p. 156) view, it is precisely this revolt that the "medical apparatus," as an agent of the "State," aims to suppress.

From the perspective of those individuals who have experienced psychiatric treatment and mental distress, the antipsychiatrists of the 1960s were not activists but dissident mental health professionals. As will be noted in the following section, the mental patients' liberation movement did not support the inclusion of sympathetic professionals within its ambit. Nevertheless, the ideas of Thomas Szasz, R. D. Laing, and David Cooper were frequently used by activists themselves to ground their critique of mental health institutions and the medical model. At the time, these ideas were radical

---

[9] The history of Liberty can be found on its website: https://www.liberty-human-rights.org.uk/who-we-are/history/liberty-timeline

if not revolutionary, and it is not surprising that they inspired activists engaged in civil rights struggles in the 1970s.

1.2.4 **The 1970s civil rights movements**

Civil rights activism in mental health began through the work of several groups that came together in the late 1960s and early 1970s in the wake of the emerging successes and struggles of black, gay, and women civil rights activists. In the United Kingdom, a notable group was the Mental Patients' Union (1972), and in the United States three groups were among the earliest organizers: Insane Liberation Front (1970), Mental Patients' Liberation Front (1971), and Network Against Psychiatric Assault (1972).[10] An important difference between these groups and earlier ones that may have also pursued a civil rights agenda (such as the NCCL) is that they, from the start or early on, excluded sympathetic mental health professionals and were composed solely of patients and ex-patients. Judi Chamberlin (1990, p. 324), a key figure in the American movement, justified it in this way:

> Among the major organising principles of [black, gay, women's liberation movements] were self-definition and self-determination. Black people felt that white people could not truly understand their experiences . . . To mental patients who began to organise, these principles seemed equally valid. Their own perceptions about "mental illness" were diametrically opposed to those of the general public, and even more so to those of mental health professionals. It seemed sensible, therefore, not to let non-patients into ex-patient organisations or to permit them to dictate an organisation's goals.

The extent of the resolve to exclude professionals—even those who would appear to be sympathetic such as the antipsychiatrists—is evident in the writings of Chamberlin as well as in the founding document of the Mental Patients' Union. Both distanced themselves from antipsychiatry on the grounds that the latter is "an intellectual exercise of academics and dissident mental health professionals" that while critical of psychiatry, did not include ex-patients or engage their struggles (Chamberlin 1990, p. 323).[11] Further, according to Chamberlin, a group that permits nonpatients and professionals inevitably abandons its liberatory intentions and ends up in the weaker position of attempting to reform psychiatry. And reform was not on the agenda of these early groups.

On the advocacy front, the mental patients' liberation movement—the term generally used to refer to this period of civil rights activism—sought to end psychiatry as they knew it.[12] They sought to abolish involuntary hospitalization and forced treatment, to prioritize freedom of choice and consent above other considerations, to reject

---

[10] In the United States, groups were able to communicate with each other through a regular newsletter, *Madness Network News* (1972–86), and an annual Conference on Human Rights and Against Psychiatric Oppression (1973–85).

[11] For a similar point, see the founding document of the Mental Patients' Union, reprinted in Curtis et al. (2000, pp. 23–8).

[12] Some activists referred to themselves as "psychiatric inmates" or "ex-inmates," highlighting the fact of their incarceration in mental institutions and their rejection of the connotations of the term "patient." This early difference in terminology—inmate versus patient—prefigures

the reductive medical model, to restore full civil rights to mental patients including the right to refuse treatment, and to counter negative perceptions in the media such as the inherent dangerousness of the "mentally ill." In addition to advocacy, a great deal of work went into setting up nonhierarchical, noncoercive alternatives to mental health institutions such as self-help groups, drop-in centers, and retreats.[13] The purpose of these initiatives was not only to provide support to individuals in distress, but to establish that mental patients are self-reliant and able to manage their own lives outside of mental health institutions. Central to the success of these initiatives was a radical transformation in how ex-patients understood their situation. This transformation was referred to as consciousness-raising.

Borrowed from the women's liberation movement, consciousness-raising is the process of placing elements of one's situation in the wider context of systematic social oppression (Chamberlin 1990). This begins to occur in meetings in which people get together and share their experiences, identifying commonalities, and reinterpreting them in a way that gives them broader meaning and significance. An implication of this process is that participants may be able to reverse an internalized sense of weakness or incapability—which hitherto they may have regarded as natural—and regain confidence in their abilities. In the mental patients' liberation movement, consciousness-raising involved ridding oneself of the central assumptions of the "mental health system": that one has an illness, and that the medical profession is there to provide a cure. In the discourse of the time, inspired by the writings of Thomas Szasz and others, psychiatry was seen as a form of social control, medicalizing unwanted behavior as a pretext for "treating" it, and forcing individuals into a sane way of behaving. By sharing experiences, participants begin to see that the mental health system has not helped them. In a book first published in 1977 and considered a founding and inspirational document for mental health activists, Chamberlin (1988, pp. 70–1) wrote of the important insights ex-patients gained through consciousness-raising:

> Consciousness-raising . . . helps people to see that their so-called symptoms are indications of real problems. The anger, which has been destructively turned inward, is freed by this recognition. Instead of believing that they have a defect in their psychic makeup (or their neurochemical system), participants learn to recognise the oppressive conditions in their daily lives.

Mental suffering and distress, within this view, are a normal response to the difficulties individuals face in life such as relationship problems, social inequality, poverty, loss, and trauma. In such situations, individuals need a sympathetic, caring and understanding response, and not the one society offers in the form of psychotropic drugs and the difficult environment of a mental health hospital (Chamberlin 1988). Consciousness-raising does not stop at the "mental health system," but casts a wider net that includes

---

the multiplicity of terms and associated strategies that will come to define activism and advocacy in mental health to this day.

[13] The earliest example of a self-help group is We Are Not Alone (WANA). Formed in New York in the 1940s as a patient-run group, it developed into a major psychosocial rehabilitation center, eventually to be managed by mental health professionals (see Chamberlin 1988, pp. 94–5).

all discriminatory stereotypes against ex-patients. In a deliberate analogy with racism and sexism, Chamberlin uses the term *mentalism* to refer to the widespread social tendency to call disapproved of behavior "sick" or "crazy." Mental patients' liberation required of patients and ex-patients to resist the "mental health system" as well as social stereotyping, and to find the strength and confidence to do so. In this context, voluntary alternatives by and for patients and ex-patients were essential to providing a forum for support and consciousness-raising.

1.2.5 Consumers/service users and survivors

During the 1980s, the voices of advocates and activists began to be recognized by national government agencies and bodies. This was in the context of a shift toward market approaches to healthcare provision, and the idea of the patient as a consumer of services (Campbell 2009). Patients and ex-patients—now referred to as consumers (US) or users (UK) of services—were able to sit in policy meetings and advisory committees of mental health services and make their views known. Self-help groups, which normally struggled for funding, began to be supported by public money. In the United States, several consumer groups formed that were no longer opposed to the medical model or to working with mental health professionals in order to reform services.[14] While some considered these developments to be positive, others regarded them as indicating what Linda Morrison, an American activist and academic, referred to as a "crisis of co-optation": the voice of mental health activists had to become acceptable to funding agencies, which required relinquishing radical demands in favor of reform (Morrison 2005, p. 80). Some activists rejected the term consumer as it implied that patients and professionals were in an equal relation, with patients free to determine the services they receive (Chamberlin 1988, p. vii).[15]

Countering the consumer/user discourse was an emerging survivor discourse reflected in several national groups, for example, the National Association of Psychiatric Survivors (1985) in the United States and Survivors Speak Out (SSO 1986) in the United Kingdom. Survivor discourse shared many points of alignment with earlier activism, but whereas the latter was opposed to including professionals and nonpatients, survivors were no longer against this as long as it occurred within a framework of genuine and honest partnership and inclusion in all aspects of service structure, delivery, and evaluation (Campbell 1992; Chamberlin 1995). [16]

----

[14] See Bluebird's *History of the Consumer/Survivor Movement.* Online: https://power2u.org/wp-content/uploads/2017/01/History-of-the-Consumer-Survivor-Movement-by-Gayle-Bluebird.pdf

[15] Mclean (1995, p. 1054) draws the distinction between consumers and survivors as follows: "Persons who identify themselves as 'consumers,' 'clients' or 'patients,' tend to accept the medical model of mental illness and traditional mental health treatment practices, but work for general system improvement and for the addition of consumer controlled alternatives. Those who refer to themselves as 'ex-patients,' 'survivors' or 'ex-inmates' reject the medical model of mental illness, professional control and forced treatment and seek alternatives exclusively in user controlled centres."

[16] Consumers and survivors aside, more radical voices persisted, continuing the discourse and activities of the 1970s groups. These voices were vehemently opposed to psychiatry

In the United States, developments throughout the 1990s and into the millennium confirm the continuation of these two trends: the first oriented toward consumer discourse and involvement, and the second toward survivors, with a relatively more radical tone and a concern with human rights (Morrison 2005). Today, representative national groups for these two trends include, respectively, the National Coalition for Mental Health Recovery (NCMHR) and Mind Freedom International (MFI).[17] The former is focused on promoting comprehensive recovery, approvingly quoting the "New Freedom Mental Health Commission Report" target of a "future when everyone with mental illness will recover."[18] To this end they campaign for better services, for consumers to have a voice in their recovery, and for an end to stigma and discrimination. They also promote community inclusion via consumer-run initiatives that offer assistance with education, housing, and other aspects of life. On the other hand, MFI state their vision to be a "nonviolent revolution in mental health care." Unlike NCMHR, MFI do not use the language of "mental illness," and support campaigns such as Creative Maladjustment, Mad Pride, and Boycott Normal. Further, MFI state emphatically that they are completely independent and do not receive funds from or have any links with government, drug companies, or mental health agencies.[19] Despite their differences, both organizations claim to represent survivors and consumers, and both trace their beginnings to the 1970s civil rights movements. But whereas NCMHR refer to "consumers" always first and generally more often, MFI do the opposite and state that most of their members identify as psychiatric survivors.

In the United Kingdom, the service-user/survivor movement—as it came to be referred to—is today represented nationally by several groups.[20] Of note is the National

----

and rejected any cooperation with services or with advocates/activists who tended toward reform. Examples include the Network to Abolish Psychiatry (1986) in the United States and Campaign Against Psychiatric Oppression (CAPO, 1985) in the United Kingdom, both of which were active for a few years in the 1980s. (CAPO was an offshoot of the earlier Mental Patients' Union.) For these groups, the "mental health system" was intrinsically oppressive and had to be abolished: attempts to reform it, merely strengthened it (see *Madness Network News*, Summer 1986, vol. 8, no. 3, p. 8). Reflecting on the beginnings of SSO (1986), Peter Campbell, a founder, wrote that CAPO and other "separatist" groups were more concerned with "philosophical and ideological issues" and that SSO was "born partly in reaction to this: they were the first part of the 'pragmatic' wing which now dominates the user movement" with an emphasis on dialogue with others (Peter Campbell on The History and Philosophy of The Survivor Movement. *Southwark Mind Newsletter*, issue 24—year not specified).

[17] Note that the reference here is to national networks and groups and not to the local groups engaged in self-help, support, education, training, and advocacy of which there are hundreds in the United States, United Kingdom, and elsewhere.

[18] National Coalition for Mental Health Recovery. Online: http://www.ncmhr.org/purpose.htm

[19] Mind Freedom International. Online: http://www.mindfreedom.org/mfi-faq

[20] National organizations are of two types: those concerned with mental health generally (discussed in the text), and those with a focus on a particular condition or behavior such as the Hearing Voices Network and the National Self-Harm network.

Survivor User Network (NSUN), which brings together survivor and user groups and individuals across the country in order to strengthen their voice and assist with policy change.[21] Another long-standing group (1990), though less active today, is the UK Advocacy Network, a group that campaigns for user led advocacy and involvement in mental health services planning and delivery.[22] A UK survey done in 2003 brings some complexity to this appearance of a homogenous movement (Wallcraft et al. 2003). While most respondents agreed that there is a national user/survivor movement—albeit a rather loose one—different opinions arose on all the important issues; for example, disagreements over whether compulsory treatment can ever be justified, and whether receiving funds from drug companies compromises the movement. In addition, there were debates over the legitimacy of the medical model, with some respondents rejecting it in favor of social and political understandings of mental distress. In this context, respondents drew a distinction between the service-user movement and the survivor movement, the former concerned with improving services, and the latter with challenging the medical model and the "supposed scientific basis of mental health services" (Wallcraft et al. 2003, p. 50). More radical voices suggested that activists who continued to adopt the medical model have not been able to rid themselves of the disempowering frameworks of understanding imposed by the mental health system. In a similar vein, some respondents noted the depoliticization of the movement, as activists ceased to be primarily concerned with civil rights and began to work for the mental health system (Wallcraft et al. 2003, p. 14).

In summary, there exists within the consumer/service-user/survivor movements in the United States and the United Kingdom a variety of stances in relation to involuntary detention and treatment, acceptable sources of funding, the medical model, and the extent and desirability of user involvement in services. Positions range from working for mental health institutions and reforming them from the "inside," to rejecting any cooperation and engaging in activism to end what is considered psychiatric abuse and social discrimination in the guise of supposed medical theory and treatment. It appears that within national networks and movements pragmatic and cooperative approaches are more common, with radical positions pushed somewhat aside, though by no means silenced. In this context Mad Pride, representing the latest wave of activism in mental health, reinvigorates the radicalism of the movement and makes the most serious demand yet of social norms and understandings. But Mad Pride, underpinned by the notions of Mad culture and Mad identity, builds on the accomplishments of Survivor identity to which I turn briefly.

1.2.6 Survivor identity

The connotations of survivor discourse are unmistakable and powerful. With survivor discourse the term "patient" and its implications of dependence and weakness are finally discarded (Crossley 2004, p. 169). From the perspective of those individuals who embraced the discourse, there is much that they have survived: forced detention

---

[21] National Survivor User Network. Online: https://www.nsun.org.uk/our-vision

[22] UK Advocacy Network. Online: http://www.u-kan.co.uk/mission.html

in the mental health system, aggressive and unhelpful treatments, discrimination and stigma in society, and, for some, the distress and suffering they experienced and which was labeled by others "mental illness." By discarding of what they came to see as an imposed identity—viz. "patient"—survivors took one further step toward increased self-definition (Crossley 2006, p. 182). In addition, the very term "survivor" implies a positive angle to this definition in so far as surviving implies resilience, strength, and other personal traits considered valuable. Morrison (2005, p. 102) describes it as the "heroic survivor narrative" and accords it a central function in the creation of a collective identity for the movement and a shared sense of injustice.

Central to survivor identity is the importance of the voice of survivors and their ability to tell their own stories, a voice that is not respected by society or the psychiatric system. The well-known British activist and poet Peter Campbell (1992, p. 122) wrote that a great part of the "damage" sustained in the psychiatric system

> has been a result of psychiatry's refusal to give value to my personal perceptions and experience . . . I cannot believe it is possible to dismiss as meaningless people's most vivid and challenging interior experiences and expect no harm to ensue.

The emphasis on the voice of survivors highlights one further difference from 1970s activism: whereas earlier activists sustained their critique of psychiatry by drawing upon the writings of Szasz, Goffman, Marx, and others, survivor discourse eschewed such sources of "authority" in favor of the voice of survivors themselves; Crossley (2004, p. 167) wrote:

> Survivors have been able to convert their experiences of mental distress and (mis)treatment into a form of cultural and symbolic capital. The disvalued status of the patient is reversed within the movement context. Therein it constitutes authority to speak and vouches for authenticity. The experience of both distress and treatment, stigmatized elsewhere, has become recognized as a valuable, perhaps superior knowledge base. Survivors have laid a claim, recognized at least within the movement itself, to know "madness" and its "treatment" with authority, on the basis that they have been there and have survived it.

Survivors are therefore experts on their own experiences, and experts on what it is like to be subject to treatment in mental health institutions and to face stigma and discrimination in society. So construed, to survive is to be able to emerge from a range of difficulties, some of which are external and others internal, belonging to the condition (the distress, the experiences) that led to the encounter with psychiatry in the first place. In this sense, survivor discourse had not yet been able to impose a full reversal of the negative value attached to phenomena of madness, a value reflected in the language of mental illness, disorder, and pathology. This is clearly evident in the idea that one had *survived* the condition, for if that is the attitude one holds toward it, it is unlikely that the "condition" is looked upon positively or neutrally (except perhaps teleologically in the sense that it had had a formative influence on one's personality). Similarly, if one considers oneself to have survived mental health institutions rather than the condition, there still is no direct implication that the condition itself is regarded in a nonnegative light, only that the personal traits conducive to survival are laudable. It is only with the discourse of Mad Pride that the language of mental illness and the social norms and values underpinning it are challenged in an unambiguous manner. Before we can examine Mad Pride discourse, it is important to examine the meaning of madness in this context.

1.3 The meaning of madness

Mad with a capital M refers to one way in which an individual can identify. In this respect it stands similar to other social identities such as Maori, African-Caribbean, or Deaf. If someone asks why a person identifies as Mad or as Maori, the simplest answer that can be offered is to state that he identifies so because he *is* mad or Maori. And if this answer is to be anything more than a tautology—he identifies as Mad because he identifies as Mad—the *is* must refer to something over and above that person's identification; that is, to that person's "madness" or "maoriness." Such an answer has the implication that if one is considered to be Maori yet identifies as Anglo-Saxon, or white and identifies as black, they would be wrong in a fundamental way about their own *nature*. And this final word—nature—is precisely the difficulty with this way of thinking and underpins the criticism that such an understanding of identity is "essentialist."

Essentialism, in philosophy, is the idea that some objects may have essential properties. These are properties without which the object would not be what it is; for example, it is an essential property of a planet that it orbits around a star. In social and political discussions, essentialism means something wider: it is invoked as a criticism of the claim that one's identity falls back on immutable, given, "natural" features that incline one—and the group with whom one shares those features—to behave in certain ways and to have certain predispositions. The critique of certain discourses as essentialist has been made in several domains including race and queer studies, and in feminist theory; as Heyes (2000, p. 21) points out, contemporary North American feminist theory now takes it as a given that to refer to "women's experience" is merely to engage in an essentialist generalization from what is actually the experience of "middle-class white feminists." The problem is the construction of a category—"women" or "black" or "mad"—all members of which supposedly share something deep that is part of their nature: being female, being a certain race, being mad. Yet in terms of the categories, there appears to be no basis for supposing either gender essentialism (the claim that women, in virtue of being women, have a shared and distinctive experience of the world: see Stone (2004) for an overview), or the existence of discrete races (e.g., Appiah 1994a, pp. 98–101), or a discrete category of experience and behavior that we can refer to as "madness" (or "schizophrenia" or any other psychiatric condition for this purpose). Evidence for the latter claim is growing rapidly as the following overview indicates.

There is a body of literature in philosophy and psychiatry that critiques essentialist thinking about mental disorder, usually by rebutting the claim that psychiatric categories are natural kinds (see Zachar 2015, 2000; Haslam 2002; Cooper 2013 is more optimistic). A "natural kind" is a philosophical concept which refers to entities that exist in nature and are categorically distinct from each other. The observable features of a natural kind arise from its internal structure, which is also the condition for membership of the kind. For example, any compound that has two molecules of hydrogen and one molecule of oxygen is water, irrespective of its observable features (which in the case of H$_2$O can be ice, liquid, or gas). Natural kind thinking informs typical scientific and medical approaches to mental disorder as evident in the following assumptions (see Haslam 2000, pp. 1033–4): (1) different disorders are categorically distinct from each other (schizophrenia is one thing, bipolar disorder another); (2) you either have a disorder or not—a disorder is a discrete category; (3) the observable features of a disorder (symptoms and signs) are causally produced by its internal structure (underlying abnormalities); (4) diagnosis is a determination of the kind (the disorder) instantiated in the individual.

If this picture of strong essentialism appears as a straw-man it is because thinking about mental disorder has moved on or is in the process of doing so. All of the assumptions listed here have been challenged (see Zachar 2015): in many cases it is not possible to draw categorical distinctions between one disorder and another, and between disorder and its absence; fuzzy boundaries predominate. Symptoms of schizophrenia and of bipolar disorder overlap, necessitating awkward constructions such as schizoaffective disorder or mania with psychotic symptoms. Similarly, the boundary between clinical depression and intense grief has been critiqued as indeterminate. In addition, the reductive causal picture implied by the natural kind view seems naive in the case of mental disorder: it is now a truism that what we call psychiatric symptoms are the product of multiple interacting factors (biological, social, cultural, psychological). And diagnosis, as the activist literature has repeatedly pointed out, is not a process of matching the patient's report with an existing category, but a complicated interaction between two parties in which one side—the clinician—constantly reinterprets what the patient is saying in the language of psychiatry, a process that permits the exercise of power over the patient.

The difficulties in demarcating health from disorder and disorders from each other have been debated recently under the concept of "vagueness"; the idea that psychiatric concepts and classifications are imprecise with no sharp distinctions possible between those phenomena to which they apply and those to which they do not (Keil, Keuck, and Hauswald 2017). Vagueness in psychiatry does not automatically eliminate the quest for more precision—it may be the case, for example, that we need to improve our science—but it does strongly suggest a formulation of states of health and forms of experience in terms of degrees rather than categorically (i.e., a gradualist approach to mental health). Gradualism is one possible implication of vagueness, and there is good evidence to support it as a thesis. For example, Sullivan-Bissett and colleagues (2017) have convincingly argued that delusional and nondelusional beliefs differ in degree, not kind. Nondelusional beliefs exhibit the same epistemic shortcomings attributed to delusions: resistance to counterevidence, resistance to abandoning the belief, and the influence of biases and motivational factors on belief formation. Similarly, as pointed out earlier, the distinction between normal sadness and clinical depression is difficult to make on principled grounds and relies on an arbitrary specification of the number of weeks during which a person must feel low in mood before a diagnosis can be given (see Horwitz and Wakefield 2007). Another related problem is the nonspecificity of symptoms: symptoms considered pathognomonic of schizophrenia such as auditory hallucinations, thought insertion, and passivity phenomena, can be found in the non-patient population, as well as other conditions (e.g., Jackson 2007).

Vagueness in mental health concepts and gradualism with regard to psychological phenomena undermine the idea that there are discrete categories with an underlying essence and that go with labels such as schizophrenia, bipolar disorder, or madness. But people continue to identify as Women, African-American, Maori, Gay, and Mad. Are they wrong to do so? To say they are wrong is to mistake the nature of social identities. To prefigure a discussion that will occupy us in Chapter 4, identity is a person's understanding of who he or she is, and that understanding always appeals to existing collective categories: to identify is to place oneself in some sort of relation to those categories. To identify as Mad is to place oneself in some sort of relation to madness; to identify as Maori is to place oneself in some sort of relation to Maori culture. Now these categories may not be essential in the sense of falling back on some immutable principle, but they are nevertheless out there in the social world and their meaning and continued existence does not depend on one person rejecting them (nor can one person alone maintain a social category even if he or she can play a major role in conceiving it). Being social in nature they are open to redefinition, hence collective activism to reclaim certain categories and redefine them in positive ways. In fact, the argument that a particular category has fuzzy boundaries and is not underpinned by an essence may enter into its redefinition. But demonstrating this cannot be expected to eliminate people's identification with that category: the inessentiality of race, to give an example, is not going to be sufficient by itself to end people's identification, in some societies, as White or Black.

In the context of activism, to identify as Mad is to have a stake in how madness is defined, and the key issue becomes the meaning of madness. To illustrate the range of ways in which madness has been defined, I appeal to some views that have been voiced in an important anthology: *Mad Matters: A Critical Reader in Canadian Mad Studies* (2013). A key point to begin with is that Mad identity tends to be anchored in experiences of mistreatment and labeling by others.[23] Poole and Ward (2013, p. 96) wrote that, by mad "we are referring to a term reclaimed by those who have been pathologized/psychiatrized as 'mentally ill.'" Similarly, Fabris (2013, p. 139) proposed mad "to mean the group of us considered crazy or deemed ill by sanists . . . and are politically conscious of this." These definitions remind us that a group frequently comes into being when individuals experience discrimination or oppression that is then attributed by them to features that they share, no matter how loosely. These features have come to define the social category of madness. Menzies, LeFrancois, and Reaume (2013, p. 10) wrote:

> Once a reviled term that signalled the worst kinds of bigotry and abuse, madness has come to represent a critical alternative to "mental illness" or "disorder" as a way of naming and responding to emotional, spiritual, and neuro-diversity. . . . Following other social

---

[23] Though note that madness here is not equivalent to a particular psychiatric category. Gorman (2013, p. 269) wrote that "'Mad' signals an identity more expansive than psychiatric consumer/survivor identities . . . more expansive in its possibility of including people who have been caught up in psy labelling beyond psychiatric hospitals and doctor's offices. Indeed, the etymology of 'mad' comes from outside of medical and scientific discourse."

movements including queer, black, and fat activism, madness talk and text invert the language of oppression, reclaiming disparaged identities and restoring dignity and pride to difference.

Pursuing a similar line of thought, Liegghio (2013, p. 122) elaborated:

> madness refers to a range of experiences—thoughts, moods, behaviours—that are different from and challenge, resist, or do not conform to dominant, psychiatric constructions of "normal" versus "disordered" or "ill" mental health. Rather than adopting dominant psy constructions of mental health as a negative condition to alter, control, or repair, I view madness as a social category among other categories like race, class, gender, sexuality, age, or ability that define our identities and experiences.

Mad activism starts with shared experiences of oppression, stigma, and mistreatment, it continues with the rejection of biomedical language and reclamation of the term mad, and proceeds by developing positive content to madness and hence to Mad identity. As Burstow (2013, p. 84) commented:

> What the community is doing is essentially turning these words around, using them to connote, alternately, cultural difference, alternate ways of thinking and processing, wisdom that speaks a truth not recognised . . . , the creative subterranean that figures in all of our minds. In reclaiming them, the community is affirming psychic diversity and repositioning "madness" as a quality to embrace; hence the frequency with which the word "Mad" and "pride" are associated.

1.4 **Mad Pride**

1.4.1 **Origins and activities**

The term "pride" was first associated with the survivor movement in 1993 with the first Psychiatric Survivor Pride day in Toronto. Lilith Finkler (1997, p. 766), one of the organizers, explained the choice of name by noting the shared oppression between survivors and members of the gay and lesbian communities.[24] However, as an expression and movement with that name, Mad Pride began in the United Kingdom in 1997 in the context of a newly emerging wave of activism. Many activists felt that by engaging with mental health services, the views of user/survivors were "absorbed into bureaucratic systems, only to be rendered powerless" (Curtis et al. 2000, p. 7). Dissatisfied with this state of affairs, and with limited progress on issues such as involuntary detention and social discrimination, some members of the organization SSO— by now folding-up—formed direct action groups. Inspired by the Gay Pride festival

[24] The objectives of the original Pride Day: "to combat stigma; to celebrate psychiatric survivors 'as active members of Canadian society'; to 'present the history and culture of psychiatric survivors from the perspective of those who lived . . . this experience'; to 'link up with other marginalized groups [including] persons with disabilities, people of colour, first nations,' in 'rejecting oppressive cultural stereotypes'; to connect with 'other community based groups in Parkdale to ensure visibility and acceptance of persons with psychiatric histories'; to 'empower those of us previously excluded, to participate in the creation and preservation of our contribution to Canadian culture" (Reaume 2008, p. 2).

in London, Mad Pride was formed in 1997, the name chosen through a questionnaire distributed in one of the final meetings of SSO. The emergence of this movement marked a new era of activism, reigniting the passion of the 1970s with a conscious attempt to put mental health on a par with other civil rights movements. The editors of the anthology *Mad Pride* wrote:

> Mad Pride is set to become the first great civil liberties movement of the new millennium. Over the last century, giant strides forward were made by those asserting their rights and self-determination in the fields of race, gender and sexuality, but "mental health" issues failed to keep pace. This is set to change. (Curtis et al. 2000, p. 7)

The new activism, the editors note, will proceed with riots, demonstrations, and medication strikes. It will work with those seeking a "complete transformation of society" and will reclaim the "experience of madness and the language surrounding it" (Curtis et al. 2000). Mad Pride will celebrate Mad identity and culture, and will abandon the victim status long associated with being "mentally ill" (Curtis et al. 2000, p. 8). In North America, Psychiatric Survivor Pride eventually changed its name to Mad Pride in 2002 (Reaume 2008, p. 2). The overall objectives included affirming Mad identities, developing and empowering Mad communities, challenging discrimination, and advocating for rights.[25]

In practice, Mad Pride consists in events that can be organized any time of the year with particular note made of July 14, now designated International Mad Pride Day and marked by a festival that can last one day to a week.[26] Events have been organized in Canada, United Kingdom, United States, Ireland, Belgium, France, and Australia, among other places.[27] Activities include displays of art made by Mad-identified individuals; theater shows; music, dancing, and poetry; picnics, demos, and bed push; discussion panels and information on issues related to the mental health system; readings by activists of their experiences and struggles. These events are defined by creativity, cooperation, the celebration of difference, and resistance to the mental health system. On this latter point, for example, the 2012 announcement of Mad Pride Toronto urged participants who are unable to attend to "orchestrate a DSM [Diagnostic and Statistical Manual] book shredding, defacing, editing, rewriting or try your hand at DSM papier mâché, origami, paper airplanes."[28]

---

[25] Consumer/Survivor Information Resource Centre of Toronto, 2015, Bulletin no. 535. Online: http://www.csinfo.ca/bulletin/Bulletin_535.pdf

[26] July 14 is the day on which French protestors stormed the Bastille fortress (1789). It is considered the beginning of the French revolution and is seen as a symbol of liberation.

[27] For records, flyers, and announcements of past, recent, and upcoming events, consult the following websites: *Toronto*: http://www.torontomadpride.com/; *Hamilton*: http://madpridehamilton.ca/; *Derby*: http://www.derbyshirehealthcareft.nhs.uk/about-us/latest-news/mad-pride-2013/; *Hull*: https://madpride.tk/; *International*: http://www.mindfreedom.org/campaign/madpride/events. See also: Mad Pride issues of the Consumer/Survivor Resource Centre of Canada Bulletin (online: http://www.csinfo.ca/bulletin.php), and *Asylum Magazine* (UK), Spring 2011, Mad Pride issue, volume 18, No. 1.

[28] Consumer/Survivor Information Resource Centre of Toronto, 2012, Bulletin no. 467. Online: http://www.csinfo.ca/bulletin/Bulletin_467.pdf

1.4.2 **The discourses of Mad Pride**

There is no one Mad Pride discourse: there are activists who emphasize the subversive aspects of madness, highlighting its connections to music and art; other activists who endorse a Marxist interpretation of society, seeing Mad Pride as part of the broader class struggle; others for whom the main alliances are with the Occupy, Environmental, and Global Justice movements; others yet for whom madness is about spirituality and connections to other worlds; and those who endorse the goals of Mad Pride and consider themselves affiliated with it but who would not necessarily identify with the term "mad." Despite this diversity, a reading of Mad Pride and affiliated publications, adverts, and manifestos reveals essential elements to the discourse:

- Mad identity and culture
- Madness, creativity, and spirituality
- Madness, distress, and disability
- Madness as a "dangerous gift"

In presenting elements of Mad Pride discourse I revert to verbatim quotes, allowing the arguments to emerge, and concluding with an account of the demands of Mad Pride.

Mad identity and culture

Central to Mad Pride discourse is a reversal of the customary understanding of madness as illness in favor of the view that madness can be grounds for identity and culture. This arises from the capacity of mad people—as expressed in what follows—to make meaning on the basis of unique experiences and phenomena. Further, a sense of solidarity and group identity arises through shared experiences of social stigma and discrimination, as well as struggles with mental health services. The coming together of self-identified ex-patients and survivors of psychiatry to share their experiences, in the context of the production and display of art and music seen to arise from a unique sensitivity and creativity, solidifies Madness as a cultural identity for those involved. The analogy with other groups seeking rights is explicitly made.

> The Mad Pride approach celebrates Mad identities, communities, and cultures including our individual and collective strengths; confronts the shame we are made to feel about our psychiatric histories and experiences of madness; resists the oppression we encounter within aspects of psychiatric/mental health systems and society; reminds us and others that as Mad people we have rights to be ourselves—just like everyone else. (Mad Pride Hamilton)[29]

> What is Mad Culture? Mad Culture is a celebration of the creativity of mad people, and pride in our unique way of looking at life, our internal world externalised and shared with others without shame, as a valid way of life. We are already an alienated sector of society, in fact the most alienated sector of society . . . we need to create our own culture in which we feel comfortable. (Sen 2011, p. 5)

---

[29] From a publicity brochure for Mad Pride Hamilton. A link to the brochure was found at: http://madpridehamilton.ca/2014

> Mad Cultures: When we talk about cultures, we are talking about Mad people as a people and equity-seeking group, not as an illness. Madness is a political and social identity that we take pride in. As Mad people, we have unique ways of experiencing the world, making meaning, knowing and learning, developing communities, and creating cultures. These cultures are showcased and celebrated during Mad Pride. (Mad Pride Hamilton)

The rejection of the language of "mental illness" and "disorder" is central to Mad Pride discourse. To replace it, the term "mad" is reclaimed, and its negative connotations replaced by more positive understandings.

> Madness is an aspect of my identity—who I am and how I experience the world—not an "illness" that is separate from me or a collection of "symptoms" I want cured . . . Canadian health care institutions are currently pushing for the public to think about Mad people as individuals with "illness." (Have you noticed all the mental health awareness campaigns?) This fails to recognize us as an equity-seeking group. We are a people who form communities and create cultures based on our unique ways of thinking, knowing, relating, organizing and living. We promote alternatives to medical ideas about madness. (Triest 2012, pp. 20–1)

> Is there such a thing as a Mad Culture? . . . Madness used to be a word used as a way to belittle people who had psychiatric experiences but these days "madness" is a word that has been reclaimed and re-possessed by the people it originally hurt. Historically there has been a dependence on identifying Mad people only with psychiatric diagnosis, which assumes that all Mad experiences are about biology as if there wasn't a whole wide world out there of mad people with a wide range of experiences, stories, history, meanings, codes and ways of being with each other. (Costa 2015, p. 4)

> Mad Pride moves away from medicalizing experiences under psychiatry to promote other sorts of framings. These Mad positive approaches do not pathologize me. Instead of being seen as someone who is "sick," I am seen as someone who diverges from our traditional narrow, exclusive, and discriminatory idea of "normal." I need the world to be different so that I can thrive as the person that I am . . . Mad Pride sees Mad people as a people and equity-seeking group similar to other marginalized populations. We are not just "individuals" with "illness." (deBie 2013, p. 7)

Mad-positive approaches: Madness, creativity, and spirituality

Mad-positive approaches and framings abound in the writings of activists. Some of these writings emphasize the uniqueness of subjective phenomena of madness: states of heightened sensory awareness, powerful voices and visions, and the ability to perceive complexity and significance in otherwise mundane everyday experiences. In the discipline of psychopathology such phenomena would be labeled as sensory distortions, hallucinations, and delusional perceptions, but for the activists they are special and valuable phenomena. The first two quotes are from the British anthology *Mad Pride: A Celebration of Mad Culture* (2000), and the third is by one of the founders of the Icarus Project:[30]

---

[30] The Icarus Project is a "support network and education project by and for people who experience the world in ways that are often diagnosed as mental illness." It aims to challenge reductive descriptions and categorizations and to "create a language that is so vast and rich that it

But Madness really turns on the colours. Man! Sanity evidently survives in an unfocused jellied miasma of black and white . . . When I was mad and ecstatic, I used to think my heart would burst against my ribcage. I'd write in one colour, then write over it in another. Layers of meaning you could decode by playing different coloured lights upon the page. (Watson 2000, p. 120)

Mad Pride offers the slogan "Madness is the new rock 'n' roll!" There really is so much that's positive and exciting about "illnesses" like "schizophrenia." All of us who've experienced "deep sea fishing" will know the sensation of heightened awareness, of consciousness enhanced far better than LSD could ever do it, of feelings of wonder and terror that can't be verbalised . . . and then have these visions which effortlessly outstrip the alienation of daily life dismissed as "delusion" by some fucking shrink. (Morris 2000, p. 207)

And the moments when I'd been soaring with eyes full of horizon and a heart branded like a contour map with the outlines of rocky sunrises and the fractal branching of so many threads of understanding: these seemed like the most important moments of my life. I didn't want to chalk them up to pathology, give them ugly labels like mania and delusion that seemed to invalidate them, make them less real. I didn't want to eradicate them all for the sake of "stability." Yet as much as I resisted their words, they were all I could find, and over and over again these incredibly limited, awkward words seemed like the barest blueprints to my soul.[31]

Elsewhere, a more "spiritual" approach is taken, emphasizing the ability to "see" unity among objects and events in the world, an ability that may harbor a capacity for wisdom and truth. Here, the slogan "breakdown can be the entrance to breakthrough" is highly relevant (DuBrul 2014, p. 267).

What do the ravings of a madman look like? Are they always incoherent nonsense with little relationship to reality? Or is there a brilliance sometimes, an ability to see phenomena as part of larger systems, to recombine the elements of daily existence through linguistic tricks and the unequivocal magic of metaphor into something that allows us to see a continuity between every little piece of dirt and every human bone that is always present . . .?[32]

Sustainable tribal cultures have elders and traditions that recognize the meaning in breakdown and the potential for the emergence of wisdom. They identify wounded healers and help train them for their new role by guiding them through the process. By contrast, mad individuals in the West are set adrift, cast aside as broken and useless. To navigate ourselves through our initiation, we have to create ourselves and a new culture as we go along.

---

expresses the infinite diversity of human experiences" (see the mission statement here: http://theicarusproject.net/mission-vision-principles/). The Icarus Project considers itself part of the Mad Pride movement; its founding member Sascha DuBrul (2014, p. 262) wrote: "At the heart of our connection is the utilization of pride around an oppressed identity to inspire political action and the understanding that when we stop being afraid of being exposed for a shamed identity, there is nothing that can stop us." Nevertheless, the Icarus Project website notes that not all members associate with the word Mad.

[31] Jacks McNamara, founding member of the Icarus Project. Statement can be found online: http://nycicarus.org/images/navigating_the_space.pdf

[32] Icarus Project: Shamanism, Psychosis and Hope for a Dying World. Online: http://legacy.theicarusproject.net/content/shamanism-psychosis-and-hope-dying-world

The key is overcoming isolation and connecting with others who have been through it too, as we explore our lives and chart new maps of return from the abyss.[33]

The uniqueness of phenomena of madness presents a potential source of creative output, a connection frequently made in Mad Pride writings by pointing out the cultural (and artistic) contributions of those deemed "mentally ill":

> Mad Pride reminds us of the great cultural contributions that those deemed mad had made in our world. When you think of madness, remember that Vincent van Gogh, Ernest Hemmingway, Emily Dickenson, and Frances Farmer were all non-conformists considered "mad."[34]

> Mad Pride is an event that will focus on the strengths of Mad people and celebrate our existence. This is a sharp contrast to the frequent depictions of our lives as tragic and not worth living or of Mad people as violent. We don't aim to glorify the suffering we endure—but rather to celebrate our skills, contributions, creativity, poetry, writing, music, art, theatre, humour, ideas, knowledge, friendships, and community. (deBie 2013, p. 8)

> [Mad Pride] allows us all to embrace each other in peace with love through laughter. We give you music, poetry, art, beauty yet we are stigmatized unto death. We need society to wake up to its responsibility towards us by taking pride in our responsibility towards ourselves.[35]

Madness, distress, and disability

This aspect of the discourse takes account of the distress and disability associated with madness/mental health phenomena. This is important in that it attempts to reconceive the apparently negative side of madness—which is, primarily, the only side seen by medicine and in public discourse—in such a way that does not contradict the foregoing positive approaches.

The first set of quotes indicate awareness of the emotional and experiential difficulties people can face:

> Fostering pride isn't always easy. It definitely isn't always loud and visible. When my life is difficult and exhausting, pride is not the first place I go. Usually I just want things to be less difficult, to experience some relief from figuring out how to navigate systems that aren't built for the way I think and feel and need to act. A lot of the time society perpetuates negative ideas about people like me so it's not unsurprising that I can feel shame for how I live and who I am. (deBie 2013, p. 8)

> I was always mad, and OK, being caught by the psychiatric system was no fun and sometimes the enhanced awareness that comes when I'm VERY mad can be a bit much to cope

---

[33] Icarus Project: Wounded Healers: Illness as Calling. Online: http://theicarusproject.net/articles/wounded-healers-illness-as-calling

[34] MindFreedom International Mad Pride campaign. Published in *Asylum: The Magazine for Democratic Psychiatry*, 2011, volume 18, issue 1, p. 20.

[35] Mad Pride Ireland. Online: http://www.madprideireland.ie/about/ (As of December 2017, the website has ceased working.)

with. But I'm still glad to be mad—beautiful, clinching evidence of concrete outsiderdom. (Morris 2000, p. 208)

Several strategies exist that deal with distress and disability. The first accepts that madness can be associated with distress, emotional and behavioral difficulties but attributes this to social and interpersonal problems rather than individual failing or pathology. Commonly cited difficulties are abuse, trauma, discrimination, oppression, stigma, poverty, and social inequality.

> . . . if we eliminated abuse, war, greed, racism, sexism, broken families, ecocide, monotonous wage labor and egoism, we would see a massive reduction in what gets called mental illness. But these bigger picture problems are overwhelming and require an enormous responsibility from all of us to fundamentally change, so instead they are often cast into the background in favor of blaming an individual's brain or genes. Thus . . . we are "Schizophrenic" and "Bipolar" not because we are traumatized or overwhelmed by the madness of our society, but because our brains are too weak to handle it. Instead of taking a ruthless moral inventory of our culture, families, societies, economics, religions, education systems, and pointing the finger outwards, we do it of and to ourselves, and now of and to our biology. (Smiles 2011, p. 8)

> We recognize that we all live in a crazy world and that too many of us struggle due to ongoing legacies of abuse, colonization, racism, ableism, sexism, and other interlocking forms of oppression. We affirm that social justice is the foundation of healthy societies and foster supportive relationships free of violence and oppression.[36]

> It is true that people labelled mentally ill may engage in behaviours that are destructive to themselves or others, but people too often assume that these choices stem only from the thought patterns; without considering that the choices may instead be a reaction to the frustration, anger and alienation that are a result of society's refusal to validate those thought patterns. (Polvora 2011, p. 5)

Another strategy, here dealing with disability, is to affirm that what gets called "mental illness" is a variation on human experience and function. These variations lead to problems in functioning because the world is not set up to accommodate them.

> Most mental illnesses are seen as disorders because they prevent the person from functioning properly in the social world we have set up for ourselves . . . If the majority of the population was bipolar, things would be set up to accommodate them, and those without bipolar "symptoms" would struggle to fit in and understand the world. Is failure to hold up to the expectations of other people really a disorder? (Polvora 2011, p. 4)

A third strategy is to accept that there are aspects of madness that are distressing—for example, aggressive voices and other terrifying experiences—and to explain this as the price one may have to pay for the special gift of madness.

"Dangerous gifts"

The Janus-faced nature of madness led to the important formulation that individual traits and sensitivities are "dangerous gifts." This idea was popularized by the Icarus

---

[36] Icarus Project: Mission, Vision, and Principles. Online: http://theicarusproject.net/ mission-vision-principles/

Project, a "network of people living with experiences that are commonly labeled as psychiatric conditions."[37] An initial statement of origin and intent declared:

> Defining ourselves outside convention we see our condition as a dangerous gift to be cultivated and taken care of rather than as a disease or disorder needing to be "cured." With this double edged blessing we have the ability to fly to places of great vision and creativity, but like the boy Icarus, we also have the potential to fly dangerously close to the sun— into realms of delusion and psychosis—and crash in a blaze of fire and confusion. At our heights we may find ourselves capable of creating music, art, words, and inventions which touch people's souls and change the course of history. At our depths we may end up alienated and alone, incarcerated in psychiatric institutions, or dead by our own hands. Despite these risks, we recognize the intertwined threads of madness and creativity as tools of inspiration and hope in this repressed and damaged society. We understand that we are members of a group that has been misunderstood and persecuted throughout history, but has also been responsible for some of its most brilliant creations. And we are proud. (DuBrul 2014, p. 259)

With the four main elements of Mad Pride discourse specified, it remains to be asked: what demands emerge from it?

Demands

From the discourse of Mad Pride emerges a clear demand, expressed unambiguously in many of the earlier quotes, and particularly in the following:

> I need the world to be different so that I can thrive as the person that I am. (deBie 2013, p. 7)

> Madness is an aspect of my identity—who I am and how I experience the world—not an "illness" that is separate from me or a collection of "symptoms" I want cured. (Triest 2012, p. 20)

> We need to create our own culture in which we feel comfortable. (Sen 2011, p. 5)

> As Mad people we have the right to be ourselves—just like everyone else. (Mad Pride Hamilton)

The expectation is for society to change in order to accommodate a unique identity and culture, one that is regarded by its holders in a positive light in that it possesses creative and spiritual potential, and can contribute to the world if allowed the cultural space to thrive. Hence, a major site of change is the reductive, discriminatory, and disrespectful language that dominates public and professional narratives, a language in which key terms all indicate deficit and pathology: disease, illness, disorder, delusion, hallucination, and, of course, "madness" itself prior to its reclamation by activists.

By demanding change in the social beliefs, norms, values, and overall practices that define madness/mental disorder—essentially society's total understanding—Mad Pride's demands lie on a par with demands for recognition long voiced by the more familiar collective identities constructed around race, gender, and sexuality. Such features constitute centers of gravity around which arise specific ways of life, perspectives, historical narratives, and shared experiences. The analogy with gay, black and women's

---

[37] Icarus Project Navigating Crisis Handout. Online: http://theicarusproject.net/wp-content/uploads/2016/08/IcarusNavigatingCrisisHandoutLarge05-09.pdf

rights is central to Mad Pride discourse and is frequently pointed out, as noted in the following:

> We need to unite to fight against society's discrimination against us, just as black people have, as women did with feminism, as gays did in the fight for equality. All these changes did not take place because society felt guilty about ostracising sections of society. The changes took place because a group of people came together and demanded change. We can never truly fight the oppression we experience every day so long as we are afraid to demand change, afraid to define ourselves as a cultural group. (Clare 2011, p. 15)

In urging cultural change, the demands of Mad Pride go beyond the equalization of civil rights *irrespective* of difference (which requires a politics of equality that rejects discrimination on the basis of morally irrelevant features) but, rather, the recognition of that difference: the distinctness of the identity in question, its claim to respect and equality. Hence, what Mad Pride want is not only to be afforded equal civil rights like everyone else; they want nothing less than a radical cultural and symbolic transformation in society that restores respect and worth to people's identities and lives.

Mad Pride is a radical discourse, and the claim that the Mad are a people whose identities are being disrespected akin to black and gay individuals is a radical claim. If true, then society has a real problem at its hands evident in public and professional stigma, discrimination, and disrespect toward mad people that would not be accepted in this day if directed toward any other group. For example, open any standard textbook of psychiatry, pick a passage on schizophrenia, then replace the term "schizophrenia" with "black" or "gay" and you are bound to feel uncomfortable in the distancing language, and the negative registers of the terms used in the descriptions. On that basis it is important to critically examine Mad Pride discourse and to resist succumbing to the powerful intuitions at play. For it is fair to say that common intuitions in this matter—that it *really* cannot be the case that madness can be grounds for identity and culture—should not be taken at face value, no matter how strong they are: similar intuitions were at play among critics of the gay liberation movement in its early days and are now widely considered to have been prejudices. On the other hand, to unquestioningly accept the discourse as valid and morally obligating is equally problematic: first, such acceptance would not satisfy the demand for substantial change in social norms, beliefs, and values, as this change requires serious engagement with the discourse in a process whose outcome cannot be prejudged; second, if it turns out that the discourse lacks validity or has limited normative force, then unquestioning acceptance can be harmful and unjustifiably burdensome on our moral obligation. A critical examination of the discourse is therefore required. Before commencing, a brief review of engagement with Mad Pride in the philosophic and psychiatric literature would be helpful in establishing the current state of thinking about these issues.

1.5 Philosophical engagement with Mad Pride discourse

Engagement with Mad Pride and mad-positive discourse in the philosophy and psychiatry literature is limited. It is concerned with restating what the discourse is trying to achieve, and providing it with a theoretical mooring in extant theories of power and social justice.

Bracken and Thomas (2005) note that Mad Pride is not aiming to improve psychiatry or fight coercion, but has the much broader and ambitious goal of initiating social and cultural change in the way "madness" and "normality" are perceived. Elsewhere they write, "what is most exciting about these groups is that they are not only reshaping the contours of mental health discourse but they are also reshaping our views of what it is to be normal, to be human and to be free" (Thomas and Bracken 2008, p. 48). Activists try to achieve this, in part, by reclaiming the power to define themselves, and to have their contributions to society recognized (Bracken and Thomas 2005, p. 80). The authors understand such activism as a struggle for full citizenship, which requires that one is "free of discrimination, exclusion and oppression" and is able "to define one's own identity and to celebrate this identity in different ways" (2005, p. 81). In addition, Thomas and Bracken (2008) provide an elucidation of Mad Pride activism in terms of Michel Foucault's theory of power and subjectivity. This is the idea that liberation requires, first and foremost, that one brings to light and resists phenomena of power by which subjectivities—persons' identities, experiences, actions, attitudes—are constituted. Given this perspective, dominant psychiatric and social narratives concerning "madness" are instances of power and must be resisted, as Mad Pride seeks to do.[38]

Radden and Sadler (2010) point toward the ethical challenges facing clinicians who are likely to find the views put forward by some mental health activists, such as those of Mad Pride, incompatible with the fundamentals of their profession. Clinicians are experts trained in treating mental disorder, and to be asked to consider such disorders as grounds for identity rather than negative states to be treated is a challenge. In such cases, Radden and Sadler (2010, p. 58) note, the clinician "cannot be required to adopt such fundamentally warring sets of assumptions" but should, nevertheless:

> try to understand, and to respect, these alternative perspectives, recognising the degree of controversy attaching to these ideas, and understanding the source of that controversy— the extent to which they rest not only on discoverable empirical realities but on deeply held moral and philosophical attitudes and beliefs.

Radden (2012) sheds further light on this controversy, providing it with a normative foundation in theories of social justice. Appealing to Nancy Fraser's two paradigms of justice—redistribution and recognition—she points out that mental health consumers (her preferred term) have a stake both in the redistribution of resources and opportunities and in the recognition of oppressed and stigmatized identities. The latter is particularly relevant at present, and provides a paradigm within which one can understand and justify activists' demands for cultural and symbolic reparation. Activists

---

[38] In a recent publication, Bracken and Thomas (2013) considered Mad Pride and related movements as presenting a challenge to the modernist, technologically driven agenda and expert-led authority of psychiatry. Such an ethos is at odds with mental health activism where there is a move to redefine madness in nonbiomedical ways, and to have much greater involvement in how services are structured and run.

have a stake in redefining and reconstructing their identity and challenging psychiatric master narratives. In doing this, as Radden astutely notes, the challenge is not merely to change the name from mentally ill to Mad Pride, but to "re-conceptualise all aspects of the way mental disorder is construed," which will inevitably have to invoke deeply held norms and values. She writes:

> . . . much is implicated in a reconstruction of cultural ideas about mental health and illness, because the beliefs, metaphors, assumptions, and presuppositions affecting patterns of representation, communication, and interpretation about this kind of disorder are entwined with categories and concepts fundamental to our cultural norms and values: rationality, mind and character, self-control, competence, responsibility and personhood. (2012, p. 3)

There is no doubt, therefore, that the radical nature and the depth and extent of Mad Pride's demands are recognized by the aforementioned scholars. Thomas and Bracken (2008, p. 48) are correct to note, as just quoted, that what's at stake is nothing less than "reshaping our views of what it is to be normal, to be human." Also important is seeing the demands in light of theories of social justice, as this would offer a foothold from where, subject to further analysis and consideration, it may be judged that Mad Pride's demands do carry normative force and the reasons they do so specified.

1.6 Next steps

From the account of Mad activism presented in this chapter, we can discern a claim and a demand: the claim that madness is grounds for culture and identity, and the demand that society should recognize the validity and worth of Mad culture and Mad identity. Parts III and IV are devoted to examining these claims by addressing the following questions: Can madness be grounds for culture or identity? Does the demand for recognition possess normative force and, if it does, how should society respond to it? To make progress with these questions, we need an account of the concepts and politics of identity and recognition. Accordingly, Part II develops an account of the concept of recognition; an understanding of the notions of social and individual identity; and a framework for responding to and justifying demands that require the recognition of what is distinctive between human beings over and above the guarantee of equality irrespective of difference. Before we can begin Part II, there are a set of problems that we need to address: Some objectors to Mad activism have argued that madness is inherently disabling and distressing, a point which they take to preclude positive or neutral evaluations and to lend support to the view that madness is a disorder of the mind and not grounds for culture or identity. Owing to the commonality and importance of these objections, I now turn to addressing them.

Chapter 2

The problem of distress and disability

2.1 **Introduction**

In their attempts to develop positive narratives of mental health phenomena, narratives that can counteract the pervasive negative views in society and the profession of psychiatry, Mad Pride and mad-positive activism faces considerable challenges.[1] The goals of Mad activism, as described in Chapter 1, include promoting the view that madness can be grounds for identity and culture, and demonstrating that phenomena of madness such as states of heightened sensory awareness, visions and voices, and the ability to perceive complexity and significance in everyday experiences are special and potentially valuable phenomena. Yet success in achieving these goals depends, in part but vitally, on the ability to deal with the fact that madness is frequently associated with distress and difficulties in social functioning. This Janus-faced nature of madness—at once a source of creativity and suffering—is recognized in Mad Pride discourse and expressed in the formulation that individual traits and sensitivities are "dangerous gifts" requiring cultivation and care (see section 1.4.2). Yet the question of distress and disability has proved to be a sticking point for Mad Pride discourse and for mad-positive approaches in general: how can one advance a positive or neutral framing of that which appears to be inherently negative?

This criticism has been expressed strongly by service users as well as academics. Clare Allan, an ex-patient who has written about her experiences with mental health services, argues that there is nothing about "mental illness" of which to be proud. While she recognizes the stigma faced by mental health patients, she understands Mad Pride as essentially a tactic to bolster the self-esteem of service users who for years have been subjected to stigma and disrespect by society and degrading treatment by services; she elaborates:

> Mental illness is not an identity. Nor is it something I wish to celebrate . . . Mental illness is ruthless, indiscriminate and destructive. It is also an illness. It is certainly not a weakness, but nor is it a sign of a special "artistic" sensitivity. It affected Van Gogh, as it does

[1] Parts of this chapter appear in: Rashed, M. A. (2018a). In Defense of Madness: The Problem of Disability. *Journal of Medicine and Philosophy.* (doi.org/10.1093/jmp/jhy016)

bus drivers, plumbers, teachers, older people and children. Winston Churchill was reportedly manic-depressive, if so, it's a diagnosis he shares with my friend Cathy, a mother of two from Peckham. Mental illness is an illness, just as cancer is an illness; and people die from both.[2]

A similar criticism can be found in the academic literature. Jost (2009, p. 2) writes that "mental illnesses" are not *different* ways of processing information or emotion; they are *disorders* in the capacities for processing information or emotion." It is absurd, she argues, to urge people to embrace such conditions and regard them positively. In making this point, Jost draws a distinction between conditions that are disabling because the physical and social environment fails to accommodate variations in traits and characteristics, and "mental illnesses" which are "inherently negative" and "will always cause suffering" even if stigma and disadvantage were to be eliminated (Jost 2009). Perring (2009) considers that for some of those who object to the movement, the analogy with black pride or gay pride—an analogy made in Mad Pride discourse—can only go so far as none of these are intrinsically disabling features of a person while "mental illnesses" tend to be seen as such. That is why, he notes, it would be equally bizarre to have a Cancer Pride movement. Such views no doubt have wide currency among many clinicians, who see every day in the clinic the effects of "mental illness": social and functional deterioration, loss of friends and family, and the distress of extreme mental states.

There is therefore a challenge facing Mad Pride discourse and mad-positive approaches: the problem of distress and disability; this chapter responds to this challenge. Disability, on an initial reading, consists in limitations to/impairments of everyday functioning and participation. Distress concerns affective states such as fear, anxiety, or sadness. Disability and distress can be connected, of course: intense fear can impact on functioning and disability can engender anxiety. This connection will be noted as required, but the two concepts raise different issues and require separate consideration. With regard to disability I develop two bulwarks against the tendency to adopt too readily the (medical) view that madness is inherently disabling. These bulwarks arise from: (1) the normative basis of disability judgments; (2) the implications of political activism in terms of being a social subject. Throughout the ensuing set of arguments on disability my purpose is not to argue against the medical model of disability as such—it certainly has its place in our thinking and practices—but against the tendency to assume it too readily in the case of madness. With regard to distress, the argument is shorter and the strategy simpler: the key point is to accommodate distress in such a way that does not undermine the idea that madness can be a positive or neutral conception of identity.

---

[2] Clare Allan. Misplaced Pride. The Guardian Newspaper. September 27, 2006. Online: http://www.theguardian.com/commentisfree/2006/sep/27/society.socialcare

2.2 **Disability**

2.2.1 **Clarifying the criticism**

The criticism of Mad Pride discourse—more generally, the criticism of attempts to construct counternarratives that remove madness from the space of psychopathology—can be stated as follows:

◆ "Mental illness" is associated with disability.

◆ This association is not contingent: disability is intrinsic to "mental illness," by which is meant that the various limitations experienced by individuals with those "conditions" are a result of the "conditions" and not the result of an intolerant or unaccommodating society.

◆ By contrast, so the argument would go, the limitations experienced by gay individuals were/are a result of a homophobic society that denied them equal rights and the right to be themselves. Once we correct for social discrimination and oppression, the limitations that gay individuals face will reduce.

In brief, the criticism can be formulated as follows: *even in a utopian world where there is absolutely no discrimination and a surplus of well-meaning regard that people show toward each other, "mental illness" will still reduce the well-being of those afflicted.* To be clear from the outset this statement cannot be intended as an empirical claim, partly because there are no studies of the fate of "mental illness" in Utopia, and partly because the proof demanded for this claim to work requires that the phenomena in question remain disabling *after* all socially discriminating and negative conditions have been removed. The problem here is that it will never be possible to assert that one has concluded the investigation, as it will not be possible to know if social conditions are the best they could be. Given that it is not intended as an empirical claim, what exactly is the basis for it? To gain some further ground here we can consider a possible response to this criticism, one that appears in the activist literature and has been raised in Chapter 1.

The response is to affirm that what is referred to as "mental illness" is a variation on human experiences and ways of being. The reason these variations may lead to problems in functioning has to do with a social world that is not set up to accommodate them and not due to some intrinsic malfunction:

> Most mental illnesses are seen as disorders because they prevent the person from functioning properly in the social world we have set up for ourselves . . . If the majority of the population was bipolar, things would be set up to accommodate them, and those without bipolar "symptoms" would struggle to fit in and understand the world. Is failure to hold up to the expectations of other people really a disorder? (Polvora 2011, p. 4)

Both the criticism and the response to it purport to specify the locus of the problem: the former locates the cause of disability in the individual—in the "mental illness" to be precise—and the latter locates it in a society designed to accommodate a particular norm. Essentially, then, the two positions here reflect a "medical" versus a "social" understanding of the limitations associated with madness. To arbitrate between them I visit the social model of disability, a framework that has been substantially worked out in disability theory and can help make sense of this dispute.

2.2.2 **Models of disability**

According to standard definitions, disability is comprised of a physical or mental *impairment* associated with long-term *limitations* on the ability to perform daily activities.[3] In light of this framework, blindness would be an impairment (or, for a less value-laden term, a variation) that ordinarily would limit the person's ability for personal and social functioning. The priority given either to the impairment or to the social and physical environment in generating limitations gave rise to a number of disability models, the most prominent of which are the medical and the social models. The medical (individual) model emphasizes variations as the primary cause of limitation and prescribes medical correction and/or financial compensation. The social model, endorsed in some form by many disability activists and theoreticians, emphasizes that limitations arise from a physical and social environment designed and conducted in such a way that excludes or does not take into account individuals with variations in traits or characteristics (Oliver 1990, 1996).[4] The social model shifts attention to restrictive and exclusionary conditions in society and prescribes various sorts of accommodations to address this. In the case of sensory impairments/ variations (e.g., blindness), accommodations can include practical adjustments such as tactile and audio signage.

It is important at this point to introduce some complexity into the notion of limitation in view of the kinds of actions involved. Nordenfelt (1997) distinguishes basic actions from generated actions. A basic action, such as moving a limb, is a simple and primary action that constitutes the first step in the chain that ends with complex, or generated, action (Nordenfelt 1997, p. 611). The latter are actions describable at the level of the person in terms of overarching goals, such as writing a book or making a chair, for example. In order to clarify what basic actions are, it helps to see them as actions that become apparent by their absence. Further, the notion of basic *action* needs to be broadened to incorporate aspects of our fundamental abilities that are not ordinarily thought of as actions. For example, a certain level of concentration is required in order to be able to focus on a task. Concentration, according to the view advanced here, is not a basic "action" but a basic "ability" that underpins much of what we do.

Ordinarily, we become aware of the basic nature of some of our abilities when we are thwarted in realizing our complex goals. Ideally, the body is the medium through which we project and realize our intentions in the world. It remains in the background as a transparent medium until, for some reason, its interference with our complex goals renders salient a particular aspect or function. It can be a painful limb, impaired concentration, poor vision, or a heightened state of anxiety. All of these can be considered within the scope of basic abilities in the sense that they are disruptions to the

----

[3] See, for example, the UK Equality Act (2010), the US Americans with Disabilities Act (1990), and the United Nations Convention on the Rights of Persons with Disabilities (2006).

[4] See Silvers (2010) for a good philosophical overview of the social model of disability.

taken for granted background of our complex activity in the world, and become salient when they hold us back.[5]

On this basis we can distinguish two levels of limitation. The first level consists in the basic inabilities (typified in disability models as impairments or variations) that become salient when our complex activity in the world is disrupted. [6] The second level consists in the disruptions to the complex activity itself: the inability to work, socialize, or go to the market. Now while an impairment constitutes a limitation at the basic level—a blind person cannot see, a broken limb cannot bear weight—it is not by itself sufficient for limitations at the level of complex activity. Complex actions are always performed in some physical and social environment, and the extent to which we can realize our goals depends, in part, on the match between the environment and our (in) abilities (see Amundson 1992, pp. 109–10). [7] So, while a blind person may be unable to see (a limitation at the level of basic abilities), his inability to realize employment (a limitation at the level of complex action) can be addressed through specially designed working quarters that take into account his specific sensory abilities. Of course, one may wish to correct for the basic inability (the impairment)—to correct for loss of

---

[5] Note that there is a difference between a person born with a sensory inability (or variation)—blindness, for example—and a person who loses sight as an adult. The latter experiences a radical change in functional capacities which may be very distressing and disabling and may take some time to adapt to. On the other hand, a person born blind may not necessarily experience blindness as a salient obstacle in everyday life. This may change, however, if that person wishes, for example, to seek employment or further his or her independence. At that point, not being able to see in the context of a physical environment that does not take this particular sensory inability (or variation) into account, may generate disability.

[6] It is possible for a particular state to become salient without resulting in disruption to daily activity; a twisted ankle may cause pain and discomfort without rendering the sufferer immobile. Similarly, one may experience sadness, paranoia or anxiety without this limiting social interaction or activity. However, the discussion in this section concerns disability, and the issue is disruption to activity.

[7] A point of clarification: A person with paraplegia and no recourse to a wheelchair may find it very difficult to move from point A to point B. Here he is clearly thwarted in realizing his goal and the obstruction is not—at least not self-evidently—a consequence of unaccommodating social arrangements. Disability theorists who endorse the social model for mobility impairments tend to begin their argument by assuming the presence of a wheelchair. Disability consists in the limitations faced by the wheelchair user in environments with limited stair-free access. Critics of this argument could object that you cannot assume the wheelchair as it is not part of a human's natural embodiment. Once you remove the wheelchair, they could argue, the extent of nonsocially imposed disability becomes evident. A response to this objection is to think of the wheelchair as a tool that improves the functional abilities of persons who cannot walk. If I come across a 1-tonne boulder and find myself unable to push it out of my path, I face a limit to my functional capacities. In order to move the boulder, I make use of tools either to break it down to smaller parts or to push it out of the way. Human beings use tools throughout the day to help them compensate for their functional capacities and to accomplish tasks that otherwise would not be possible. The wheelchair is a tool in this sense, and it is acceptable to assume it as a given in arguments concerning the social basis of disability.

vision or hearing, for example—but where that is not possible (technologically) or desired (e.g., Deaf Pride), then the variation/environment interaction can be scrutinized for impediments to the realization of some specific complex goals.

Another helpful way to cash out the distinction between these two levels of limitation is in terms of the extent to which disadvantages are conditional on/produced by the social context. Amundson and Tresky (2007, p. 544) define the terms as follows:

> Conditional Disadvantages of Impairment (CDIs): Disadvantages that are experienced by people with impairments, but which are produced by the social context in which those people live.

> Unconditional Disadvantages of Impairment (UDIs): Disadvantages that are experienced by people with impairments, but which are produced irrespective of their social context.

Mapped onto the two levels of limitations specified earlier, basic inabilities would be unconditional while disruptions to complex activities would be conditional. While I see a place for the distinction, I would not put it this strongly as the notion of an absolutely unconditional disadvantage does not work (except for some kinds of pain and psychological distress). As I argued previously, a basic inability is made salient in the context of failing to achieve a complex action. The latter itself is relative to physical and social environmental contexts and hence is, in part, conditional upon them. So it is more accurate to see this distinction as a matter of degree and not kind; as a distinction concerning the proximity of a particular description of disadvantage to one's physical and mental states as opposed to the environment in which one is pursuing goals. [8]

The importance of the distinction between conditional and unconditional disadvantages is that it serves to limit the "oversocialization" of the radical form of the social model of disability, which appears to deny a role for impairment in generating disadvantage (Terzi 2004, p. 153). With this distinction in place it becomes possible to argue, for example, that while a deaf person may be unable to hear and may not be able to listen to music, these particular "limitations" flow from the impairment/variation and are separate from the restrictions he or she may face in finding employment or watching the news when no alternative form of communication, such as sign language, is made available.[9] The former are basic inabilities—whether or not they are undesirable—and the latter are the limitations caused by an unaccommodating social environment. As Amundson and Tresky (2007, p. 544) note, in disability rights unconditional disadvantages "are taken as brute facts of human variation" and are not considered within the scope of disability claims and campaigning. Similarly, the social

---

[8] Note that the focus here is on the generation of disadvantage (limitation) and not the factors implicated in the genesis of the variation/impairment in the first place, which can include various psychological, biological, and social factors.

[9] Unconditional disadvantages are referred to in the disability literature as "impairment effects." These include the discomfort, pain, and inabilities which disabled people face, and which are distinguished in the literature from the disadvantages experienced as a consequence of social restrictions and discrimination (Thomas 2004).

model—writes Mike Oliver (2004, p. 22), the person credited with its introduction— "is not about the personal experience of impairment but the collective experience of disablement."

Having made this distinction, it is important to note that there is no hard and fast way of drawing the line between unconditional and conditional disadvantages. The distinction is worked out in practice, leaning heavily on disabled peoples' experiences, and on what exactly the demand for social accommodation is about in the context of wider debates on these issues (see Amundson and Tresky 2007, p. 553). Yet the problem with the medical model of disability, and with the criticisms of Mad activism described earlier, is that this distinction—if it is made at all—appears to lean too heavily on one side, with all or most limitations considered to arise from the impairment/variation. Such medical models conflate the two levels of limitation discerned earlier, or recognize them as distinct but put too much emphasis on basic inabilities over disruption to complex activity. The area of contention then lies precisely at the boundary where what is put forward by disability rights activists as a conditional disadvantage is seen by advocates of the medical model as an unconditional disadvantage flowing from, or intrinsic to, the impairment itself. It is the latter, medical view which I consider problematic and to which I now turn.

2.2.3 **Naturalism, normativism, and disability**

Critics of the medical model of disability have argued that the claim that limitations are "caused" by the impairment—that, say, not being able to access information is caused by a person's sensory impairments—presupposes a naturalistic view of function (Amundson 2000). Naturalism is the view that norms of physical and mental functioning can be objectively determined. Two well-known naturalist accounts have been put forward by Christopher Boorse and Jerome Wakefield. For Boorse (1997), a normal function of a part or process of an individual is a statistically typical contribution by it to the individual's survival and reproduction. Statistically normal function is determined relative to the individual's reference class, which is the appropriate segment of the species as defined by age and sex.[10] For Wakefield (1992, p. 384), the natural function of a mechanism is the function for which it has been designed (selected) in evolution; it is "part of the evolutionary explanation of the existence and structure of the mechanism." For example, the heart pumps blood, the legs move our body, and the visual system conveys perceptual information about the world: these are natural functions of the respective organs; they are what the organs were designed to do.

Based on their accounts of natural function, Boorse and Wakefield can then purport to specify physical or mental dysfunction in value-free terms as deviation from natural function. Both also recognize that that is not sufficient by itself to delineate the conditions that should be treated. For Boorse and Wakefield a further evaluative component is required, which consists in the evaluation of this dysfunction as harmful in light of personal, social, and medical norms (Boorse 2011, p. 28; Wakefield 1992). In

---

[10] Reference classes are included by Boorse to account for the wide variation of function within *homo sapiens*: normal function in a newborn is not the same for an 8-year-old child.

Wakefield's formulation, disorder becomes a *harmful dysfunction*, or—which amounts to the same thing for our purposes here—a harmful *impairment*. With this kind of reasoning, a blind person would have a dysfunction/impairment in the visual apparatus which, if associated with harm, would qualify the condition as a disorder. And given that according to naturalistic accounts function is a matter of objectively determined natural facts—with dysfunction being a deviation from normal function—then the limitation, the harm, that may arise from this is referred back to the dysfunction and not to a deficiency in the design of the physical and social environments relative to the functional abilities of different persons. This is because the person with a dysfunction, on this view, lies outside the range of normal functional abilities, and he or she lies outside this range not due to some discriminatory value judgment, but by the facts of human nature.

The foregoing view requires naturalism about function, but the problem is that attempts to define dysfunction in value-free terms have not been successful. The arguments here have been well rehearsed by several philosophers and I will only state their conclusions.[11]

Since its inception, Boorse's theory has been subject to a lively interchange and many objections. Of particular relevance here are accusations of implicit normativism in both the notion of statistically normal function and the reference class against which this is to be assessed. With regard to the former, Bolton (2008, p. 113) points out that statistical (ab)normality does not by itself tell us at what point on a continuous distribution curve "deviance from the mean become(s) subnormal function." Factors that do in fact underlie this judgment are those associated with the value component: harm and functional limitations as judged by personal and, more broadly, social values and norms. As a principle purporting to provide a factual basis for discerning normal from subnormal function, statistical normality does not work. With regard to reference classes, Kingma (2007, 2013) argues that Boorse's account requires that he specify the reference classes appropriate to an assessment of health. Otherwise, any condition can be rendered healthy if we devise a reference class that shows it in a good light. For example, if we were to allow for a reference class of "uncommonly heavy drinkers," then liver functions that would otherwise be considered abnormal would no longer be so, and those heavy drinkers, according to Boorse's account, would be considered healthy (Kingma 2007, p. 128). Boorse therefore needs to provide an account of the appropriate reference classes, and to do so in a value-free, noncircular way; that is, without introducing values into what is supposed to be a fact-based definition of normal function, and without presupposing the distinction he is trying to prove between health and disease. As Kingma (2007, 2013) argues, Boorse's account cannot provide this.

---

[11] There are many critiques of naturalist accounts of (dys)function; the following are particularly helpful: Boorse (2011, pp. 26–37) for a summary of the theories and the objections; Bolton (2008) for a short critique of Boorse's theory and a substantial analysis and critique of Wakefield's; Kingma (2013) offers an overview of both theories and a general critique of naturalist accounts of disorder.

Wakefield's *harmful dysfunction* analysis of disorder has also met with serious objections. Dysfunction, as noted here, is deviation from the natural function of a mechanism, the function that explains, in evolutionary terms, the mechanism's existence and design.[12] For our purposes here, the most relevant objection to Wakefield's analysis of dysfunction questions its presumed factual basis. For Wakefield, the norms underpinning function are natural (evolutionary) norms to be contrasted with social (cultivated) norms (Bolton 2008, p. 124). The former underpin the objective status of dysfunction and the latter feature in the harm component. According to Bolton (2013), it is no longer possible to maintain a clear distinction between what is natural/innate and what is social/cultivated. It is now generally accepted that psychological functions are a product of an interaction between several factors: socialization processes, genetic inheritance, and individual differences and choices (Bolton 2013, pp. 442–3). These factors are not separable through the science we currently possess (Bolton 2013). Yet without a clear distinction, Wakefield's account cannot tag exclusively onto a fact of our evolutionary nature in its bid to provide a value-free account of dysfunction.

If we accept the criticisms of these two leading naturalist theories, we can conclude that it has not proven possible to define function and dysfunction in value-free terms. We may accept this conclusion yet continue the search for a value-free, theoretical concept of function. An alternative position is to take seriously the value-ladenness of the relevant concepts and see where this may lead us. It will lead us to various forms of normativism about function. Here, descriptions of normal function are made in terms of what is good or bad, desirable or undesirable for an agent in the context of specific life-situations and environments, in the present or a projected future. Those descriptions, though not pretending to have an objective standpoint in nature, are not any less "real" than naturalistic accounts: the core values that inform our lives, the projects we engage in, and the futures we plan are very serious matters. It is a reflection of their seriousness that we tend to refer to those aspects of our abilities that may prevent us from pursuing them as *diseases* or *disorders*. But the apparent objectivity of these terms should not obscure that they signal a normative and not a natural limit; they signal the limit of what a person and/or society considers normal, valuable, or good. These latter notions are set against a background of abilities that are considered the norm, in the sense of being the taken for granted foundations of a particular way of life in a particular social and physical environment. This has implications on how we can talk about disability.

It will help at this point to recall the problem that led us here. It was borne out of the need to arbitrate between the medical and social views on the origin of the limitations associated with variations in function. Advocates of the medical model consider the majority of the limitations to be unconditional (i.e., intrinsic to the dysfunction/impairment/variation itself). Given the prior analysis, we have a different way of understanding this claim. When we witness a person struggling to achieve some

---

[12] One problem with Wakefield's approach is that even if we assume that it is correct, it has limited clinical utility: it speculates the existence of complex evolved mechanisms in the absence of ready-to-hand models that could enable a clinician to judge whether the patient in the consultation room has a relevant evolutionary dysfunction as opposed to a design/environment mismatch (Bolton 2007).

complex goal, we may refer this back to some dysfunction in his or her abilities. Now we can see that the limit drawn by our reference to dysfunction is a normative and not a natural limit. Hence, when we say that a dysfunction (or an impairment or variation) is intrinsically disabling, we need also to give an account of the norms, values, and contexts by which we were driven to make this claim, and to come to terms with *that* being the basis of our judgment. The importance of remaining cognizant of this point is that in its absence we would not occasion the need to perhaps examine those norms, values, and contexts and see if they can be modified in such a way that would reflect positively on that person's ability to function and thrive in society through various sorts of adjustments. This would act as a bulwark against the gratuitous individualization of the difficulties others face, and the powerful tendency to medicalize their predicament instead of coming to terms with the social solutions that can be put in place, bearing in mind that that is what activists are asking for.

Before proceeding, a final clarification. The argument for a normative reading of disability judgments does not entail that we must in each case employ the social model, evidently not; in many cases addressing limitations through medical correction or, more generally, intervention at the personal level will be recommended. What it does mean, however, is that the judgment as to whether we should intervene at the individual or social level cannot be made through recourse to some account of natural function and dysfunction, but by pragmatic as well as ethical factors including considerations of efficiency, safety, equality, and justice to name a few.

2.2.4 **Applying the social model to madness**

Having established the normative nature of disability judgments, and having developed the first bulwark against the tendency to view certain variations/impairments in functioning as inherently disabling, it remains to be seen just how the social model can be applied to madness. In the ensuing discussion, note that the concern is with conditions that are long-lasting, have a substantial effect on daily activity, and where treatment is either not desired or not possible (i.e., we are concerned with "disabilities" and not acute or self-limiting problems).

Applying the social model to madness is not new; activists and academics have written about the potential and the problems of doing so. The disability movement has achieved some progress in making salient the contributions of the physical and social environments to generating limitations, with many accommodations to address this now enshrined in law. Developing a social model of madness in keeping with the social model of disability is seen as a way of counteracting the "medicalized individual approach" that is dominant in society and mental health institutions (Beresford 2005; see also Mulvany 2000). Resistance to this proposal has come from both sides. Some psychiatric survivors/service users refuse to be associated with disability discourse as they do not consider themselves to have an impairment, nor do they want to be associated with the "pathologizing" implications of the term impairment (see Beresford 2000; Beresford et al. 2010). Conversely, others actively endorse the term disability as it creates a sense of community across the survivor/service-user/mad and disability movements (Price 2013). Some are reluctant to use "disability" for fears of being accused that they are not disabled enough; that they do not have the appropriate lifelong impairments (Spandler and Anderson 2015, p. 24). The reluctance of some within the Mad movement to accept the social model of disability and adopt its terminology has been interpreted by a physically disabled activist as reflecting the "disablism" prevalent within sections of this movement (Withers 2014). That is, in refusing to be referred to as disabled, and in asserting that unlike disabled people they have no tangible, "real" impairments, these activists are contributing to the idea that disability is a fixed thing and not an outcome of the interaction between individual capacities and specific social/physical contexts. Fears of increased stigma are another stumbling block for a shared discourse and activities between the disability and the Mad movements. Each group faces its own distinctive stigma in society, and to take on the term "madness" or the term "disability" is to take on an extra challenge (Withers 2014).

While noting that these are important issues, the key point for the argument here is the underlying framework and not the terminology in place: what is of essence in the medical/social model framework is an account of the relation between the individual and society in relation to the production of limitations on everyday activity. With regard to naming, one may eschew the problematic term "impairment" for the less-loaded one "variation," and one need not use the word "disability" at all. On the question of what constitutes a mental variation, we do not need to assume some account of natural function by which mental functions (and variations thereof) can be specified—the idea of natural function has already been problematized.[13] Given the argument presented earlier, a relevant mental variation is that which is made salient when our complex activity in the world is disrupted. It would not be "schizophrenia" or "psychosis," but the features that typically underlie these diagnoses such as voices, paranoid beliefs, anxious feelings, difficulties understanding social behavior, mood fluctuations, impaired attention and concentration, and others. These features can impose a range of limitations on the ability of individuals to realize their goals and to participate in everyday social situations and interactions. A few examples will illustrate.

---

[13] There have been recent calls to adopt the discourse of neurodiversity as a positive replacement for the language of impairment (Graby 2015; see also McWade et al. 2015). Advocates of this move believe that this would bring about a positive change: instead of *impairments* we would have a diversity of *minority neurotypes*, which stand alongside so-called normal neurotypes as real and valid neurological types. These neurotypes, it is argued, should be accommodated as an element of diversity like race or ethnicity. A major problem with the neurodiversity discourse is that it assumes that existing categories and identities (e.g. Autism, ADHD, Normal, Bipolar, Mad) can be traced back to a shared neurology. But our identifications and categorizations of behavior—as is now generally accepted in the domain of mental health—do not "cut nature at the joints" or reflect natural discontinuities. If so, then there is not much sense in the claim that there are distinct neurological types essentially different from each other. Further, neurodiversity raises several difficult questions, for example: What exactly is a normal neurotype? Do all "normals" share one neurotype? Do all people with autism share one neurotype? Neurodiversity may be important from an activism point of view, but as an argument it does not work.

◆ A person who experiences chronic anxiety (or paranoia) finds it difficult to negotiate the long, crowded, bright lanes of the local mall and heads home without
shopping. We can look at this disruption to activity from two vantage points: as
a problem with the world or as a problem with one's mental state. Wherever we
start, the other vantage point is implied: the difficulty of negotiating the mall makes
salient my anxious feelings; my anxious feelings make salient the difficulty of negotiating the mall.

◆ A person hears voices and converses with them as she finds this helpful and affords
her a measure of control. When she does this in public people give her strange looks
and sometimes walk away from her. Due to this, on many days she feels unable to
leave the house and her social isolation is increasing. Here, as with the previous
example, the disruption to activity (social isolation) can be seen as a consequence
of one's behavior or due to negative social responses, with each view made salient
by the other.

◆ A person experiences fluctuations in mood; when feeling high he can work for
many hours on end, frequently overnight. Such episodes are followed by several
days of rest during which he feels tired and low in mood. Due to this he is unable to
keep consistent employment as his line of work cannot accommodate the requirement for erratic working hours. In this case, disruption to activity (employment)
can be seen as a consequence of his mood fluctuations or due to unaccommodating
working arrangements.

In each case, once a specific mental variation is identified, it becomes possible to reflect
on the variation/environment mismatch and to formulate more precisely what exactly
needs to change: modify the mental state/behavior, alter the environment, or some
combination of the two.

The issues are different when the variation in question consists in a strongly held,
nonconsensual belief: a "delusion." For the sake of exposition consider two paradigmatic examples: the belief that one is persecuted by certain agents (persecutory delusion), and the belief that one's spouse has been replaced by an impostor (Capgras
delusion). On the basis of such beliefs, the person holding them may, respectively,
barricade himself at home, or avoid the spouse.[14] For an outside observer who can
see that both beliefs are false, those individuals are subjecting themselves to unnecessary limitations; they are disabled by their beliefs. But for the believers themselves,
this insight would not arise as long as they continue to hold the requisite belief with
conviction.[15] For them the problems they experience are facts about the world—that
one *is* unsafe and that one's spouse *is* an impostor—and not the beliefs per se. In terms

----

[14] Not all "deluded" individuals act on their beliefs, a phenomenon known as double bookkeeping
(see Sass and Pienkos 2013, pp. 646–50). An oft-used example is that of the man incarcerated
in an asylum who believes he is Napoleon yet does nothing towards exercising his regal powers.

[15] This can change if the person develops primary insight into the delusional nature of the belief;
if he or she is able to see that it is false; that he is not persecuted and that her husband is not an
impostor. In such cases the person loses conviction in the belief and is able to see that it really
was determining behavior in limiting ways.

of the basic idea underlying the social model, as argued in the previous section, what is made salient by what appears to be disruption to daily activity is not one's mental state, but facts about the social world. If I refuse to leave the house because someone is waiting outside for me with a gun, I am not disabled; I am sensible. If I am convinced that I am under threat despite there being no threat, then others may consider me disabled by my belief, but I would not. In this specific respect, "delusional" beliefs are outside the scope of the social model. They are brought back within it, however, in a different manner.

The "delusional" person may experience limitations of a different sort. He may experience disqualification and ridicule for the very fact of holding the belief(s) in question. In this respect, the disqualification in question would be no different to that which some religious minorities or sects face, except in relation to the question of numbers; the delusional person goes it alone, while sects tend to have a larger following. Here we are brought back within the scope of the social model, as the person is subjected to disqualification and ridicule due to the beliefs that he holds. A remedy could be to change the belief or, alternatively, to change the social environment by making it more accepting and tolerant.[16]

These examples show that even though the issues are complex and will require conceptual work and ingenuity, it is possible to apply social model thinking to at least some mental variations and related behaviors. In fact, this approach to mental variations has made its way to a number of publications by academics, policymakers, and charities in the United Kingdom and elsewhere.[17] These publications have

---

[16] Making society more tolerant is a solution that tends to be pursued in communities that advance liberal notions of free-speech and multicultural acceptance. The flip side of this tolerance is for the groups in question to develop secondary insight (a point which also applies to the "delusional" person). Secondary insight refers to subjects' abilities to see their beliefs from the point of view of dominant social values and norms, and in doing so to see that others may find those beliefs unusual or bizarre. The benefit of secondary insight is that it introduces appreciation of what others' views are without requiring agreement with those views. It allows contrasting beliefs to exist side by side, with both groups remaining aware that it will be difficult to reconcile those beliefs with each other. This is to be contrasted with primary insight, which requires that the person concedes the falsity of her ("delusional") beliefs and demonstrates awareness that she is "ill."

[17] See Thornicroft et al. (2008), Goering (2009), the UK Department for Work and Pensions (DWP 2009), the mental health charity Rethink (2012), and Heron and Greenberg (2013). Of note is that the UK Department of Health now recognizes a mental health condition that lasts more than 12 months and affects normal day-to-day activity as a disability. Among the listed conditions that may lead to disability are schizophrenia, depression, and bipolar disorder. By being classified a disability, a mental health condition falls under the protection of the Equality Act (2010) and the United Nations Convention on the Rights of Persons with Disabilities (2006), which the United Kingdom ratified in 2009. According to these acts, the state is under an obligation to provide individuals with disabilities the chance to participate fully in all aspects of life through the provision of reasonable adjustments that promote access to and engagement with the environment. This now also includes mental health conditions that qualify as disabilities.

issued recommendations on reasonable adjustments in the work place for people with "mental disabilities." Underlying this is the understanding that by contrast to physical impairments, mental variations tend to be less visible, have a more significant impact on the social rather than the built environment, and hence require adjustments that focus on social interactions and relationships (DWP 2009). Among the recommendations are: time-out if one feels anxious or paranoid; flexible hours; reduced workload; quieter workspace; private rather than open-plan working arrangements; availability of contact with a support worker or friend if someone feels particularly paranoid; working conditions matched to a person's tolerance for contact with large numbers of people; and combating stigma among colleagues at work. Rethink (2012, p. 9) go further, stating that stigma and negative attitudes of colleagues "can undermine adjustments which would otherwise be effective."

Rethink are exactly right to point toward stigma as a major issue: without some significant change in how people think about madness/mental health problems, any proposed adjustments are likely to be superficial with limited effectiveness. Further, stigma and negative perceptions can impact on individuals' self-esteem and psychological well-being, thus creating further barriers to participation.[18] Yet in pushing to alter such attitudes, the cited work, including Rethink's, advances or supports the line of thought that mental health problems are illnesses akin to physical illnesses, in the sense that they occur for reasons outside a person's control (which arguably reduces blame), can be treated, are not to be feared, and are not a sign of weakness. However, as an antistigma strategy, this is problematic on two counts: first, some studies have shown that the argument that "mental illness is an illness like any other" does not reduce stigma but in fact is associated with perceptions of unpredictability, dangerousness, and fear (Read et al. 2006); second, this argument is antithetical to the demand for recognition of Mad identity where concerned groups do not see themselves as ill and where aspects of madness are reformulated in a positive light or, at least, neutrally. Rethink are correct in pointing out that negative attitudes can genuinely hamper a person's ability to partake in the work environment; the difficult question is to specify what lies at the root of the problem in society at large.

To put this differently, impaired concentration, anxiety, paranoia, and social withdrawal are experiences that are commonplace enough not to generate any severe or unique discrimination from others. We are familiar with these experiences—think of sleep deprivation, jet lag, or a bad hangover—and readily find excuses for each other for them and, if we are generous, accommodate each other for them. What generates particular challenges in the case of madness is precisely the association of such experiences with phenomena that generate fear and distrust in others. To be anxious or paranoid due to effects of alcohol overuse is not the same as having those experiences due to hearing voices or harboring fears that one is persecuted by government agencies or by invisible beings. The latter are phenomena that, for most people, defy simple if any meaningful explanation and from there engender a certain kind of disqualification, and possibly distrust, grounded in the apparent unintelligibility of these phenomena. At the point where this occurs, it is hard to sustain a social interaction in

---

[18] This is referred to in the disability literature as psycho-emotional disablism (see Reeves 2015).

which the unique variations and traits of that person are noted and respected by way of creating for him or her a more accommodating environment. More likely than not, when unintelligibility sets in we move from a position of accommodation to one of seeing the person before us as the main cause of their struggles. Intelligibility, therefore, is an important concept and merits a further look.

2.2.5 Intelligibility and the limits of social accommodation

There is no doubt that the variations discussed in the previous section differ in some significant respects when compared to mobility and sensory variations in relation to the question of social accommodation. One difference, noted by Pilgrim and Tomasini (2012, p. 634), is that at the heart of the social reaction to "mental health problems" is an "attributed loss or lack of reason." By contrast, with mobility and sensory variations (physical disability more broadly), that capacity is not at stake. Assumed lack of reason, they continue, underpins the disadvantage and discrimination that characterize the social response to madness; it underpins fear and distrust as well as paternalistic limitations of autonomy. Unreason here is used quite broadly and ranges from not being able to meet social obligations (due to anxiety or depression), to failures in intelligibility exemplified by individuals whose behavior is underpinned by voices, bizarre delusions, thought disorder, or other states that for some may resist everyday understanding.[19] Intelligibility emerges as a helpful concept in marking out more precisely an important, if not central, factor that determines the limits of the social accommodation of difference: the point at which we cease to consider discourses of the social adjustment in favor of those that describe, in various ways, some sort of failure in the individual, for example, that he or she is "mentally ill."

Consider the experience of hearing voices and its impact on behavior. A "voice-hearer" (Woods 2013) may at times converse with the voices and be distracted by them. In some social contexts, as indicated earlier, behaving in this way may generate negative responses from others, which may lead the voice-hearer into isolation and fears of appearing in public. In this example, developing social narratives in which voice-hearing is normalized or marked out as a unique experience may engender a measure of intelligibility and tolerance of the associated behaviors, and this in turn may improve social inclusion for the voice-hearer. As Spandler and Anderson (2015, p. 19) note, this is what the Hearing Voices Movement has been seeking to do: to effect a shift from the view of voices as symptoms of illness to that of voices as meaningful phenomena. Intelligibility will depend on the kind of narrative put forward to create this meaningfulness. Some narratives draw connections between voice-hearing, spirituality, and nonhuman agents such as spirits. Other narratives see voices as denoting aspects of

---

[19] In each of these cases intelligibility means something different. With voices, the issue may be that such experiences are completely alien, given my worldview. With bizarre delusions I may be struck by how patently false these claims are or fail to understand why this person is holding them. With thought disorder there may be a more basic inability to grasp any meaning at all. The point here, however, is not to parse out the different forms of failure of understanding (for more on this, see Rashed 2015a).

self and hence as offering a means for a more profound understanding of one's past and identity.

For the voice-hearer's interlocutor, intelligibility will depend on the extent to which he or she is able to accept the assumptions supporting the different narratives. And this underpins the challenge of expanding our limits of the social accommodation of difference and our ability to conceive social adjustments: madness asks us to question our total worldview; to question our beliefs, values, sense of self, ideas of rationality, and personhood.[20] The change required here is not to install a ramp or an alternate sign, it is to change notions fundamental to us as persons, and to broaden the idea of what is possible. This is most evident in cross-cultural encounters. Consider, for example, a person who barricades himself at home upon hearing the voice of a spirit threatening him with death if he leaves the house. Whether we consider this an "illness"—after all it appears to be a paradigmatic example of "action failure"—or a genuine threat, will depend on the extent to which we take the cause of the obstruction as real.[21] In cultural contexts where spirits are considered to exist and to have a say in human affairs, that person's self-imposed incarceration may appear to be a sensible course of action until the spirit is dealt with. In cultural contexts where the "spirit" is understood as alienated mental content—objectified aspects of self—that person may be considered "ill."

While we are on the theme of cross-cultural encounters, we can consider other phenomena that appear to *really* defy intelligibility across cultural contexts. Such phenomena (e.g., thought disorder) do not enjoy the collective reasonableness and positive-reframing achieved by, say, the Hearing Voices Movement (Pilgrim and Tomasini 2012, p. 642; Spandler and Anderson 2015, pp. 18–19). Jones and Kelly (2015, p. 47), mental health activists and academics, assert that

> the struggles of a distressed individual who can nevertheless communicate with others, can and must be distinguished from an individual with thought disorder so severe that he or she can no longer be understood, even in the most basic of ways.

For Jones and Kelly the limit of intelligibility is thought disorder, which is the limit it would appear of thought itself. For other less accommodating individuals the limit lies much earlier, being evident for them in the slightest eccentricity in belief or behavior. The limit of intelligibility lies at different places for different people and, as indicated previously, marks out the point at which we begin to consider the limitations experienced by an individual to flow from the variation itself. At this point we cease to consider changing social behavior in favor of changing the individual.

---

[20] Whereas mobility and sensory impairments ask us, primarily, to question our embodiment. I say primarily because many physical conditions also generate huge stigma—HIV, for example, or leprosy—and hence also implicate the self of patient and other.

[21] It would constitute action failure in so far as it is a negatively evaluated experience of incapacity, where incapacity is defined as a failure of intentional action (Jackson and Fulford 1997, p. 54). The example provided fulfils the two requisite elements for action failure: (1) There is a failure of intentional action (the person is unable to make his will effective and not due to an external cause). (2) This incapacity is negatively evaluated. (See Rashed 2010, pp. 189–90.)

There are two bulwarks against this move or, at least, against assuming it too readily. The first has already been mentioned, and concerns the need to specify the values and standards by which one was driven to regard a particular variation as intrinsically disabling. In doing so, one may give more thought to the possibility of changing those standards in a way that would permit a broader accommodation of difference. The second bulwark arises from political activism; from the very demand for social justice.

2.2.6 Political activism and the social subject

The demand that society should change to accommodate a broader range of variations as a matter of justice or fairness, implies that the person making this demand is a *social subject*. What is meant by social subject will become apparent in due course, but as an approximation it can be taken to mean a human being who sees oneself and sees others as engaged in a shared project in which each individual's well-being is at stake and matters equally. Now at first sight this claim may appear paradoxical, for a popular view in both lay and scholarly accounts is that a central aspect of madness (or of "schizophrenia") is the *dis-sociality* of the subject; a sign of mad subjects' madness is their withdrawal from society. For example, a person with severe paranoia may have a radical, sometimes global, loss of interpersonal trust. For that person, others appear not as coparticipants in a shared project but as a threat to one's existence. In a related manner, the phenomenological psychopathology literature describes the "schizophrenic person" as having a crisis of intersubjectivity, a disruption to the two fundamental poles of social reality: *sensus communis* and attunement.[22] Other times the "schizophrenic person" is described as having a disorder of consciousness and self-awareness, an ipseity disturbance characterized by hyperreflexivity and diminished self-affection.[23] (The latter view also concerns the

---

[22] This account is found in several works, particularly the work of Giovanni Stanghellini (2004). According to Stanghellini, at the basis of intersubjectivity are two phenomena: *sensus communis* and attunement. The former are tacit rules and axioms of everyday life shared by a social group, and which make it possible to "experience the different phenomena of the world as solid realities whose meaning is taken for granted" (Stanghellini 2004, p. 67). *Sensus communis* underlies our shared interpretations of social situations, objects, and behavior. Attunement is "non-propositional knowledge consisting in the emotional-conative-cognitive ability to perceive the existence of others as similar to one's own, make emotional contact with them and intuitively access their mental life" (2004, p. 10). According to this account, schizophrenic *dissociality* is underpinned by disorders in self-consciousness and attunement which lead to loss of the tacit, self-evidence of *sensus communis*. The latter is replaced with a conscious effort to work out the basics of social interaction and interpretation of others' behavior.

[23] This account is found in the work of Louis Sass, Joseph Parnas, and others. Ipseity is understood as the enduring sense of self that enables us to exist as a "subject of experience that is at one with itself at any given moment" (Sass and Parnas 2007, p. 68). Disturbed ipseity has two complementary aspects: hyperreflexivity and diminished self-affection. Hyperreflexivity is a type of exaggerated self-consciousness in which the subject becomes aware of sensations and experiences that normally remain tacit in the background of awareness; diminished self-affection is a decline in the implicit experience of existing as a unified subject of awareness. As Sass and Parnas (2007, p. 77) explain: "if something normally tacit became focal

"schizophrenic person's" dis-sociality, but starts from subjectivity rather than inter-subjectivity.) These accounts may seem to invalidate the idea that the "schizophrenic person" can be a social subject in the sense described earlier. If one accepts this conclusion, how do we make sense of those making the demand for social justice? One (cynical) approach is to claim that Mad activists are not really mad at all. Another approach is to argue that the issue here is a matter of scope: the phenomena referred to by phenomenological psychopathology are at the far end of the spectrum of sociality and are not representative of all "schizophrenic," "psychotic," or mad experiences.[24] I reject the first approach, and accept a qualified version of the second, as will be evident in what follows. But first I return to the idea of the social subject implied by the demands of activists.

Implied by the demand for the accommodation of a broader range of variations as a matter of justice are, at least, the following:

◆ An understanding of oneself as an individual among others.

◆ An understanding that individuals are different in some respects from each other (i.e., human diversity).

◆ An understanding that individual well-being depends, in part, on the sustenance provided by social interactions and arrangements.

◆ The ability to see oneself as part of a smaller group that is part of wider society.

◆ An understanding of oneself as a person who possesses rights and whose claims merit attention.

◆ An understanding that others too possess rights (this is already implied by the way in which the demand is couched in the language of justice and fairness).

In short, what is implied by the demand is a view on social justice and an understanding of society. Returning to the limits of intelligibility discussed in the previous section, we can say that by virtue of making this demand—notwithstanding the unintelligibility of specific experiences or behaviors—the person should be seen as a candidate for the social accommodation of difference rather than the medical (individual) correction (treatment) of behavior; the demand should act as a bulwark against the prioritization of an individual approach. The reason this is so is that the demand trumps the objection against social accommodation. In the terms raised here, this objection can be put as follows: mad individuals are, as it were, outside society, and to argue for accommodating their behaviors and mental variations is to risk losing society altogether, grounded as it is in shared rules and assumptions. The political demand

---

[hyper-reflexive awareness], one might, as a result, no longer feel as if one were inhabiting the tacit medium [diminished self-affection]; but if, for some reason, one no longer had a sense of inhabiting the tacit medium, this could lead to hyper-reflexive awareness of what is normally tacit." Volitional forms of hyper-reflexivity alienate and objectify mental life, leading to more hyper-reflexive attention and culminating in aspects of the self experienced as wholly detached and alien (Sass 2003).

[24] A third approach is to cast doubt on the methodology by which the conclusions of phenomenological psychopathology are reached (see Rashed 2015a).

demonstrates the person's sociality and appreciation of the shared meta-project that is society, and hence refutes this objection.

I return now to the point I made earlier, which is that I accept with qualification that on the question of sociality there is an issue of scope: some mad (or "schizophrenic") experiences appear incompatible with sociality, a point made in phenomenological psychopathology. I see those whom phenomenological psychopathology describes as suffering with a crisis in intersubjectivity to be those subjects who are yet to see their situation in terms of identity, diversity, and social justice; who are yet to be brought to a conception of themselves as social subjects. Here, the principle of consciousness-raising which is described in the activist literature and discussed in Chapter 1 is instructive. This is the process by which people get together, share stories, see similarities in their situations, and interpret their predicaments as arising from discriminatory and difficult social conditions rather than individual pathology. Once this is achieved a demand is made to change those conditions. Given this, a key goal within activist communities is to support individuals such that they are able to make that demand. In this endeavor, creating "collective reasonableness" in relation to particular phenomena is also crucial. It may not be possible for some individuals to make the demand despite such support, and others may not wish to make it, opting instead for a more individual, illness-based discourse and intervention. But for those who are able to make that demand—or who cannot make it today but might be able to make it in the future—the political act itself suggests that the individuals concerned are candidates for the social accommodation of difference rather than the individual correction of behavior.

2.3 **Distress**

Whereas disability concerns limitations to/impairments of everyday functioning and participation, distress refers to affective and emotional states such as anxiety, sadness, fear, and paranoia. In the previous discussion, such states were relevant to the extent that they impacted on functioning. Here what's at stake is the unpleasantness and unmanageability of such states irrespective of their impact on function. Auditory hallucinations (voices), passivity of thought and action, and other disturbing and unusual somatic sensations are frequently unexpected, terrifying, and unpleasant. Intense affective states, much like pain, are discomforting and (most) people would want to be rid of them whether or not they are disabled by them. In addition, in light of dominant psychological and behavioral norms, such states may engender the worry that others may question one's sanity, which in turn may compound isolation and fear; this point was referred to earlier as psycho-emotional disablism (Reeves 2015). Given these rather negative registers, distress can arise as a problem for mad-positive approaches, including Mad Pride. At the very least, critics can point out that urging acceptance of madness as a positive or neutral conception of identity is challenged by the negative nature of the distress associated with madness.

In the activist literature, reviewed in Chapter 1, the problem of distress is dealt with in two ways: the first is to attribute distress (anxiety, sadness, paranoia, in addition to the distress of unusual experiences) to social and interpersonal difficulties such as abuse, trauma, oppression, and poverty; the idea is that such experiences, in some causally significant way, arise from those difficulties, rather than from some individual deficiency or weakness. Here the slogan is that madness is a sane (understandable) and creative response, or adjustment, to an insane world. In the academic literature concerned with developing social approaches to distress, something resembling this strategy is worked out in detail. Tew (2005, 2015) argues that distress and apparently dysfunctional behaviors, such as self-harm, can be understood as a response to difficult life experiences, either as a coping or survival strategy, or as an expression of underlying social stressors and conflicts. A social model, he writes, "locates experience within an understanding of social relations in which power plays a determining role" (Tew 2005, p. 23). Several writers have unpacked how power differentials, inequality, and discrimination can result in distress and dysfunctional behaviors in the case of childhood abuse (Plumb 2005), racism (Keating 2015), sexism (Diamond 2014), and homophobia (Carr 2005). Instead of being seen as resourceful or unavoidable responses to extreme challenges—the argument proceeds—distress and (apparently) dysfunctional behaviors are (wrongly) elected as symptoms of illness, obscuring the social problems that lie at their origin, and the social solutions that are required.

Even though there is much to be commended in this argument, it offers only a partial response to the problem of distress. To describe distress as a reasonable or understandable response to difficulty is to potentially attribute positive qualities to the person. There are hints here of survivor discourse (see section 1.2.6), of ingenuity and bravery in the face of difficulty, and of resistance to oppression and inequality. Of course, positive attributes are not entailed by the argument that one's experiences are responses to difficulty, but it remains a possible, positive spin on that argument. Yet even in the case of adopting this positive spin, the argument is insufficient as a response to the problem of distress, as it leaves the actual experiences negatively evaluated. If a person experiences paranoid feelings, it is possible to understand this as a response to continuing experiences of racism and racial mistrust in his case. It may even be possible to feel solidarity with that person, and to see his experience of paranoia as a sign of resistance; an indication that he has not fallen for an unbalanced accommodation with the perpetrators of racism. But this narrative, assuming it makes sense, has not touched upon the experience of paranoia as such, only at the qualities of the person having this experience. The experience itself remains a problem, and the point of the argument is to elect oppressive social conditions, rather than individual failing and pathology, as its cause.

A full response to the problem of distress will have to contend with the experience itself: to show how the experience can be accommodated within a broader, positive narrative. The activist literature offers a second strategy to deal with the problem of distress, which is to accept that some aspects of madness are distressing, but to understand this as part and parcel of the special gift of madness; this is the discourse of the "dangerous gift" (section 1.4.2). Here, creative forms of expression, the global search for meaning, and inward thinking/reflection are one face of madness, the other being, respectively, manic states, paranoid experiences, and melancholy; creativity and distress are intertwined and indispensable to each other. Another possible strategy is to see distressing experiences as necessary conditions for valued and worthwhile goals. For example, the religious ascetic embarks on a spiritual journey beset with psychological, emotional, and material difficulties, but he or she does this in order to achieve a higher mode of being. The twelfth-century Muslim scholar Al-Ghazali (2010, p. 16) expresses something along those lines when he writes:

> For instance, if a man ceases to take any interest in worldly matters, conceives a distaste for common pleasures, and appears sunk in depression, the doctor will say, "This is a case of melancholy, and requires such and such prescription." The physicist will say, "This is a dryness of the brain caused by hot weather and cannot be relieved till the air becomes moist." The astrologer will attribute it to some particular conjunction or opposition of planets. "Thus far their wisdom reaches," says the Koran. It does not occur to them that what has really happened is this: that the Almighty has a concern for the welfare of that man, and has therefore commanded His servants, the planets or the elements, to produce such a condition in him that he may turn away from the world to his Maker.

This teleological approach renders the phenomena valuable in the broader context of the worthwhile goal or achievement for which it is a necessary condition. For example, if I want to compete at and win a marathon, I will have to go through a long and grueling training process in which I will experience pain and physical challenges. The pain here is not an annoyance that obstructs my attempts, but a necessary condition of the training required to place me at a competitive advantage or to allow me to compete at all. In summary, the "dangerous gift" narrative and a teleological approach to suffering are two examples where we can see that a phenomenon can be distressing and valuable, and this despite distress or, in some cases, because of it.

2.4 **Conclusion**

Along the decades, different groups have campaigned and struggled for respect and rights; some have been successful at achieving symbolic and cultural reparation, others less so. The enlarged scope of Gay rights in a few select communities around the world is usually cited as a success story. It is now pointed out that societies need to come to terms with the rights of Transgender individuals and the respect they may be owed. Yet Mad individuals, and madness more broadly, are yet to feature in the conversation on respect and identity, a conversation still dominated by framings that emphasize the medical idiom and the notions of distress and disability. This chapter addressed the problem of distress by demonstrating that a phenomenon can be distressing and valuable. The chapter also addressed the problem of disability by erecting two bulwarks against the tendency to assume, too readily, a medical interpretation of the limitations experienced by individuals with the kind of variations in mental function that fall under the umbrella term "madness."

The first bulwark arose from an analysis of the disability model that revealed the normative basis of disability judgments: when we say that a variation (or impairment) is intrinsically disabling, we need to accompany this judgment with an account of the values, norms, abilities, and contexts that underpin it. This requirement, though it may appear too subtle to make a difference, actually brings about a profound change in perspective: instead of seeing the limit of our ability to understand and accommodate difference as an indication of a (natural) problem with the difference itself, we come to view it as a normative limit constituted by values, norms, and abilities that go so deep they appear natural. With this insight in place, it becomes possible to resist medical-izing difference, and to reflect on what possible social solutions can be put in place to accommodate it.

The second bulwark arose from reflection on the implications of political activism. To demand, as a matter of social justice, that society changes to accommodate a broader range of variations in function is to be a social subject; it is to be a candidate for the accommodation of difference rather than for the individual (medical) correction of behavior.

There is no question that effecting the recommended change in perspective is a challenging endeavor. Although applying social model thinking to mental variations (to madness) is possible—as I have demonstrated—it raises issues different to the kind of variations in physical function for which the social model of disability was initially developed. A key difference is the way in which madness presents a challenge of intel-ligibility; it asks us to question and broaden our values and beliefs with respect to fundamental notions such as our sense of self and overall worldview. Difficult though as that may be, at least we can now come to view this (apparently) insurmountable difference for what it is: as a radical challenge to norms and concepts constitutive of who we are. Whether we should attempt to examine these norms and concepts in order to accommodate a broader range of experiences, behaviors, and identities—whether, that is, society ought to respond positively to Mad activism's demand for recognition—is a further question to be considered. Toward an answer to this ques-tion, Part II of this book develops a perspective on the philosophy and politics of identity and recognition, a resource that will enable us to understand the nature and the normative force of demands for recognition in general and in the specific case of madness.

Part II

Recognition

Chapter 3

The concept of recognition and the problem of freedom

3.1 Introduction

Recognition is a multifaceted concept; not only does it have technical philosophical usages, it has managed to acquire a politics of its own—*The Politics of Recognition*—yet remains a commonly used conversational term. In order to reconstruct the concept, it would be helpful to begin by specifying some meanings of recognition.[1] In common parlance, recognition can refer to identification: I recognize this object as a pen, this pen as my father's, that day as our anniversary. To identify something as being such and such is to *re*-cognize it; it is to have known it or its type before, recognition being an affirmation of that knowledge. Another meaning of recognition is evident when we talk about, for example, the international community recognizing the sovereignty of a newly formed state. Here something like affirmation of a status is involved, a status that can equally be withdrawn. Another related sense is where a people recognize a particular date as the start of the illegal occupation of their land, while the occupiers recognize that date as the day they finally acquired their own state. Here there is disagreement over the significance that should be attributed to that date. With recognition of persons all these meanings are relevant but in a special way.

Unlike pens and anniversaries, people respond to how they are identified by others (though pens and anniversaries tend to have people objecting on their behalf if they are misidentified). You see a person walking down the road and you *re*-cognize that person as a man on the basis of assumptions about grooming and dress. As he approaches you, you realize you were wrong. You can be wrong in several ways: you may have *perceived* wrongly, for example, by failing to see other "signs" that that person was not a man. You may also have *assumed* wrongly, that is, the problem is not with your ability at the identification of physical features, but with the assumptions that guide your interpretation of these features as denoting one social identity and not another. People form an understanding of who they are, which we can call their identity, and this understanding may be appropriately recognized by others, it may be misrecognized or not recognized at all. In other words, people may be *socially visible* in just the right way, they may be visible in a way that does not correspond to how they see themselves or, in extreme, they may be invisible.

---

[1] For a discussion of the different meanings of recognition, see Margalit (2001) and Ikaheimo (2002, 2007).

Social invisibility is a state associated with the history and, in some contexts, the reality of servitude and slavery. Taking a cue from Ralph Ellison's novel *The Invisible Man*, Axel Honneth (2001a) reminds us of a historical anecdote in which the nobility, who before their equals had strict rules of propriety, found it natural to undress in front of their servants. What is happening here is that others are overlooked because they are deemed to be socially meaningless: they are not considered the kind of subjects before whom shame is possible, let alone persons whose self-understanding matters. Less extreme, and more common, are situations in which persons are visible but not in the way they wish to be. The problem is not that they are socially overlooked but that they are looked upon in the wrong way; it is not a problem of the complete lack of recognition but of *misrecognition.* Many social struggles today are struggles for recognition, for transforming social norms and practices by which people's identities are not recognized—interpreted, valued—in the right way.

A key example of a struggle for recognition is the topic of this book: individuals who are subject to powerful societal discourses and practices that present them as disordered or mentally ill, and who are demanding recognition of madness as grounds for identity or culture and not as a disorder of the mind. Part III of this book examines the claim that madness can be grounds for identity or culture, while Part IV responds to the demand for recognition of Mad identity by asking whether or not it possesses normative force and, if it does, how society should respond to it. In order to be able to consider these questions, we need to have a theory and politics of identity and recognition that we can work with. Toward this end, Part II examines the following: the concept of recognition (Chapter 3); identity and the psychological consequences of recognition (Chapter 4); the normative and political frameworks by which we can justify, adjudicate, and respond to demands for recognition in general (Chapter 5).

In order to put together a theory and politics of recognition we need to begin at the beginning and examine the concept of recognition. The main aim of this chapter is to reconstruct the concept by tracing its dialectical development in Hegel's *Phenomenology of Spirit.* Hegel was not the first to discuss recognition—Fichte and Schelling had done so before him—but he was the first to offer an account of the concept that fully realized its meaning and potential. Among the various writings of Hegel, it is the presentation in Chapter 4 of the *Phenomenology* that tackles the concept in its fundamental structure, an account that can be abstracted from the systematic and historical issues that Hegel dealt with and which may not be relevant for us today. Further, contemporary theoreticians of recognition, such as Axel Honneth and Charles Taylor, ground their work in key Hegelian ideas, and in order to understand their work better and be able to critique it we need to grasp these ideas.

The dialectic of recognition (section 3.3) can be read as a sustained exploration of the problem of freedom: How can a subject affirm its independence amid other subjects; can it do so alone without taking account of anyone outside of it? The dialectic takes us through the tribulations of a subject that attempts, in many different ways, to do just that. Ultimately, it fails at sustaining this view and arrives at the realization that dependence on the recognition of others is a condition of its own freedom. Stated more fully, the central claim of this chapter—or rather my interpretation of what Hegel was up to in Chapter 4 of the *Phenomenology*—is this: a subject can only become a free agent once it engages with other subjects in uncoerced relations of mutual recognition by which is confirmed for it as objectively true its own self-conception as a free agent. As reconstructed here, the concept of recognition is therefore an answer to the question of "the nature and the very possibility of freedom" (Pippin 2000, p. 155). It is not an empirical concept of identity formation, nor is it a metaphysical concept describing the basic ontological structure of social existence; it is a philosophical account of what it is to be a free agent, an account that offers a conceptual resolution of the tension between, on one hand, individual autonomy and, on the other, social and natural necessities (section 3.4). It is with an outline of that tension, and its formulation by Immanuel Kant and Hegel's response, that I shall begin.

3.2 **What is it to be a free agent? Moral duty vs. ethical life**

What is it to be a free agent? A free agent is able to see its actions as the product of its own will and not directly an imposition by external authorities or other dependencies. On its own this is insufficient, for a state in which the agent *only* seeks to free itself from the forces of social or natural necessity, without giving attention to the motives and the values (or the principles) under which it should act, would not be evincing freedom but a chaotic and unpredictable state (see Pinkard 2002, p. 48). A free agent, therefore, must be a self-determining (autonomous) agent; it must act under a conception of what it considers to be good. What conception should that be and from where can the agent derive it? A well-known answer to this question can be found in Kant's moral and practical philosophy.

In the *Groundwork of the Metaphysics of Morals*, Kant seeks to establish the "supreme principle of morality" from where we ought to act. For Kant, an autonomous will must not act out of desires, inclinations, or interests—it must act out of duty. A person who acts in this way evinces a good will, a will that is good in itself and would have that value without limitation irrespective of specific circumstances (Kant 1998, pp. 7–8). The reason we can consider a will to be good in this absolute manner is that the value in question arises from the *motive* under which the person acts, and not from what the will "effects or accomplishes" (1998, p. 8). An autonomous will must act on the basis of principles, but in order not to be subject to the will of another those principles must be of its own making. Autonomous beings legislate for the very principles that they bind themselves to by their own will. The principles by which we can discover what we ought to do are given to us by reason, for if they are to be absolute (unconditioned by contingency and universal) they cannot derive from anything empirical—including the demands or needs of particular communities—and must be derived a priori. Reason leads us not to several but to one "supreme principle of morality"—the categorical imperative—albeit with three formulations, including: "act only in accordance with that maxim through which you can at the same time will that it become a universal law" (Kant 1998, p. 31). On the Kantian account, to act freely is the same as to act morally, which is to stand outside of the *phenomenal* realm—our inclinations, desires, communities, traditions—and formulate maxims for action that would pass the test of the categorical imperative. Moral principles are thus grounded in the *noumenal*, transcendent realm of pure reason. For Kant, then, to be a free agent is to be a moral agent acting under the formal requirements of reason.[2]

In the *Phenomenology of Spirit*, Hegel takes issue with Kant's moral theory (without naming Kant as such). His critique can be construed as a general problem with Kant's transcendental method, and a related specific problem with Kant's notion of unconditioned yet action-guiding moral principles (Hegel 1977, pp. 252–62). The general problem is one that we will encounter in much more detail in section 3.3. In the *Phenomenology*, Hegel is critical of the modern epistemological tradition—including Kant's critical philosophy—that set out to examine the possibility and bounds of knowledge by *standing outside* of knowledge and examining our intellectual faculties. It is precisely that withdrawal from some aspect of the world that is at issue here.[3] Ethical-certainty is the term Hegel (1977, p. 254) employs to refer to reason's withdrawal from the world in order to formulate absolute principles for moral conduct. Hegel wants to argue that ethical-certainty fails as it does not account for fundamental aspects of the situation: the societies, traditions, relationships, and commitments in which we are embedded and that precede our existence as autonomous subjects. The Kantian could respond by arguing that without disengaging from these practices we would not be able to exercise our autonomy by rationally deliberating on what we ought to do. Granted, but the question here is this: Where do we withdraw to? According to Kant we withdraw to the noumenal realm and appeal to reason to formulate maxims for action. Such withdrawal, Hegel would argue, is problematic since a standpoint where all social and individual contingencies and concerns are eliminated—assuming such a standpoint is possible—can only produce *formal* principles, for example, the categorical imperative, that become *contingent* the moment we begin to apply them in the world in order to guide action. This final point refers to a set of problems with Kant's moral theory that have been extensively debated (e.g., Anscombe 1958; Korsgaard 1996), yet which have been noted by Hegel in the *Phenomenology* a mere twenty-two years after publication of the *Groundwork* in 1785.

---

[2] As an example of the categorical imperative, consider the following: suppose I am inclined to act under the maxim "I will lie in order to secure what I want." In order to test this maxim I need to universalize it into the following law: "everyone ought to lie in order to secure what they want." But a world in which everyone lies to secure what they want is a world where no one can lie to secure what they want since it will be a world where the practice of taking others at their word could not exist, and my initial maxim requires that such a practice exists. The maxim is therefore contradictory as its universalization undermines a necessary condition for its possibility. Since you cannot rationally will that the maxim "I will lie in order to secure what I want" become a universal law, you must not act on it.

[3] This problem will confront us twice again in this chapter with sense-certainty and self-certainty (section 3.3). Sense-certainty is a form of knowing that seeks determinate knowledge of objects without taking any responsibility for knowledge (i.e. without applying concepts and only by registering what is before it *here* and *now*). It fails and, ultimately, leads us to self-consciousness. Similarly, self-certainty—the first attempt by self-consciousness to know itself—withdrew from the world, seeking to establish self-knowledge without taking proper account of other subjects. It fails and, ultimately, leads us to mutual recognition.

Briefly, the problem here arises from the requirement that moral principles be unconditioned yet action-guiding. This means that they must be universal and absolute while possessing sufficient content such that they can be applied in concrete situations. Consider the moral law "everyone ought to speak the truth." When we examine how such a law can be applied we immediately find that it needs to be qualified in some way. At the very least, as Hegel (1977, p. 254) notes, we need to add the clause "everyone ought to speak the truth *if he knows it.*" And qualifications need not stop here as many other conditions apply: everyone ought to speak the truth if he knows it, if the other person would understand it, if telling the truth would not result in significant harm, and so on. The point is that the more we qualify a law, the less universal and the more contingent it becomes; it ceases to be a *law* as such and becomes relevant to the contingency in question. Yet without qualifying it, it remains merely formal, lacking in content, and cannot guide action (Hegel 1977, p. 256).

What emerges from the foregoing argument is that moral principles acquire content not through the demands of reason—which only produce the form of the law—but from the very practices that Kant argued we must withdraw from in order to know what we ought to do; as Hoy (2009, p. 161) points out: "if the universal law formula has some content, that content does not follow from the idea of pure duty (*Moralitat*) [moral duties], but from more empirical practices (*Sittlichkeit*) [ethical life] that are tacitly presupposed by the moral point of view."[4] Given this, we can argue that it is no more possible to formulate principles for moral action by fully distancing oneself from the contingences of social practices (ethical-certainty's illusion), than it is to know objects without applying a conceptual scheme (sense-certainty's illusion), or to acquire self-knowledge by withdrawing fully from the world outside of us (self-certainty's illusion).[5] If that is the case, our conception of freedom as rational autonomy is incomplete. Earlier I pointed out the Kantian's retort that disengaging from social practices is necessary if we are going to be able to exercise our autonomy, our rational moral agency. Now we can see that what we withdraw to is not a noumenal realm where "each person can individually rise above the contingencies of space and time and act purely from the moral law" (Hoy 2009, p. 155); we withdraw to shared social practices that, to a greater or lesser extent, can allow us to become free subjects. Our updated conception of freedom has to take this into account.

We can now re-ask the question we began with: What is it to be a free agent? The first feature identified at the beginning of this section remains: a free agent is self-determining (autonomous).[6] Whatever conception of freedom we arrive at has to

---

[4] Solomon (1983, pp. 489–90) expressed a similar point when he wrote that Hegel rejected "the bloodlessly formal structure of Kant's theory, in which *principles* ("laws") alone formed the basis of morality, apart from any public or communal concerns and apart from the interpersonal interactions which gave these principles their moral significance."

[5] Both sense-certainty and self-certainty are discussed in section 3.3.

[6] Contrary to some interpretations, Hegel was never opposed to individual autonomy; what he was opposed to was the attempt to ground it in a noumenal realm of transcendent freedom, and what he tried to accomplish was to bring it back into the social world as actualized freedom. The concept of mutual recognition is his attempt to do so. Indeed, in Charles Taylor's

preserve this since to lose it is to lose the notion of freedom altogether. The principles under which an autonomous subject ought to act, and by which it can experience its freedom, cannot be adequately grounded in the notion of pure moral duty. In pure reason, the subject only finds the form of the law. If the subject cannot find satisfactory confirmation of its principles and motives in pure reason, it has no choice but to seek this confirmation in the shared social practices in which it exists. However, the subject might not "see" itself in those practices; it might be alienated from them. If this is to be overcome then some sort of reconciliation has to be achieved such that social practices conform with the subject's autonomy, and the subject's autonomy conforms with social practices, and this in a way that takes all agents into account, and in a manner that is rational in order that it can be assented to. In other words, some kind of balance between individual self-determination and the inevitability of social dependence has to be arrived at. Hegel refers to that balance as *ethical life* (to be contrasted with Kant's pure moral duty), a term which he defines in the *Philosophy of Right* as "the concept of freedom which has become the existing world and the nature of self-consciousness" (Hegel 1991, p. 189). How can we aim at ethical life? In accordance with what must individual autonomy and social practices be structured? The answer that would be offered by Hegel, if he had put the question in those terms, would be the concept of mutual recognition. The claim is that mutual recognition is the only position that can rationally reconcile individual autonomy with social dependence. In what follows I reconstruct the concept of recognition with the aim of elucidating the arguments underpinning it and the distinctive conception of freedom that it provides.

3.3 **The conceptual structure of recognition in the *Phenomenology of Spirit***

In Chapter 4 of the *Phenomenology*, Hegel (1977, p. 110) made this claim: "*Self-consciousness achieves its satisfaction only in another self-consciousness.*" This remarkably compact statement marks a major turning point in the book and contains the basis of Hegel's concept of recognition.[7] In order to unpack what it means, and to understand the problem that Hegel is grappling with here, it is necessary to venture briefly into the project of the *Phenomenology* as a whole.

3.3.1 **The project of the *Phenomenology***

The *Phenomenology of Spirit* is an introduction to Hegel's philosophical system. Despite the complexity of its arguments, its aim is straightforward: to establish the standpoint

----

(1979) *Hegel and Modern Society*, the central theme running throughout is that Hegel's ultimate philosophical motivation and ambition was to achieve a synthesis between, on one hand, radical autonomy and, on the other, expressive unity with nature and society.

[7] Hegel also discussed the concept of recognition in the *Jena Manuscripts* and in *The Philosophy of Right* (where it features in the context of Hegel's political philosophy), and in the *Encyclopaedia Philosophy of Spirit* (where it features in a broader, systematic account of "spirit"—or social and cultural existence). See Williams (1997) for a comprehensive account of the concept of recognition in the writings of Hegel.

from where speculative, a priori thought can begin. Hegel considered this standpoint unattainable if one remained within the epistemological tradition beginning with Plato, passing through Descartes, and culminating in Kant's critical philosophy. With the appearance/reality distinction at its heart, modern epistemology was concerned with examining our faculties to see whether or not they can give us access to true knowledge of reality. Different answers to this concern generated the debate between empiricists and rationalists; the former consider all knowledge to derive from the instrument of sense-experience, and the latter regard thought as the medium through which we can access true knowledge. The problem with this procedure is that it ends up generating skepticism about the world; for whether we regard our intellectual faculty as an instrument or as a medium we can no longer receive the truth as it in itself, as it will either be altered by the effects of the instrument or will arrive to us "as it exists through and in this medium" (Hegel 1977, pp. 46–7). Modern theories of knowledge thus deepen the division between the knowing subject and the object that is known, a division that found its culmination in Kant's critical philosophy. Recognizing that neither empiricism on its own nor rationalism can account for knowledge, Kant sought to mediate these two approaches, reconciling experience with pure reason. The result was synthetic a priori knowledge: the basic concepts that are a condition of our experience and, hence, cannot themselves be derived from that experience. But Kant's placement of a priori knowledge on a secure footing came at the huge price of cutting us off from the objects of our experience, since they can only be known as mediated via the concepts of understanding and never as they are *in-themselves*.

Hegel considered this result lamentable since it left us with the self-defeating outcome that even though we had started out seeking the truth, our very method left us with an unbridgeable gulf between thought and object. Yet it is a result that we are not obliged to accept, especially that the method that led to it is premised on unexamined assumptions (Hegel 1977, pp. 47–8). The critical project of setting out to examine our intellectual faculties in order to demonstrate the prior possibility and bounds of knowledge lands us in a paradoxical situation. If the critique itself is knowledge, as it must be, then how is this knowledge itself justified? If the epistemologist posits another critical faculty that examines the first, then that faculty will itself stand in need of examination, and so on ad infinitum (see Stern 2002, p. 38). To posit a critical faculty that lies outside of knowledge and stands in no need of justification is a dogmatic assumption that places Kant "in the position of (uncritically) knowing before he (critically) knows" (Williams 1992, p. 31). Hegel (1892, p. 17) put the issue like this:

> But the examination of knowledge can only be carried out by an act of knowledge. To examine this so-called instrument is the same thing as to know it. But to seek to know before we know is as absurd as the wise resolution of Scholasticus, not to venture into the water until he had learned to swim.

Hegel's solution is not to abandon speculative thought but to adopt a different method that would justify the philosophical standpoint without being dogmatic and without begging the question against other forms of knowledge. His solution, unlike Scholasticus', is to venture straight into the water; it is to introduce phenomenology into the inquiry. For the only way to proceed without assuming a problematic, unexamined first principle is to let knowledge appear by itself. It is to abandon Kant's transcendental, ahistorical approach, and venture into the world of experience. The *Phenomenology* is a survey of ever more complex forms of knowing, or shapes of consciousness, each of which frustrates its own truth by itself, on its own criteria, and leads to a more developed form of knowing.

Underlying the text as a whole is a view on the basic structure of phenomenal knowledge: consciousness distinguishes itself from the object outside of it while at the same time relating to it such that it can know it; knowledge is a relation. On the basis of this relation, the object has two aspects: (1) the true nature of the object—how it is independently of how it appears to us, and (2) how it appears to consciousness in the activity of knowing. The criterion by which true knowledge can be determined—by which the appearances of the object can be judged—is the true being of the object. But where does this criterion come from? As Hegel (1977, p. 54) points out, we cannot get "behind the object as it exists for consciousness, so as to examine what the object is *in itself.*" This leads to the point that both aspects of the object are internal to consciousness: the object as it is in itself is the *concept* of the object which consciousness projects onto the world, while the object as it appears to us is how it emerges in the activity of knowing. In this way, "consciousness provides its own criterion from within itself, so that the investigation becomes a comparison of consciousness with itself" (Hegel 1977, p. 53). If those two moments do not match—if the concept of the object fails to account for the various aspects of the experience of the object—then that particular form of knowing would have failed on its own terms.

For example, sense-certainty, the first form of knowing discussed by Hegel, is the most elementary way in which mind can relate to world: it is immediate knowing, unmediated by concepts. For sense-certainty, its concept of the object (what it regards the object to be in itself) is that of a singular, determinate item. Yet upon examination, this concept does not survive its demonstration in experience. Sense-certainty seeks determinate knowledge through the simple immediacy of what is before it without altering anything in the object or having to know anything else besides this immediacy (i.e., without applying any concepts). But in its experience, it finds itself in possession of what is simply present *here* and *now* which keeps changing as here becomes there, and now becomes a different moment. "Here" and "now" are conceptual realities (universals), and we are "made aware of their conceptual status, precisely because [their] singular content is continually changing" (Harris 1997, p. 216). Sense-certainty, therefore, is unable to realize its understanding of the object as a determinate item and finds itself, instead, conscious of universals.[8] Sense-certainty's failure constitutes the basis

---

[8] Note that in the midst of this process, consciousness does not yet behold the impact of its conceptual activity. That is, in moving from one concept of the object to another, consciousness registers that the world before it has changed, but it does not understand this change to involve a developed conceptual understanding of the truth of the object. What it considers to have happened is that it had learned something about the world that it had not known before. The truth of the object always stands, for consciousness, as a fact about the world external to its cognitive activity. It is the phenomenological observer who can witness a conceptual progression occurring as consciousness learns from its experience. As Harris (1997, pp. 187–8)

for a more developed concept of the object and the transition to a new form of knowing: perception. Perception takes over what was gained through the failures of sense-certainty—the idea that the object must, in some way, incorporate a conceptual aspect (or universals). Perception thus regards the object to be a thing with properties (i.e., universals such as red, hard, round, and so on). However, perception also fails at realizing its idea of the object in experience. This process of examination, disappointment, and movement to a more developed form of knowing is the process of the education of consciousness, and continues until we arrive at the philosophical standpoint, the point at which there are no further internal contradictions to resolve between our concept of the object and our experience of the object.

A note before continuing: the dialectical development of self-consciousness—and indeed of all the different shapes of consciousness which Hegel discusses—are to be understood as conceptual developments and not social/historical ones. This is in spite of the fact that Hegel frequently develops the dialectic with reference to concrete historical ideas and events such as Stoicism, Greek tragedy, Christianity, and the French Revolution. Many Hegel scholars agree on this point: Solomon (1983, pp. 436–7) notes that the *Phenomenology* is a "*conceptual* progression, to be understood in terms of the adequacy of forms, not the circumstantial emergence of humanity in history"; it is not concerned with "childhood or human development [but with] the conceptual preconditions and presuppositions of self-consciousness." Similarly for Houlgate (2003, pp. 10–11), the book "does not examine how human consciousness has actually changed through time into modern self-understanding, but shows how certain general "shapes" of consciousness necessarily transform themselves, because of their very structure, into further shapes." Siep (2014, p. 87) regards the shapes of consciousness in the *Phenomenology* as '"ideal' forms of human beings' intercourse with one another and with the world." According to other interpretations, this distinction, for Hegel, is merely one of perspective, as his overall position held that reality, including history, has a rational, conceptual structure, and he therefore considered it a given that the conceptual progression which he describes will be evident in history. We can leave aside, for now, the systematic context in which Hegel composed the dialectic of self-consciousness and recognition, and reconstruct it as a conceptual progression. How to interpret the concept that results will be addressed in section 3.4.

3.3.2 The concept of self-consciousness

Upon arriving to self-consciousness, the dialectic of consciousness had exhausted its possibilities. Consciousness in the form of sense-certainty, perception, and the understanding was passive, and sought to validate its view of the truth of the object without taking note of its own conceptual activity in determining knowledge. With self-consciousness, this activity itself becomes the object of reflection: consciousness now turns to examine what it can know of the world in knowing itself. That is why

---

put it, "we [consciousness] know that we learn things, and that as we put them together, our standpoint changes. But we are not aware that we are constructing a 'concept' of the world, into which our experience fits."

upon turning to self-consciousness we have entered, as Hegel (1977, p. 104) puts it, the "native realm of truth," even if we are on the very first step of it. This shift is central to the *Phenomenology* and marks a move that defines the rest of the book and much philosophy to follow: the move from theory to practice, from passive apprehension to active engagement, from consideration of an isolated subject to intersubjectivity. Crucial to understanding this shift, and the concept of recognition that arises from it, is an understanding of the concept of self-consciousness.

In turning to itself, consciousness relates to itself and hence has a doubled structure: the relation and what is related to must be distinguished from each other, even though they are both internal to consciousness. The nature of the relation is similar to that described earlier between subject and object, but now consciousness is *both* subject and object. Accordingly, consciousness holds a particular conception of what it takes itself to be, and seeks to realize that conception in the world as reflecting its true nature. In Hegel's terminology, self-consciousness is both *for-itself* (it conceives of itself in a certain way) and *in-itself* (what it is objectively, its truth). As will be seen, the *satisfaction* of self-consciousness occurs when it finds itself at home in the world, which is when its self-conception is confirmed/realized in the world outside of it as true. This confirmation, to anticipate the endpoint, cannot arise solely from the subject and is a matter of what is considered valid within particular social practices; the dialectic of recognition is a conceptually articulated account of the process by which such satisfaction can be arrived at.

If we consider a subject's self-conception as its certainty of what it is, and how it finds itself in the world as the truth (or otherwise) of that certainty, then satisfaction, or self-identity, exists to the extent that certainty and truth correspond. This identity has to be mediated, for otherwise it cannot be described as self-consciousness. Early on in the dialectic, Hegel rejects the case of a pure relation of consciousness with itself to the exclusion of everything outside of it. His target here must be Descartes' *cogito* and virtually all theories of self-identity, up to Fichte, that posit a subject able solely through introspection to gain self-knowledge in an immediate manner (or in Hume's case to find no such knowledge).[9] What these theories leave us with, Hegel (1977, p. 105) admonishes, is not self-consciousness but "the motionless tautology of: 'I am I.'"

The relation of consciousness to itself is mediated via its relation to an other. This is not accidental—it is necessary for self-consciousness to be possible at all: "the self needs opposition to define itself" (Solomon 1983, p. 433). In turning to relate to itself, consciousness left behind the world of experience—the world of sense-certainty and perception—and hence "is essentially the return from *otherness*" (Hegel 1977, p. 105). It is through this movement and the contrast afforded by what is other than it, that it can arrive at a consciousness of itself. Mediation is therefore necessary. The challenge is how to reconcile the necessity of mediation—and therefore of potential dependence— with the subject's initial conception of itself as absolutely independent. The latter is the self-conception with which the dialectic begins, a general, rather bare notion of

---

[9] Hegel does not cite Descartes or Fichte but is clearly alluding to their philosophy. In fact, Hegel is notorious for raising and then rejecting in a few terse sentences whole philosophical positions without attributing those positions to specific philosophers.

independence consisting in sovereignty with regard to one's beliefs and will. This means that the subject determines what to believe and how to act completely "undetermined (or unconstrained) by anything—whether the world or other subjects—that is not itself": it is a self-sufficient subject (Neuhouser 2009, p. 40).[10] Self-consciousness, therefore, seeks to affirm as true its conception of itself as absolutely independent while at the same time relating to what is other than it in order to know itself at all. If that self-conception is to be true, then that other must be made to conform with it; Harris (1997, p. 320) expresses it as follows:

> The world *appears* to be something other than myself. It must appear so, in order for me to be certain of myself at all. But if that certainty of self is what is absolutely *true*, then the "otherness" has to be an appearance only; and *that* must be made apparent by changing what appears so that it expresses the self.

Desire is the movement in which self-consciousness seeks to affirm its sovereignty by demonstrating that the object has no independence and is subject to its beliefs and will. As an object of a practically oriented self-consciousness, it is merely there to satisfy the subject's desires and has no self-sufficient status of its own: "desire's aim . . . is to show not that nothing else *exists*, but that nothing else has the kind of being that imposes constraints on it (on its will and belief)" (Neuhouser 2009, p. 43). Self-consciousness accomplishes this by superseding (negating, consuming) the object, hence Hegel's use of the term "desire" which, as Houlgate (2013, p. 65) points out, has the connotations in German [*Begierde*] of "greedy consumption" and of "wantonly destroying things, for no other reason than to affirm one's sense of self." However, the negation of the object does not satisfy self-consciousness; it does not allow it to confirm its self-conception as true and this for two reasons (see Hegel 1977, p. 109).

First, in order to affirm its self-conception of absolute independence, self-consciousness depends on the object, as it is only by negating the object that it can prove the truth of its self-conception. Yet that dependence belies its claim to self-sufficiency, and its self-conception is challenged. Second, by negating the object in order to affirm its self-conception, self-consciousness has lost the very thing that it needs to affirm itself, which is an independent object it can use to prove its self-sufficiency. Hence, it searches for another object in order to repeat the process and, once again, be able to affirm itself. This movement has to be repeated endlessly and the subject cannot find a stable and satisfactory confirmation of its self-sufficiency.[11]

---

[10] Note the parallels with sense-certainty's attempt to gain determinate knowledge without any mediating conceptual activity; self-consciousness begins with a similarly extreme—though in this case polar opposite—position: it wants to gain absolute self-certainty without having to accommodate, in any way, the object outside of it.

[11] Neuhouser (2009, p. 44) clarifies the double-bind in which self-consciousness is caught as follows: "the very moment at which Desire satisfies itself is also the moment at which it loses what it sought. This loss engenders the need to seek out a new object in relation to which self-consciousness can prove its self-sufficiency, and so, as long as it continues to conceive of self-sufficiency in the same way, it is caught in an unending cycle of satisfaction and emptiness, followed by the renewed search for another object in relation to which it can once again demonstrate its sovereignty." In a helpful analogy, Neuhouser (2009) argues that the fate of

The question to ask at this juncture is what kind of modifications would address these problems such that the subject's self-conception can be affirmed as true (see Siep 2014, p. 90). Clearly, it has proven necessary that the object must have a degree of independence in order for the subject to be able to affirm its self-sufficiency. Further, in order for self-consciousness to absolve itself of the repetitive movement of "desire," the object has to effect the negation from within itself, that is, it must by itself deny any claims concerning its own independence in such a way that confirms the subject's absolute independence. And the only object that can fulfill these two conditions—that can negate itself without losing all standing—is another subject: "*Self-consciousness achieves its satisfaction only in another self-consciousness*" (Hegel 1977, p. 110).[12]

Now this modification to the object requires modification to the conception of independence that has animated the dialectic so far. By admitting dependence on another subject, the conception of what it is to be self-sufficient will have to be updated. Arriving at a conception of independence that can be realized in the world is the point of this exercise, but that fully developed conception will have to await completion of the dialectic. To anticipate, the endpoint will be arrived at when the conception of what it is to be independent includes the idea that "only another [independent] subject can provide self-consciousness with a satisfying confirmation of its own self-sufficiency" (Neuhouser 2009, p. 45).

So far, the term "self-negation" has been used to describe the activity of the object, now subject, in the dialectic of self-consciousness. Self-negation and recognition are two ways of describing the same action: every act of self-negation is an act of recognition, and every act of recognition is an act of self-negation. To self-negate, that is, to voluntarily restrict one's agency in order to allow the other to be, is to *recognize* the other's claim to independence. At the beginning of the dialectic of recognition, to be discussed in the following section, the second subject negates itself fully such that the first subject can affirm its absolute independence. It becomes "nothing but a reflection of the first"; it sets itself aside and, in a helpful metaphor, turns itself "into a mirror for that other" (Houlgate 2013, p. 67). Yet this initial concept of recognition is one-sided and unstable.

....

self-consciousness in the mode of "desire" is similar to that of a serial seducer. A seducer seeks to confirm his image of himself as a person able to entice whomever he chooses into a romantic encounter. The seducer requires a person who provides him with resistance, and his ability at confirming his image of himself lies precisely in his ability to undermine that person's resistance. But once he has successfully seduced that person, that person no longer offers the required resistance and is of no value to the seducer. In order for the seducer to once again affirm his self-conception he needs another person who can offer the required resistance.

[12] To negate oneself—to set oneself aside in order for another to be, even though it is a forfeiture of independence, is still an act performed by the negating subject, and hence that subject is self-determining: it is not a thing that can be consumed as in "desire."

3.3.3 **The concept of recognition**

> Self-consciousness exists in and for itself when, and by the fact that, it so exists for another; that is, it exists only in being acknowledged [recognized]. (Hegel 1977, p. 111)

This thesis, with which Hegel begins the dialectic of recognition, is actually the result of the dialectic but is stated at the outset to indicate where things are heading. For something to exist "in and for itself" is for it to be "completely developed" (Solomon 1983, p. 280). In the terms explicated in the previous section, it is to be able to realize one's self-conception in the world: it is not just to conceive of oneself as independent, it is to actually be independent. It is not just, say, to (subjectively) believe that one owns a property or is a talented actor, but to (objectively) have this confirmed through the recognition that one is the owner of said property, or that one is an accomplished actor in the views of one's peers or audience. At that point certainty and truth would correspond. As we have seen, however, my certainty has to go through others before it can return to me as my truth: it has to be mediated through my relation with others. That relation, as the dialectic intends to show, is one of mutual recognition. This insight is not yet explicit at this stage of the analysis; the dialectic continues, now with two self-consciousnesses confronting each other; the first continues to affirm its absolute independence while the second only recognizes the first.

"Self-consciousness is faced by another self-consciousness; it has come *out of itself*" (Hegel 1977, p. 111). In having its self-conception affirmed through recognition by another self-consciousness, it becomes explicit for the first self that this affirmation cannot come through its action only—as the attempt had been in "desire"—but depends on the action of the second, recognizing self. As Hegel (1977, p. 111) argues, this is significant in two ways: first, self-consciousness has thereby "lost itself." What this means is that even though it has found affirmation of its self-conception out there in the world, accepting this is to acknowledge its dependence on the second affirming self, which undermines the very self-conception for which recognition was sought. Second, by seeing the other self repudiate any claims to independence (in self-negation), it ceases to regard that self as a being in its own right and sees it merely as a passive reflection of it, and hence as an entity incapable of offering the required recognition: "it does not see the other as an essential being, but in the other sees its own self" (Hegel 1977, p. 111).

This dilemma cannot be solved without modifying the self-conception at play. Consider: if self-consciousness, in an attempt to solve the first problem, were to deny the second self's independence in order to maintain its conception as absolutely sovereign, it would thereby lose the recognition it needs to affirm its self-sufficiency and achieve satisfaction; we would be back to the fruitless pattern of "desire." What emerges from this is that the second self must be regarded as sufficiently independent in order for its recognitional activity to satisfy the first self. For this to be possible, it is necessary to modify the notion of independence evident in the self-conception that has animated the dialectic up to this point. Self-consciousness cannot be absolutely sovereign; it cannot be unconditioned by anything outside of it. This does not mean that independence is repudiated, but that its meaning must be modified such that dependence on the recognition of an independent other is a necessary condition of being an independent agent. With that developed notion, the first self-consciousness, as Hegel (1977, p. 111) puts it, "lets the other again go free," for it becomes explicit to it that the other self has to be genuinely independent. Note, however, that this minimal recognition of the second self's independence is consistent with its treatment as less than an equal. The independence in question is that which merely makes the other self a being that can confer recognition. Further steps are needed before we can arrive at genuinely mutual recognition.

Another layer of complexity is required to make sense of the process of recognition. Recall that in order to escape the repetitive movement of "desire," the object had to effect the negation within itself: it had to, through its own action, deny any claims concerning its independence. This self-negation cannot be forced upon it; it must be uncoerced in adopting such a position. The reasoning behind this is that coercion would undermine the independence of the second self and hence the value of the recognition offered, since that value arises precisely from the fact that it is offered freely by a being like oneself. Hegel (1977, p. 112) here reminds us that the second self "is equally independent and self-contained, and there is nothing in it of which it is not itself the origin." The second self is therefore not an object to be denied as in "desire," but an independent existent in its own right; the first self "cannot utilize [it] for its own purposes, if that object [the second self] does not of its own accord do what the first does to it."[13]

Recognition, therefore, must be reciprocal and uncoerced: it requires the joint, free action of two self-consciousnesses. In order for the concept of recognition to achieve its ideal realization, recognition must also be *equal*. The ideal in question consists in what Hegel (1977, p. 110) describes as "the unity of the different independent self-consciousnesses which, in their opposition, enjoy perfect freedom and independence: 'I' that is 'We' and 'We' that is 'I'." This unity, which Hegel refers to as *spirit*, need not be conceived of as some bizarre metaphysical substance, but as a social conception of self-sufficiency in which "individual subjects renounce their claim to absolute sovereignty" and where equal value is accorded to "all individual subjects that compose" the social collectivity in question (Neuhouser 2009, p. 53). At that point all subjects would be fully aware of mutual dependency and equality as conditions of freedom.[14] To further clarify what equality means here consider the converse of this ideal: the master/slave relation.

Immediately following the dialectical analysis of the concept of recognition, Hegel (1977, p. 112) proceeds to describe how the "pure Notion of recognition . . . appears to self-consciousness." This is where the concept takes on more determinate forms beginning with Hegel's well-known account of the life and death struggle and the

---

[13] Some commentators have noted that there is an elementary notion of morality here: treat others only as an end and never as a means for the satisfaction of one's desires (Williams 1992, p. 157; see also Honneth 2012, pp. 15–16). Hegel's argument, however, is not directly moral but conceptual.

[14] Elsewhere, Hegel (1971, p. 171) expressed this insight as follows: "I am only truly free when the other is also free and is recognised by me as free."

master/slave relation. What is relevant to my point here is the nature of the master/slave relation, which is a relation of absolute inequality in that one self is "being only *recognised*, the other only *recognising*" (1977, p. 113). To be more precise, the master does recognize the slave in the minimal sense required for the slave's recognition of the master to count as valid. But the master does not recognize the slave as a being equal to it such that [the slave's] satisfaction also counts. As Hegel (1977, pp. 115–19) describes—and which I will not recount here—such an unequal relation is inherently unstable in the sense that it ultimately fails to provide satisfaction for the subjects involved.

Equality, then, involves something like symmetry of interaction, clearly demonstrated in this description of the recognitive encounter:

> A and B here meet one another with the attitude of conceiving of themselves and their interaction partner as autonomous self-consciousnesses. The interaction thus implies on the one hand the recognition of the free self-determination of the respective other, so that the interaction implies a self-confinement on both sides. On the other hand, because A and B conceive of themselves as such autonomous agents, this attitude contains the request towards the other to confine himself in order to let room for the other. (Quante 2010, pp. 98–9)

In such a symmetrical interaction, each partner is aware that it is recognizing the other and that it is being recognized by the other. Each partner is acting in such a way that would satisfy the other, while being aware that the other is acting in such a way that would satisfy it. As Hegel (1977, p. 112) puts it: "They *recognise* themselves as *mutually recognising* one another."

3.4 **What kind of concept is the concept of recognition?**

The foregoing reconstruction of the dialectic of self-consciousness and recognition can be summarized as follows:

> The subject can only become a free agent once it engages with other subjects in uncoerced relations of mutual recognition by which is confirmed for it as objectively true its own self-conception as a free agent. To this we can add a thesis concerning the stability of such relations which require equality in the sense of symmetry of interaction.

With such a conception of freedom we can see many possible openings in relation to several areas of inquiry such as social ontology, normative political theory, philosophical anthropology, and moral theory. Important strands in contemporary politics of recognition take Hegel's concept of recognition as a fundamental grounding notion, both as a normative guide for moral and political action, and as a psychological theory of self-formation (e.g., Honneth 1996; Fraser and Honneth 2003). Despite these obvious attractions, care must be taken in how to understand the concept and how to employ it in more concrete discussions such as will be attempted in the following chapters. A key question here is to ask: What kind of concept is Hegel's concept of recognition? Is it, as Siep (2011, p. 135) asks, "an empirical concept in the sense of a common trait of social phenomena, is it a norm generated by human valuations or evaluative experiences, or is it a hermeneutical hypothesis for understanding the development, the order and the acceptance of historical social institutions?". In order to address this issue, I return to Hegel's philosophy, now with a broad view of its main presuppositions. The purpose is to arrive at an interpretation of his philosophy that we can accept and from there to come to a view on how to regard the concept of recognition.

3.4.1 Interpretations of Hegel's idealism and implications for the concept of recognition

Hegel's philosophy is a form of idealism. At the very least, idealism is the epistemological thesis that material objects can only be known through the constituting activity of conscious minds. This thesis can be taken to imply several ontological positions—views on the nature of those objects and the extent to which they depend for their very being on the activity of the human mind. For example, Kant's idealism was a deduction of the a priori forms of intuition and categories of understanding to which objects must conform if they are to be experienceable by human subjects. The transcendental nature of this process meant that we can never have access to things-in-themselves, but only to objects as mediated via the categories. The price to pay for the necessity and universality of a priori thought was therefore the logical impossibility of knowing the object as it is in itself. However, Kant was not an ontological idealist, for he regarded objects as independent of mind though unknowable in so far as their true nature was concerned.

Hegel also held that objects are ontologically independent, though he differed from Kant in that he rejected the separation between thought and object, a separation which Hegel considered a lamentable and avoidable result of Kant's method and presuppositions (see section 3.3.1). Hegel's solution to this problem—the phenomenology of different forms of knowing—culminates in absolute knowing: the point at which no further contrast can be drawn between our conceptual frameworks and objects in the world (Pippin 1989, p. 91). Absolute knowledge is not some mysterious God's eye perspective on things; it is knowledge that is "unbiased, undistorted, unqualified, all-encompassing, free from counterexamples and internal inconsistencies" (Solomon 1983, p. 274). A tall order, no doubt, but the idea is to arrive at an adequate conception of knowledge. Its adequacy lies in that it solves for (Kantian) skeptical doubts without falling into subjectivism: upon arriving to absolute knowing, consciousness finally grasps the role of its own self-determining (conceptual) activity in constituting the world, while rejecting both skepticism (that there is a way the world "really" is that is inaccessible to us) and subjectivism (that the world has no existence independently of our cognitive activity) (see Westphal 1989).[15] This amounts to closing the gap between thought and being, and with it the distinction between epistemology and ontology.

This compact account of Hegel's idealism as it emerges through the *Phenomenology of Spirit* can be interpreted in several ways; I will mention two prominent

---

[15] Hegel (1977, pp. 56–7) put it like this: "In pressing forward to its true existence, consciousness will arrive at a point at which it gets rid of its semblance of being burdened with something alien, with what is only for it, and some sort of 'other', at a point where appearance becomes identical with essence."

interpretations: the conceptual realist view (metaphysical Hegel), and the post-Kantian view (nonmetaphysical Hegel).[16]

Conceptual realism

According to some contemporary interpretations, Hegel's idealism is a form of "conceptual realism": the view that reality has a rational, conceptual structure (e.g., Wartenberg 1993; Houlgate 2005; Stern 2009). To describe Hegel as an idealist–realist may sound like an oxymoron, but begins to make sense once we consider his claim that "every philosophy is essentially an idealism" (Hegel 1969, pp. 154, 155). If we accept Kant's Copernican revolution, it has to be, for every inquiry into objects in the world is an inquiry into our concepts and the basic structures of our minds. Unlike Kant, Hegel's conceptual realism arises from the manner in which he believed he had solved the problem of the inaccessible thing-in-itself, and that he had, in that way, closed the gap between thought and being. Having achieved this, speculative thought can begin, for if we accept the identity of thought and being it becomes possible to discern "the structure of being from *within* thought itself" (Houlgate 2005, p. 65). That is what Hegel proceeded to do in his later work in three areas: the general structure of being (*The Science of Logic*), and the two specialized domains of nature (*The Philosophy of Nature*) and social/cultural existence (*The Philosophy of Spirit*). This is the sense in which Hegel is an idealist–realist. It is also a picture in which Hegel can be thought of as an ontologist, out to describe the necessary structure of being as such and not only of thought.

Post-Kantian view

An alternative view of Hegel's idealism aligns it more closely with the Kantian project even as it recognizes Hegel's criticisms of Kant (e.g., Pippin 1989, 2010; Pinkard 1994). We have already seen in section 3.3.1 Hegel's reliance on Kant's formulation of knowledge as a relation between subject and object, where the subject projects onto the world the conceptual structures that enable an experience of the world. Those conceptual structures, in being necessary for any possible experience, cannot therefore be derived from, nor refuted by, experience (Pippin 1989, p. 8). From there we can see that both Kant and Hegel agreed that "contrary to the rationalist tradition, human reason can attain nonempirical knowledge only *about itself*, about what has come to be called recently our "conceptual scheme," and the concepts required for a scheme to count as one at all" (Pippin 1989). Hegel, however, went beyond Kant in two ways.

First, he rejected, as already mentioned here, Kant's skeptical doubt that such conceptual schemes have a legitimate claim to truth in an absolute manner (i.e., encompass the whole of reality). For Hegel, according to Pippin (1989, p. 250), such

---

[16] In addition to these two positions, there are earlier, traditional metaphysical interpretations where the *Phenomenology* is described as an account of how, through rational introspection, we can arrive at knowledge of the Absolute Spirit, God or some such cosmic substance. Such accounts, though they do have some evidence in certain of Hegel's pronouncements, do not fit with the overall aims of his philosophy, nor with the fact that he had taken seriously Kant's critical turn which ended the possibility of dogmatic metaphysics.

skeptical doubts though they are logically coherent, are "epistemically idle." Hegel argued this by demonstrating that there is no external standpoint from where we can judge that some aspect of reality—the thing-in-itself—is foreclosed to us. Contrary to the conceptual realist position, the identity of thought and being does not equate the ontological thesis that conceptual frameworks *determine* the content of natural, social, or ethical life. The thesis here is that such conceptual frameworks are adequate to the *investigation* of reality without us having to harbor skeptical doubts as to their adequacy. This makes Hegel not so much an ontologist describing the necessary structure of being, but a critical philosopher engaged in a demonstration of the conditions required for being self-conscious knowers. And it is in this latter sense where he, again, went beyond Kant.

Second, Hegel extended Kant's account of apperception—of the possibility of self-conscious experience—by placing the subject in the natural and social worlds. We have seen this with the concept of recognition, and in Hegel's rejection of those accounts that posit a pure subject of experience reflecting on the world and itself to the exclusion of everything outside of it. The necessary conditions for being self-conscious knowers turn out to include engagement with other subjects in relations of recognition. Self-knowledge cannot be accounted for in terms of a transcendental relation between subject and object or a subject with itself, but in terms of participation in social practices.

Returning to the original question—What kind of concept is the concept of recognition?—it is clear that the answer will vary on the basis of the interpretation of Hegel's idealism that we adopt. If reality has a rational, conceptual structure, then the examination of those concepts—as Hegel attempts in his work—would not only tell us about the dialectical development of rational thought, it would tell us about the ontology of social reality. In this sense, recognition would be an ontological concept that tends toward realization in social life. According to this interpretation, what we need to do socially and politically is to ensure that this process can proceed without disruption. But this interpretation is one that we cannot accept.

The issues here are complex and, in part, exegetical, and it would take us too far off course to attend to them in detail. Suffice to say that to interpret Hegel as a conceptual realist is to engage in a metaphysical project that engenders significant skepticism: the idea that we can specify the necessary structure of reality in accordance with the structure of the concept is one that, today, is impossible to accept. It may even be considered as a return to the kind of metaphysical theorizing which Kant had declared dead. It is, that is, to slip into a pre-Kantian, dogmatic kind of metaphysics where philosophers believed that they could, in an a priori manner, produce an account of the fundamental and necessary structures of being. Kant's innovation, of course, was to limit a priori endeavors to an examination of the conditions for being self-conscious knowers rather than the nature of being itself. We are left, then, with the post-Kantian interpretation outlined earlier. In my view, that interpretation avoids the problems just mentioned while presenting us with a positive account of recognition. Both Hegel and Kant were concerned with a conceptual articulation of the conditions required for being self-conscious knowers, but whereas Kant proceeded deductively, Hegel proceeded dialectically. The resulting concepts are ones that we can use to investigate subjectivity and social reality. According to the interpretation developed in what follows, recognition is not an empirical or metaphysical concept; recognition is a philosophical concept that indicates how we ought to think about freedom and ethical life.

3.4.2 **Recognition as affirmation of a normative status**

In what direction does the concept of recognition suggest we ought to think about freedom and ethical life? What is it to be a free agent in light of the concept of recognition? The short answer: to be a free agent is to be recognized as a free agent and for this to issue from those whom I in turn recognize as free agents. Recognition, therefore, is affirmation of a normative status (of being a free agent), and this has to be distinguished from views where the concept of recognition is understood as an empirical or a metaphysical concept. As Pippin (2008b, p. 62) explains:

> Hegel's argument for a particular sort of original dependence necessary for the possibility of individuality—recognitional dependence—is not based on a claim about human need, or derived from evidence in developmental or social psychology. It involves a distinctly philosophical claim, a shift in our understanding of individuality, from viewing it as a kind of ultimate given to regarding it as a kind of achievement, and to regarding it as a normative status, not a fact of the matter, whether empirical or metaphysical.

The idea of recognition as a "normative status" can be further clarified through Pippin's (2008b) analogy between recognition of what is mine in a material sense and what is mine in a psychological sense. He begins by noting that a fundamental starting point of "modern political reflection" is the distinction between what is mine, yours, and ours. To affirm that a property belongs to you—and not to me or to us—is to affirm a normative status involving a right, not an empirical fact that can be "read directly off the social world" (Pippin 2008b, p. 65). It is to affirm a sphere of what is rightfully yours, here pertaining to property, and in which consists an aspect of your freedom as a person. Freedom is not limited to ownership and extends to being regarded as a successful agent, an agent able to "own" her mental states. Here we can talk about what is rightfully mine in a psychological sense; what does that mean? I can claim a piece of land, but I cannot be properly said to own it until I am recognized as the owner (by my peers, the government, or an entity capable of offering that recognition). Similarly, I can claim to be the best pianist in the world, but I cannot be cognizant of myself in the right way until I am recognized as the best pianist in the world. In fact, in the absence of recognition, my insistence that I am the best pianist in the world could amount to delusion or, at least, self-deception. A person who is deluded is not regarded as a successful agent: they are wrong about who they think they are. From this we can see that my self-conception can only be rightfully and genuinely mine—in the sense of being truly who I am—if affirmed through recognition. One's success as an agent requires that others:

> (1) recognise me as having the social status and identity I attribute to myself; (2) recognise the deed as falling under the act-description that I invoke; and (3) recognise me as acting on the intention I attribute to myself. In general, this success requires that I am taken by others to have the intentions and commitments that I take myself to have, and so *to be doing* what I take myself to be doing. (Pippin 2008b, p. 67)

What is it to be a free agent? Now the long answer: as we established in section 3.2, as a free agent I am able to define a sphere of what is rightfully mine in terms of self-conceptions and reasons for action (and in that sense I am self-determining). Given that I cannot withdraw from social life in order to affirm for myself the validity of my self-conceptions and reasons for action, this affirmation can only come from others whose free bestowal of recognition is a condition of my freedom as an agent, and this mutually. It is in this sense that we can understand the claim, first noted in section 3.2, that the concept of mutual recognition is the only position that can rationally reconcile individual autonomy with social dependence: through mutual recognition, a provisional, unrealized notion of autonomy can become a concrete notion of freedom in the social world: freedom cannot be conceived of properly except as a socially achieved state.[17]

3.5 What reasons do we have to accept the concept of recognition?

In the conclusion to section 3.4.1 I noted that recognition is a philosophical concept that indicates how we *ought* to think about freedom and ethical life. From where does this ought derive normative force? Why should we accept the concept of recognition and the view of freedom it suggests—can't we, for example, see freedom as some kind of capacity people have *irrespective* of whether or not they are recognized as free? I present two answers; the first arises from the dialectic of recognition and the second from intuitions pertaining to failed self-conceptions.

3.5.1 The dialectic of recognition and the meaning of necessity

Why should we accept the concept of recognition? The first answer to this question requires that we refer ourselves back to the dialectic of recognition presented in section 3.3. The dialectic just is an argument for the concept of recognition, an argument that demonstrates how all attempts by the subject to affirm its independence without taking account of other subjects fail, culminating in the realization that dependence on the recognition of others is a condition of its own freedom. The extent to which we accept the dialectic as a valid argument is the extent to which we accept that we ought to think about freedom through the concept of recognition. And our acceptance of the argument hinges crucially on how we understand the sense of necessity it is supposed to possess; recall that throughout this chapter I have been referring to recognition as a *necessary* condition for freedom, and that a subject can *only* be free if recognized as free. What does "necessary" mean here?

First we can look at what "necessary" *does not* mean in the dialectic of recognition. Ordinarily, a necessary proposition is one that could not have been false; it must be true under any and all conditions. Such a proposition is knowable a priori since in

---

[17] This is to be distinguished from the practical conditions under which a particular agent can become free. What we are considering here are matters to do with the nature of freedom as such.

being necessarily true it cannot depend on facts about the world which can only tell us what is, rather than what must/must not be, the case. For example, analytic propositions are of this sort as their truth is a matter of the meaning of the concepts involved; "all bodies are extended" is a proposition whose denial is logically contradictory as "extension" is part of the meaning of the concept "body." This cannot be the sense of necessity intended in the claim under examination; for Hegel was not merely offering an analysis of the concept "self-consciousness," but an account of the conditions for self-consciousness. This suggests that perhaps the proposition is not analytic but synthetic, the latter being a proposition where the predicate is not contained in the subject. An example would be Kant's (1952) thesis in the *Critique of Pure Reason* that the concepts of Space and Time are not empirical concepts derived from experience, but exist in the mind as the a priori grounds of the possibility of all experience. Again, if we look at the manner in which Hegel derived his thesis, we find that it was not deduced in the way that Kant derived the forms of intuition and the concepts of the understanding. In fact, there is no straightforward deduction of this sort in the arguments and transitions of the *Phenomenology*.[18] What, then, is the sense of necessity invested in the dialectic?

According to one view, the necessity in question is similar to that which we perceive in a work of art. John Findlay (1962, p. 71) writes that despite what Hegel says about the necessary character of the transitions in the *Phenomenology*, they are "only necessary and inevitable in the rather indefinite sense in which there is necessity and inevitability in a work of art." Quentin Lauer (1993, p. 35) considers this view an unacceptable weakening of the force of the *Phenomenology* and suggests strengthening the notion of artistic necessity:

> In the contemplation of a great work of art . . . there is an awareness on the part of one who with taste looks long and hard that "nothing else will do"; each detail *demands* each other detail. It would be difficult (impossible) for the observer to formulate reasons *why* the details are demanded, but the details reveal themselves as "necessary" to the long, hard look.

The problem with such accounts is that they restate what needs to be explained: granted that necessity in the *Phenomenology* is comparable to *artistic* necessity and things have to be this way, just what is it that makes that the case? To answer this we need to distinguish between two kinds of moves that Hegel makes in the *Phenomenology*. On one hand, we have the macrotransitions from one shape of consciousness to another—from sense-certainty to perception, or from self-consciousness to reason, or from religion to absolute knowing. On the other hand, we have the microtransitions that are internal to each shape of consciousness.

---

[18] Another meaning of necessity is when we say, for example, that "water is necessary for life." Here we are stating a fact which could have been otherwise in another world—and hence is not logically necessary—but in ours it is a proposition that accords with robust empirical evidence. But this, again, cannot be the sense of necessity in the dialectic, for Hegel was not affirming the conclusions of empirical observation.

The macrotransitions are Hegel's grand vision of the process of the education of consciousness to the philosophical standpoint, or "absolute knowing" as he refers to it (see section 3.3.1). The transitions that make up this process are to be accounted for in terms of the telos of the education of consciousness. Hegel believed that all aspects of reality have a developmental plan aimed toward the telos of self-actualization. Development is a temporal process, and one way in which this process can be seen as rational—that is, "as capable of explanation"—is to know the telos it is intended to achieve (Wartenberg 1993, p. 108). For example, if a plant's goal is to produce fruit, then we can understand the different stages in the plant's development as both necessary and rational in light of the accomplishment of this goal. The telos of the education of consciousness can be described from various vantage points, though in each case it amounts to the same logic: the actualization of our conception of the world as a whole is achieved in the unity of concept and object (the "absolute idea"); the actualization of human existence is achieved by the full consciousness of freedom in spirit (or social and cultural life). This feature of Hegel's thought accounts for the distinctiveness of his philosophy, a philosophy that is always going somewhere—moving forwards toward an endpoint, and moving backwards from that endpoint to justify the progression of human consciousness through history. But this feature of his philosophy is also responsible for one of its most fundamental shortcomings. For it becomes clear that the necessity invested in the macrotransitions is a teleological necessity that stands or falls on the basis of whether or not we accept the claim that self-actualization is the telos of human nature. Apart from certain religious traditions, no one really accepts today that human beings have an ultimate telos; it strikes us as an unjustified essentialist claim.[19] Siep (2014, pp. 6–7) puts this whole issue in no uncertain terms:

> In today's culture, the claim to "absolute knowledge" and a complete understanding of religion and history necessarily presents itself as untenably hubristic. Practically no one in philosophy shares this project anymore ... Nature is not a logically structured totality, and neither is there a rational telos that tends towards its own realisation.

Given this, doubts are cast on Hegel's argument that human thought *necessarily* progresses along the shapes of consciousness that he describes, for in the absence of the telos of self-actualization, there is no reason why those particular transitions have to occur and in that order.[20] This leaves us with the second kind of transition I mentioned earlier, the microtransitions internal to each shape of consciousness. Do these dialectical transitions constitute valid arguments?

Microtransitions are best thought of as attempts to solve philosophical puzzles. These puzzles are grounded in particular assumptions, have an unrefined starting point, and are governed by specific rules. The dialectic of self-consciousness and recognition reconstructed in sections 3.3.2 and 3.3.3 is an example of such a puzzle and demonstrates a set of microtransitions. The puzzle in this case, as stated at various points throughout this chapter, is the possibility of freedom in the midst of other

---

[19] However, see Ikaheimo (2011) on Hegel's normative essentialism.

[20] Note that the point of contention here is not teleological explanation as such, but the notion that there is a human "nature" and that the telos of this nature is "self-actualization."

subjects. The grounding assumptions are: (1) the distinction between subject and object for knowledge to be possible at all: knowledge is a relation; (2) the necessity of mediation for self-knowledge to be more than a tautology: the relation of consciousness to itself is mediated via its relation to an other. The puzzle therefore becomes: how can the necessity of mediation (and of potential dependence) be made consistent with the subject's initial (and unrefined) conception of itself as absolutely independent? In trying to answer this question within the constraints of the grounding assumptions and without introducing new principles, the dialectic proceeds in microtransitions. Each transition involves demonstration of a contradiction in the conception of independence that animates the dialectic, followed by incremental modifications either to that conception and/or to the conception of the object (the other) that mediates the relation of self-consciousness to itself, until an adequate solution is arrived at.

Microtransitions, given the view just articulated, are not animated by a telos grounded in human nature; they are animated by the assumptions and constraints inherent in a particular shape of consciousness in the context of trying to solve the puzzle in question. What, then, of the claim that such transitions are necessary? Given the various meanings of necessity surveyed in this section, they are not. However, this does not mean that the dialectic of self-consciousness is no longer valid. Pippin (1989, p. 108) offers the view that we should understand a particular transition from, say, conception A to B not in the strong sense that B is the *only* way to resolve the inadequacies in A, but in the sense that B, as a matter of fact, "*does* resolve the inadequacies of A in the appropriate way, and issues a challenge to any potential objector to provide a better resolution." What this means is that a potential objector must consider the dialectic of self-consciousness and recognition and attempt to provide a better solution for the puzzle it raises given the constraints in question. In the absence of a competing account, the dialectic of self-consciousness and recognition remains a valid argument (or the best argument we possess) for reconciling individual autonomy with the social world. If it is a valid argument, then the concept of recognition is a concept that we ought to employ in thinking about freedom and social relations.

3.5.2 Intuitions about self-conceptions

The second reason I want to consider for why we should accept the concept of recognition has to do with our intuitions pertaining to what can be described as failed self-conceptions (identities). These are identities where persons wholly forsake recognition or wholly forsake their autonomy. In the former case autonomy is unrealized, in the latter it is nonexistent. In both cases, we would not consider the lives in question to have attained a free, successful existence. This, I maintain, suggests that we already consider the concept of recognition to possess normative force.

Queen Nefertiti who is not Queen Nefertiti

Nadia believes that she is Queen Nefertiti. She does not merely think that we have got her name wrong when we refer to her as Nadia; she actually considers herself to be Queen Nefertiti and the rightful heir to the throne of Egypt. She conducts herself in a manner consistent with her regal status—she dresses accordingly and expects people to acknowledge her power. Her circumstances are by no means regal; she lives in a poor neighborhood of Cairo and her neighbors oscillate between feeling sorry for her and infuriated at her. But Nadia continues in her belief and conduct, seemingly disinterested in any social confirmation of her idea of herself.

The man without qualities

The man without qualities[21] has no identity of his own; he is what everyone else wants him to be. His reference points are all determined by the circumstances in which he finds himself. Whatever idea or value is presented to him becomes, immediately, a guiding light until, that is, something else comes his way. For him, being socially accepted is of paramount importance and conformity is the only motivation for his conduct.

These two admittedly extreme examples are nevertheless illuminating in several ways. Depending on the perspective we adopt, the first example demonstrates a person who is denied recognition or has wholly forsaken any interest in social confirmation. The second example demonstrates a person who has wholly forsaken any interest in individuality. One constructs and carries through her self-conception outside society, the other constructs it wholly within society. Our intuitions regarding these two examples are clear. With regard to Nadia we have several descriptions that would generally be invoked: she may be described as living an illusion, as a deluded individual who is refusing to accept reality. On the other hand, the man without qualities would not strike us as a person who has a rich and fulfilling life. Even if we value conformity—of which he clearly is top champion—we *choose* conformity and hence are exercising our autonomy in that very choice; he does not choose. Neither Nadia nor the man without qualities would be considered successful agents. And the lack of that success agrees with what we have learned in reconstructing the concept of recognition. The subject of recognition seeks confirmation of his identity in the world. His certainty of who he is must pass through others before it can return to him as his truth. We regard with importance that we come to our own idea of our individuality *and* realize that idea in the social world. It is precisely the juxtaposition of these two notions that creates the tension that animates and problematizes social relations as conceived through the concept of recognition.

This final point takes us to the heart of the problem of recognition, the problem that is the central concern of this book in the case of Mad activism. The key issue here is how to resolve the tension between individual autonomy and the social world, a tension brought to light by the many movements struggling for recognition. Do we repair social relations such that persons receive the recognition they are demanding for their identities, or do we insist that the identities in question must be rejected in the terms they are presented since they are incoherent or morally objectionable? This is a critical issue to come to a view on and we will revisit it throughout the ensuing chapters.

The analysis of the situation of Nadia and the man without qualities drives home another important point. It shows that recognition, as argued previously, is not an empirical theory of the conditions under which people form identities but a normative standard of successful agency. People form identities under all sorts of conditions;

---

[21] This character is inspired by Robert Musil's novel with the same title.

Nadia was able to convince herself that she is Queen Nefertiti irrespective of the facts around her and in the absence of recognition from others that she is in fact who she claims to be. The reason we can see that she is not a successful agent is because we have prior intuitions to this effect, intuitions expressed in the concept of recognition. Having drawn this distinction, we must nevertheless note the interaction between the normative and the empirical (psychological) considerations. To be related to as a successful agent is very likely to have psychological consequences. To have one's views on one's identity and the meaning of one's actions confirmed by others as true is likely to engender a certain kind of confidence in who one is. Conversely, to be denied such recognition is likely to undermine one's confidence and esteem. The use of the term "likely" is intended to convey the uncertain nature of this process: for some people, no amount of positive recognition can counteract deeply seated insecurities; for others, no amount of misrecognition can shake off their singular belief in themselves. Still, the idea of the psychological consequences of (mis)recognition is important and will come to play a role in Chapters 4 and 5.

In conclusion, on the basis of the force of the arguments for (the dialectic of) recognition, and on the basis of our intuitions pertaining to failed identities and the value of achieving a balance between individual autonomy and social confirmation, the concept of recognition ought to inform our thinking about freedom and ethical life. Just how it can practically inform social relationships and political institutions is a separate question that I consider in Chapter 5.

3.6 **Conclusion**

The main aim of this chapter had been to reconstruct the concept of recognition in Hegel's *Phenomenology of Spirit*. This reconstruction, which sided with the "post-Kantian" interpretations of Hegel's philosophy offered, primarily, by Robert Pippin and Terry Pinkard, gave us a distinctive conception of freedom: being a free agent requires that one's self-conceptions, beliefs, and reasons for action are socially recognized as valid, and for this recognition to issue from those whom one considers capable of offering it. Such affirmation, therefore, cannot arise solely from the subject and requires participation in social practices: "a subject cannot be free alone" (Pippin 2008a, p. 186). The ideal of recognition has been described in several ways: we can think of it as the moment when one's certainty of who one is corresponds to the truth about who one is as the latter arises in social practices. We can also think of it, in an evocative metaphor, as the point at which the subject is able to find itself *at home in the world*. This metaphor offers a powerful means of distinguishing between Kant's and Hegel's views on freedom. If I may take the liberty of modifying this metaphor we can say that for Kant, to be free is to find oneself at home in *reason*, while for Hegel it is to reconcile one's autonomy with the social world in which one exists. Autonomy becomes concrete freedom through reciprocal, interpersonal recognition: being free is an achieved state, not a presocial given.

The concept of recognition, as reconstructed here, is neither an empirical nor a metaphysical concept. It is not a psychological theory of identity formation, even if affirming or denying a person's status as a successful agent can have psychological consequences (more on this in Chapter 4). Recognition is a philosophical concept that offers an account of what it is to be a free agent. In so far as we accept the dialectical arguments that underpin the concept, and in so far as we can appreciate the intuitions pertaining to the value attached to a successful identity—an identity that achieves the double-requirements of individuality and social confirmation—then the concept of recognition ought to inform our thinking about freedom and social and political life.

Chapter 4

Identity and the psychological consequences of recognition

4.1 **Introduction**

The examination of the concept of recognition and the problem of freedom in Chapter 3 led to the following claim: to be a free agent (a successful agent) is to have my identity, reasons for action, and beliefs recognized by others as valid, which is for the way that I take myself to be to correspond to how others take me to be, and for this recognition to issue from those whom I consider capable of offering it. These interactions occur against the background of collective practices that determine the standards against which identities, reasons for action, and beliefs can have a measure of validity. If I claim that I am a successful pianist, there are certain standards against which the truth of that claim can be measured; if I claim that I am praying in order to bring about rain, others may doubt the validity of my reasons for action. Truth and validity, here, are to be understood in social terms—Pinkard (1994, p. 53) expressed this point:

> The standards for what counts as authoritative reasons should be seen as the outcome of a process of a community's collectively coming to take certain types of claims as counting *for them* as authoritative, a process best understood in historical and institutional terms—that is, in terms of participation in social practices.

Given this, a person is more likely to be related to as a successful agent the more her identity corresponds to standards of validity in a given social context. That person would have to be a well-adjusted member of society with an unproblematic point of view on the world, and this over the course of life since recognition is not a one-off bestowal but an ongoing interpersonal interaction. That kind of ideal situation, as we all know, is not always obtained. What is evident when we consider the many movements demanding recognition, and by reflecting on our own personal difficulties in finding ourselves at home in the world, is that identity is complex, contested, and the site of ongoing struggles for self-definition and acceptance.

This complexity and contestation has to be seen against the background of distinctly modern conceptions of identity. Identity is contested because it is no longer a given; almost all self-definitions previously considered "natural" are now being questioned. Identity constitutes an orientating framework for deliberation and action, and is expressive of my individuality. Somehow, the personal vision that arises needs to be affirmed in social interaction: we have already anticipated the dual importance of individuality *and* social confirmation in section 3.5.2 through an analysis of two examples of failed identities; the first concerned wholly with individuality, the second concerned only with social affirmation. The concept of recognition—and our intuitions (arguably) agreed—required that individuality and social affirmation are juxtaposed, neither dominating and taking over the other. While there is importance in finding my own way of being human by taking a personal stance in relation to the collective categories in which I find myself, I cannot just "go it alone" and forego any need for social confirmation. If I do so I would be like Nadia who thinks herself Queen Nefertiti while we think her "deluded." Yet social confirmation is not always forthcoming, and people do end up with devalued, misrecognized identities. To be recognized as a successful agent is something that cannot be taken for granted. Sometimes achieving it will require working to transform the social standards that fail to recognize or that misrecognize the identity in question. Sometimes, that is, it will be necessary to engage in a struggle for recognition.

This is the first part of the exposition that I attempt in this chapter (sections 4.2 and 4.3). The second part has to do with the psychological consequences of recognition. Recognition is not just a normative status—an affirmation of agential success—it is also of psychological importance. To be related to as a successful agent is likely to have positive psychological consequences that make it more likely for you to be related to as a successful agent. Among the theorists of recognition, it is Axel Honneth who develops the most sophisticated account of the psychological consequences of recognition and of the harms of misrecognition. Section 4.4 outlines his approach, indicates some problems with it, and highlights its normative potential for social and political action.

4.2 **Identity**

4.2.1 **A primer on identity**

The term "identity" has become ubiquitous in academic research. A Google Scholar search for all publications with the word "identity" in the title reveals 220,000 results. In most of these results—180,000—it appears in the phrase "identity politics."[1] In many discussions in the humanities today, that phrase has become somewhat unacceptable, and unity in condemnation of "identity politics" a point of agreement among many academics. It is pointed out that engaging in political activity on the basis of a shared identity as a group places pressure on individuals to conform to particular ways of behaving, hiding power struggles within the group in favor of the appearance of homogeneity. Further, the focus on group identity tends to encourage separatism; the fragmentation of our social existence into ever more subtle (and small) groupings, thus losing sight of common and shared human concerns. Unfortunately, in the midst of these criticisms (aspects of which I look at in section 4.2.4) something tends to be lost from the notion of identity, now that it is reduced to the *sociopolitical*: ethnicity, race, nationality, gender, and so on. In this section I want to step back from the sociopolitical dimensions and consider a more fundamental question: what is identity?

---

[1] For those reading this book in the distant future (assuming it has survived several reprints), "Google" was the most popular internet search engine in the first two decades of the twenty-first century. "Scholar" was Google's dedicated academic research portal.

To answer this question, it is necessary to begin with some reflections on the nature of human agency, for identity—the question of who I am—has to ultimately be characterized as an articulation of notions central to me as an agent. Charles Taylor (1985, 1989) has done important work toward an account of identity in those terms. In his essay *What is Human Agency?* Taylor (1985) argues, along with Frankfurt (1971), that an essential feature of human agency is the ability to form second-order desires, which are evaluations whose object is a first-order desire. We are able to evaluate our desires, to rank them in some way, to outlaw some, and to allow others to be effective in action. For example, you have a strong urge to have chocolate cake now, but you resist this urge as you are having dinner with friends in one hour and don't want to ruin your appetite. Taylor further divides our capacity to evaluate desires with respect to the nature, or depth, of the evaluation in question. In the foregoing example you arrived at a decision by a process of weighing, and the enjoyment of chocolate cake now paled in comparison to the pleasure to be derived from a hearty appetite later. Taylor calls weighing of this kind "weak evaluation." By contrast, you might refrain from having chocolate cake—though desirous of it—not because that might ruin an anticipated, greater pleasure at a later time, but because you want to live a life of moderation; you don't want to succumb to every appetitive urge that comes your way. Here, something more than simple weighing is going on, for the concern is not so much, or solely, with optimizing outcomes but with the qualitative worth of the desire itself (1985, p. 16). Taylor (1985, p. 18) calls evaluations of this kind "strong evaluations":

> In weak evaluation, for something to be judged good it is sufficient that it be desired, whereas in strong evaluation there is also a use of "good" or some other evaluative term for which being desired is not sufficient; indeed some desires or desired consummations can be judged as bad, base, ignoble, trivial, superficial, unworthy, and so on.

The difference between strong and weak evaluations can be further clarified in light of the contingent nature of the latter. I refrain from keeping a fifty pound note I found in the office, though needing it, not because I will be caught—no one can find out—but because it is wrong to take someone else's hard-earned money. For the weak evaluator, endorsing or rejecting the desire may be contingent on the possibility of getting away with it, whereas for the strong evaluator it is not contingent on that. Strong evaluations, then, are "discriminations of right or wrong, better or worse, higher or lower, which are not rendered valid by our own desires, inclinations, or choice, but rather stand independent of these and offer standards by which they can be judged" (Taylor 1989, p. 4).

Taylor (1989, p. 27) argues that strong evaluation is a central feature of human agency, that we would not recognize—or would recognize as extremely shallow and distorted—a human agency for whom qualitative distinctions pertaining to the worth of desires and motives never arose. For that person, the only consideration in relation to desires is satisfaction and optimization of outcomes and, should he exist, is likely to be rare; even hedonists value the hedonistic lifestyle as such (i.e., they also are engaged in strong evaluations). Strong evaluations are about the standards we have set ourselves, the kind of persons we are or want to be, and the values in accordance with which we want to structure our lives. In this way, they constitute an orientation to the good (Taylor 1989, p. 47), where "good" is to be understood broadly to encompass the ethical, moral, esthetic, and social. At this point we arrive to the notion of identity:

> To know who I am is a species of knowing where I stand. My identity is defined by the commitments and identifications which provide the frame or horizon within which I can try to determine from case to case what is good, or valuable, or what ought to be done, or what I endorse or oppose. In other words, it is the horizon within which I am capable of taking a stand. (Taylor 1989, p. 27)[2]

When people get to know each other in what is expected to be more than a passing acquaintance, questions of identity in the sense defined here loom large. On a first encounter we are, as it were, trying to get a sense of the other person. We typically ask questions like "where are you from" and "what do you do" as a first and admittedly rather imprecise guide to their values, what they care about, what they stand opposed to, and so on. But they are a starting point. We may learn that the other person is a teacher, moreover one who takes a strong stand against the teaching of Creationism in schools. Another may emphasize that her job is only a source of income and not defining of who she is, her real passion lying in a creative pursuit.[3] We may learn that a person comes from a Muslim background, a fact that by itself may not tell us much, but which can be very informative once we learn from that person how he regards it. This points out that what is crucial in the question of identity is not so much a list of markers such as religion, background, profession, ethnicity, and others, but, as Taylor (1985, p. 34) notes, the *way* in which these properties "figure in my identity." Consider, for example, my own relationship with Islam: I grew up in predominantly Muslim and, in some ways, rather different communities in Egypt and the United Arab Emirates. During my late teenage years and early twenties I reacted strongly against religion in general. Today, even though I would not refer to myself as a religious individual (in so far as being religious involves doctrinal commitments and ritual practices, neither of which I believe or engage in), religion played a huge role in defining my identity. We frequently get the most perspicuous vision of who we are and what matters to us in the process of distinguishing ourselves from ideas and expectations which previously were at the forefront of our lives.

If identity involves, as discussed, an orientation to the good, then the way I am situated and situate myself in relation to the relevant collective categories is also how I arrive at an idea of the life I want to live.[4] What kind of person do I want to be, what kind of father, son, partner, and friend, what kind of teacher and philosopher? By no means is any of this straightforward: we can spend significant periods of our lives struggling to articulate just what it is that matters most to us,

---

[2] Understood in this way, "identity" becomes a central structuring element in our life. This is thrown into relief when we reflect on situations where identity is threatened: an "identity crisis."

[3] Even inquiries about culinary preferences may reveal important values; a person may prefer Colombian coffee for the taste, and also because it is fair-trade.

[4] The use of the active and passive senses of situate—to situate oneself versus to be situated—is intended to bring to light the play of individual autonomy and social givens (see section 4.2.3).

our difficulties sometimes manifesting in paralyzing ambivalence, and other times finding unexpected resolution. All of this occurs in a space of questions "which touch on the issue of what kind of life is worth living, or what kind of life would fulfil the promise implicit in my particular talents, or the demands incumbent on someone with my endowment, or of what constitutes a rich, meaningful life" (Taylor 1989, p. 14).

We can recognize something universal in these questions. As Taylor points out in *Sources of the Self* (1989) and in the more recent *A Secular Age* (2007), human beings have always been concerned with the possibility of a full, worthwhile life. But the conditions under which this occurs have undergone significant historical change. This change is presaged by the collapse of the idea of a single, self-evident master narrative; today there are multiple orientations to the good, and no single narrative can expect to simply command our allegiance or appear as solely true (Taylor 1989, p. 17). Connected to this is the modern understanding of individuality and the importance accorded to the discovery of one's own "moral horizon" (1989, p. 28). In the context of these changes it becomes possible to deal with questions of the worthwhile life in personal terms; returning to the example I used earlier, in relating to Islam as a young man I was establishing its meaning for me. Religion itself was under question, and not a master narrative against which I can assess the worth of my life or determine what is good.

The contrast here is between an attitude in which orientations to the good constitute the standard against which I can measure the worth of my life, as opposed to those orientations being elements toward which I need to situate myself in my own way. Taylor's method for bringing up this contrast is predominantly historical, comparing earlier and modern periods of what he refers to as the Western thought tradition. Another way of doing this is to compare attitudes across cultural contexts instead of through time. Consider the following excerpts from a piece of research I had conducted a few years ago (Rashed 2012). The descriptions refer to a rural community in the Dakhla Oasis of Egypt:

> Individual time is synchronised with society at large through cyclical repetition embodied in regular prayers five times a day and longitudinal anchor-points in the form of non-negotiable views on the mile-stones of adult life: work, marriage, and bearing and raising children being the most prominent. At the base of all this lies a narrow view on what constitutes moral, physical, and mental integrity. Life here is not—as the existentialist ideal would have it—a personal project but a striving towards fulfilling these fundamental goals, and within acceptable time-frames too: failure to do so damages the person's worth, sometimes permanently.

> To the extent that the norms and values of an ideal life favour repetition, stability, and conformity over flux, uncertainty, and uniqueness it is to be expected that the subject may not have had the opportunity to attend vigorously to what she—as a project-creating individual—would want out of her life, over and above what is socially prescribed. This is not to eliminate individual agency, for there will always be reactions against these dominant norms. Yet within this attitude, when a problem occurs—a problem that challenges the fulfilment of expected goals—the natural response would not be to question the purpose and meaning of one's life—something that requires

an ability to see one's life as a malleable creation—but to focus on where and why the failure had occurred. Drifting into your late twenties without getting married is not an occasion to question whether you want, at this point, to get married but an occasion to inquire into the reasons behind the failure to fulfil this important milestone. Much like a child failing to walk at the appropriate age invites speculation as to his constitution and health.

In this passage we can discern an ideal that emphasizes the importance of aligning one's life with a preset trajectory. This is in contrast to the ideal articulated by Taylor where life, identity, is seen as something personal to be discovered and articulated. It is this latter ideal—the ideal of authenticity—that is central to contemporary political demands for recognition, and to which I now turn.

4.2.2 **Identity and authenticity**

As noted in the introduction, central to the political question of recognition is the problematization of identity; the question "who I am" no longer has a pregiven answer but is an open question to be addressed in my own way. The ideal animating this modern understanding of identity can be referred to as the ideal of authenticity. It may be tempting to think of authenticity as a meta-ideal: an ideal whose object are other ideals. The temptation comes from the fact that contrary to other ideals, it does not offer concrete advice on how to live save for the guiding principle of making the question of how to live answerable in personal, authentic terms. This temptation should be resisted, for no matter how thinly specified, the ideal of authenticity is still an orientation to the good, and it too is constituted by strong evaluations of the kind described earlier. The ideal of authenticity is

> the understanding of life which emerges with the Romantic expressivism of the late-eighteenth century, that each one of us has his/her own way of realising our humanity, and that it is important to find and live out one's own, as against surrendering to conformity with a model imposed on us from outside, by society, or the previous generation, or religious or political authority. (Taylor 2007, p. 475)

In *The Ethics of Authenticity*, Taylor (1991) credits two thinkers in particular as having been the first to describe the ideal's central motifs. The first is Rousseau who held that our capacity to realize true and independent being requires that we recover contact with ourselves. Such contact is threatened by certain of our passions key among which is *amour propre*, a form of self-concern that induces us to seek admiration and regard from others. *Amour propre* consigns us to dependence on the favorable opinions of others; we become subject to their will since it is only through them that we can satisfy this passion. Such a dependent, conformist mode of existence can be remedied by recovering, as Taylor (1991, p. 27) puts it, "authentic moral contact with ourselves."

The second thinker who contributes to modern understandings of the ideal of authenticity, as discussed by Taylor, is Herder. While Rousseau articulated the importance of self-contact, Herder increased this importance by linking it to originality in self-realization:

> There is a certain way of being human that is *my* way. I am called upon to live my life in this way, and not in imitation of anyone else's. But this gives a new importance to being true to

myself. If I am not, I miss the point of my life, I miss what being human is for *me* . . . Being true to myself means being true to my own originality, and that is something only I can articulate and discover. (Taylor 1991, pp. 28–9)

The two facets of the ideal of authenticity—self-contact and originality—can be discerned in the examples and discussion toward the end of the previous section, specifically in a person's endeavor to situate herself in her own personal way toward the various orientations to the good, or identity categories, or ways of life that are on offer. In order for this attitude to be possible, she needs to step back and recover contact with herself, as opposed to losing herself in those categories or ways of life. And in order for this attitude to be successful, she needs to fashion or discover her identity.

As described here the ideal of authenticity raises some worries. The problems raised by the term "authenticity" will be addressed in the following section. For now I want to consider the consternation that may be caused by the use of the term "ideal." To talk about an *ideal* of authenticity is perhaps to be overly concrete about it. For the term ideal implies some clear-cut notions to which people subscribe; we talk about the ideal of beauty being a certain height, weight, symmetry, and so on (relative, though, as these may be). The term appears overly cognitive, demanding when we mention it that we specify its elements. Indeed, this is what Taylor had done as presented previously: he teased out the elements of the ideal of authenticity by tracing key developments in the history of ideas. We know, of course, that people do pick out what they consider beautiful without necessarily being able to immediately articulate the ideal behind their choice. In a similar way, people may take an attitude of discovery toward their life without necessarily having a set of clearly articulated ideas that motivate them in this way. That being said, unless you are a behaviorist, the question is one of articulacy and not redundancy; that is, talk of ideals is not optional: attitudes and choices if they are going to be that cannot be random, and hence have to be informed by some overarching notion of what is important and valuable. It is hard to imagine how without some notion of the value of being true to oneself being operative in a person's moral and psychological life—no matter how poorly articulated this notion is—that she would approach her life as a project and try to make it her own; anymore in fact than we can imagine a person following to the letter the dictates of the Bible or the Qur'an in the absence of a broader conviction that the Divine Plan is the best blueprint to one's life. Ideals are not optional and, no matter how poorly articulated, are there orientating us to the good. But there is another criticism of the ideal of authenticity: the problem of essentialism.[5]

---

[5] A third criticism of the ideal is that it may encourage narcissism and self-indulgent forms of individuality (see Taylor 1991). However, a proper understanding of the concept of recognition would show that forms of individuality that regard the other merely as a means for confirming one's superiority, or that pay no attention to the well-being of others, fall short of the structure of recognition that we are concerned with (and which was described in Chapter 3).

4.2.3 **The problem of essentialism**

In articulating the ideal of authenticity, Taylor has been criticized for committing an error of philosophical anthropology. Anthony Appiah (2005, p. 107) argues that authenticity presupposes an essentialist view of the self, the view that the authentic "real self" is buried in there waiting to be dug out and expressed.[6] He contrasts this with the view that developed after Romanticism where the "self is something that one creates, makes up, like a work of art." Appiah (2005, pp. 17–18) argues, rightly in my view, that neither idea is correct: "The authenticity picture is wrong because it suggests that there is no role for creativity in making a self, that the self is already and in its totality fixed by our natures," and the creativity picture is wrong "because it suggests that there is *only* creativity, that there is nothing for us to respond to, nothing out of which to do the construction." He offers a middle-ground solution where "we make up selves from a tool kit of options made available by our culture and society," and while we do make choices, "we don't, individually, determine the options among which we choose" (Appiah 2005, p. 107).

While an essentialist view of self is incorrect, it is a view to which Taylor in fact does not subscribe. The essentialist view is monological in the sense that it makes identity the product of introspection and not interaction, but Taylor's account of identity is dialogical through and through: "The crucial feature of human life is its fundamentally *dialogical* character. We become full human agents, capable of understanding ourselves, and hence of defining our identity, through our acquisition of rich human languages of expressions" (Taylor 1994a, p. 32). These languages are not limited to the spoken word and encompass various other communicative practices such as ritual, art, and so on (Taylor 1994a). Languages are shared social practices and hence to be "inducted into personhood" one is "initiated into a language," which places oneself from the start and throughout life in a "common space" of meanings and significances (Taylor 1989, p. 35). We may, later in life, challenge certain understandings and come to a newer view on what matters to us, but this always occurs, as Taylor (1989, pp. 35–6) notes, "from the base in our common language." All of which is to say that there is no zero point to which we may retreat, as it were, and through introspection define who we are; our identity is defined in interaction with others.

If identity is dialogically constituted then what do we make of authenticity, a term that, it must be admitted, does have essentialistic overtones? Appiah (2005, p. 107) argued that "we should acknowledge authenticity in our political morality" only if we are able to develop an account of it that is not monological. I agree, and I think it is possible to provide such an account. To more precisely identify the problem, recall that the ideal of authenticity has two facets: self-contact and originality. "Self-contact" does not cause any major problems of philosophical anthropology, for it merely denotes an

---

[6] Tempelman (1999) makes a similar point by referring to "primordialist strands" in Taylor's conception of cultural identity. By this is meant that Taylor takes identity to possess "(quasi-) natural features" that are fixed and form the basis of our " 'authentic' moral and social frameworks" (Tempelman 1999, p. 21). For a contrasting view, see Novotny's (1998) defense of Taylor's views on identity against the charge of essentialism.

attitude of looking closely, critically at oneself. "Originality" seems to be the problem here and merits examination.

In ordinary usage the term "original" is understood in two main ways. We say of something that it is original if it is what it claims to be in terms of origin; that it is *authentic*. "Original" has another meaning that denotes *creativity* and uniqueness, as when we say that a work of art, an idea, or a novel are original. Applied to persons, originality as authenticity can be understood not in the untenable sense of a self waiting to be uncovered, but in the moral-psychological sense of those aspects of a person that are central to his or her identity. If you are to shed all that you are able to conceive of as contingent, you would arrive at certain features of your identity which you can no longer exclude without ceasing to recognize yourself.[7] For many people, sex, gender, and sexual orientation will emerge as central features; for others, race and ethnicity may play a big role; many would consider their religious affiliation to be of fundamental importance; vocation may feature for some, parenthood for others. Recovering "authentic moral contact with ourselves," as Taylor phrases it following Rousseau, would then mean directing our gaze inwards and asking if aspects of what we have previously considered central to our identity should be regarded as contingent, as something we have not chosen, something that constrains rather than enriches our life and hence calls for revision. For it may be the case that we have never questioned that aspect of our identity, perhaps because we were brought up to be of a certain religion or to conceive of gender roles in a certain way. Or perhaps because we have, up to that point, taken for granted a scheme of values prevalent in our social environment and unquestioningly measured the success of our life against it.

This activity of reflection takes us to the second meaning of originality as creativity. It is creative in the sense that it seeks to fashion an identity in which one feels at home by ridding oneself of what comes to be seen as an unchosen burden. But the creativity here is not boundless, for in fashioning an identity and seeking a clearer vision of what is authentically hers, the person can only appropriate from the ideas, values, and ways of life available, even as he or she innovates upon and challenges established norms.[8]

---

[7] This can be carried through as a thought experiment where you sort out the importance and priority of your identifications. Of course, the sorting out itself will occur from the vantage point of your more fundamental beliefs and values as there is no zero point from where to assess what is important to you. For some people such insights come by means rather more testing than a thought experiment. Frequently we come to awareness of what is central to our identity if we are prevented from, punished for, or more insidiously made to feel ashamed of, expressing it. Alternatively, we may discover that aspects of our identities were central to who we are in the very process of losing them, say in the midst of acculturation or an "identity crisis."

[8] Consider a teenager discovering that he is attracted to members of the same sex in a society where such attraction is considered a sin or a crime. He may fail to articulate that aspect of himself and come to terms with it or, even worse, he may endorse negative social scripts concerning his sexuality and turn against himself in self-hatred. Or if he manages to articulate his sexual identity through his exposure to more benign, if isolated, discourses he might be forced to pass as straight in order to avoid expected repercussions in that particular community. Far from being there waiting to be discovered, identity is subject to the social

And this applies even in the most extreme case, that of the "hero" going it alone against the grain of society:

> Taking the heroic stance doesn't allow one to leap out of the human condition, and it remains true that one can elaborate one's new language only through conversation in a broad sense, that is, through some kind of interchange with others with whom one has some common understanding about what is at stake in the enterprise. A human being can always be original, can step beyond the limits of thought and vision of contemporaries, can even be quite misunderstood by them. But the drive to original vision will be hampered, will ultimately be lost in inner confusion, unless it can be placed in some way in relation to the language and vision of others. (Taylor 1989, p. 37)

Originality, therefore, can be understood in two connected senses, neither of which are suspect from a philosophical-anthropological point of view: authenticity and creativity. A person's identity is authentic to the extent that it consists in elements that he is able to endorse as central to who he is. A person's identity is creative to the extent that she actively seeks to define who she is, or wants to be.[9]

So far I have been defending the ideal of authenticity against the accusations it may face in virtue of being an *ideal* and in virtue of the term *authenticity*. Underpinning the discussion as a whole has been the notion of individual identity, what it is and the ideals that animate it. It is time now to return to an issue I left at the beginning of section 4.2.1, which is the social (or sociopolitical) dimension of identity: how does this relate to individual identity?

4.2.4 The relation between social identity and individual identity

When it comes to the political expression of demands for recognition, we find that such demands are always presented as applying to social identities based on race, gender, sexuality, religion, ethnicity, and cultural affiliation, to name some key categories. Yet so far in Part II, the exposition of the concept of recognition and of the notion of identity centered on the individual subject. This is not incidental; as I have argued in Chapter 3, the concept of mutual recognition is an attempt to reconcile individual autonomy with social practices. Our starting point, therefore, is the individual and their ability to find themselves at home in the social world. How do social identities come into this? Social identities are important to the individual in two ways: (1) as

---

conditions—including the available scripts—to which this young man can appeal to in articulating his sexuality. Yet his sexuality, in a significant sense, can be understood as belonging to his originality, and the congruence between this and the self-understanding that he develops will be an important measure of the extent to which he is at home in the social world.

[9] A separate objection to this line of thought is that it presupposes an agent free of social influences and free of the power-relations embedded in our languages of expression. While it may seem to you that you are being creative and authentic—the objection can continue— you are taking part in social practices that perpetuate your subjection by getting you to endorse roles that do not serve you but serve society. For a response to this objection see section 4.3.

an aspect of an individual's self-definition such that recognition of a social identity is required for recognition of the individual; (2) as an organizing principle for social action aimed at addressing misrecognition.

Appiah (2005, 1994b) draws a helpful distinction between two dimensions of our individual identity: a personal dimension evident in various features of importance such as intelligence, kindness, charm, and so on, and a collective dimension that consists in the intersection of the social identities that a person takes to be central to who she is such as being an African-American, heterosexual woman. Now the features that constitute the personal dimension, as Appiah (1994b, pp. 151–2) notes, do not make up a social group as this is ordinarily understood: "there is a logical but no social category of the witty, or the clever, or the charming, or the greedy." Social identities, on the other hand, do not "belong" to the person even if they are central to his or her individual identity; they are social categories that already provide norms and scripts for how a person belonging to such a category should behave (Appiah 1994b, p. 159). That is not to say that the scripts provided are fixed or uncontested; as Appiah (2005, pp. 22–3) observes:

> There is not just *one* way that gay or straight people or blacks of whites or men or women are to behave, but there are ideas around (contested, many of them, but all sides in these contests shape our options) about how gay, straight, black, white, male, or female people ought to conduct themselves. These notions provide loose norms or models, which play a role in shaping our plans of life. Collective identities, in short, provide what we might call scripts: narratives that people use in shaping their projects and in telling their life stories.

To the extent that I identify with a specific social identity and find (or make) it central to my individual identity, it becomes important to me how this identity is publicly valued and understood: "my being, say, an African-American among other things, shapes the authentic self that I seek to express. And it is, in part, because I seek to express my self that I seek recognition of an African-American identity" (Appiah 1994b, p. 153). The connection between individual and social identity means that misrecognition of social identities through stigma, disrespect and, in general, promoting negative narratives concerning others, extends to individual identity. The work of recognition is to fashion positive narratives pertaining to the social identities in question. The way this goes with the Gay rights movement is familiar:

> An American homosexual after Stonewall and gay liberation takes the old script of self-hatred, the script of the closet, and works, in community with others, to construct a series of positive gay life-scripts. In these life-scripts, being a faggot is recoded as being gay: and this requires, among other things, refusing to stay in the closet. And if one is to be out of the closet in a society that deprives homosexuals of equal dignity and respect, then one has constantly to deal with assaults on one's dignity. In this context, the right to live as an "open homosexual" will not be enough. It will not even be enough to be treated with equal dignity despite being homosexual: for that would suggest that being homosexual counts to some degree against one's dignity. And so one will end up asking to be respected *as a homosexual*. (Appiah 2005, pp. 109–10)

We can see here that even if one did not identify as gay to begin with, by being subject to discrimination for being homosexual and by taking part in the kind of social action that addresses civil rights and discrimination, one can come to develop such an identification; being gay may assume importance for that person's sense of who he is.

In addition to being key components of individual identity, social identities as group identities are important as a means of organizing for social action.[10] Yet the idea of group identity is problematic. It has been argued that emphasizing group affiliation as a means of addressing misrecognition may end up generating further instances of misrecognition through the reification of identity. Nancy Fraser (2010, p. 215) expressed this worry, noting that the "need to elaborate and display an authentic, self-affirming and self-generated collective identity"—as frequently required by group-based political action—puts pressure on individuals to conform, discourages cultural dissidence and criticism in the name of group loyalty, and obscures power dynamics and divisions within the group in the name of homogeneity. The effect of this is the imposition of a "single, drastic simplified group identity which denies the complexity of people's lives, the multiplicity of their identifications, and the crosspulls of their various affiliations" (Fraser 2010). Thus, what began as a means of establishing more viable, genuine, and respectful societal understandings of one's identity, ends up forcing people into tight scripts that cannot conceivably correspond to their sense of who they are. Appiah (1994b, p. 163) recognized this predicament, warning of the risk of replacing "one kind of tyranny with another." It is true, as Appiah notes, that if one were black and gay, one may choose the world of Black Power and Gay Liberation over the world of "Uncles Tom's cabin" and the "Closet" (Appiah (1994b). And it will also be true for some people, as Appiah again observes, that one may wish such a choice did not have to be made, that there was sufficient freedom to decide for oneself the extent to which such categories are defining of identity.

These are important criticisms, but they need to be placed in the context of the perennial concern with reification and simplification in political organizing in general. On the one hand, some degree of homogeneity is necessary for any political action to be possible, otherwise we would have as many political parties as there are citizens. That is not a justification for one-party totalitarianism, any more than identity-based political activity should lead to simplified identities that dictate the *only* way a certain kind of person must behave. If that occurs, then we would have certainly crossed over from the "politics of recognition" to the "politics of compulsion" (Appiah 1994b). To avoid this, a mature understanding of the subtlety of individual identity and of the cross-pulls of people's different affiliations is required. The latter are those intersectional identities where the person, say, is both disabled and gay, and where the two identities may conflict with one other. This has to be balanced with pragmatic

---

[10] Note that this role of social identities can come apart from the first role as a component in individual identity. It is conceivable that I join an affiliation based on features that I share with others—say a specific disability—in order to pressurize the government to provide accommodations in the work place, without this requiring or implying that a disability identity is an important part of my self-definition, only that it was necessary in the present context to organize around it in order to make claims upon the government. This suggests that not all identity-based organization is actually about identity.

considerations such as the viability of political action: the more the categories of identity are refined and divided such that they correspond more faithfully to people's understanding of themselves, the smaller the group becomes and the weaker its organizing and campaigning power (the problem of "separatism"). Conversely, the bigger and more united the group becomes, the more its campaigning power but the price to pay is the potential reification of identity and the pressure on others to conform. These are inevitable risks that need to be carefully noted and addressed; they do not, in themselves, undermine identity-based political activity, but call for care and maturity in conducting such activity.

In the foregoing account of identity there is frequent mention of the *demand* for recognition (indeed, the title of the book features the same). We have made some progress toward understanding the nature of the gaps in social validation under which such a demand can become possible: individuals who are unable to find their self-understanding reflected in the social categories with which they identify and who are demanding social change to address this; what motivates people to seek this kind of social change—what motivates them to struggle for recognition?

4.3 **The struggle for recognition**

4.3.1 **The motivation for recognition**

There are, at least, four possible sources of motivation for recognition. One of these sources has already been identified in the discussion of Hegel's teleology (section 3.5.1). In accordance with this, the struggle for more equal and mutual forms of recognitive relations is driven forward by the telos of human nature which is the actualization of freedom: if *that* is the ultimate goal, then the dialectical development of consciousness' understanding of itself will lead to an awareness of mutual dependency as a condition of freedom. But this account has been considered and rejected on the grounds that positing an ultimate, rational telos for human beings that tends toward realization is a problematic assumption, with connotations to the kind of metaphysical theorizing that Kant's critical philosophy had put to rest. The metaphysical source of the motivation for recognition must be rejected.

Another possible source is empirical and has to do with the psychological nature of human beings. In the *Struggle for Recognition*, Axel Honneth (1996) provides such an account through the empirical social psychology of G. H. Mead. According to Mead (1967) the self develops out of the interaction of two perspectives: the "me" which is the internalized perspective of the social norms of the generalized other, and the "I" which is a response to the "me" and the source of individual creativity and rebellion against social norms. It is the movement of the "I"—the impulse to individuation— that shows up the limitations of social norms and motivates the expansion of relations of recognition (see Honneth 1996, pp. 75–85).

In a later work Honneth (2002, p. 502) rejects his earlier account; he begins by noting: "there has always seemed to me to be something particularly attractive about the idea of an ongoing struggle for recognition, though I did not quite see how it could still be justified today without the idealistic presupposition of a forward-driven process of Spirit's complete realization." Honneth thus rejects the teleological account that we, also, found wanting. He then goes on to render problematic his earlier proposal to ground the motivation for recognition in Mead's social psychology:

> I have come to doubt whether [Mead's] views can actually be understood as contributions to a theory of recognition: in essence, what Mead calls "recognition" reduces to the act of reciprocal perspective taking, without the character of the other's action being of any crucial significance; the psychological mechanism by which shared meanings and norms emerge seems to Mead generally to develop independently of the reactive behaviour of the two participants, so that it also becomes impossible to distinguish actions according to their respective normative character. (Honneth 2002, p. 502)

In other words, what Mead describes is a general process that is always occurring behind people's backs in so far as it is a basic feature of the human life form. His theory explains how shared norms emerge and why they expand but deprives agents' behaviors toward each other of normative significance. They become unwitting subjects of this process rather than agents *struggling* for recognition. To struggle for recognition is to perceive oneself to be denied a status one is worthy of, and not to mechanically act out one's innate nature. And this remains the case even if our treatment by others engenders feelings of humiliation and disrespect. To experience humiliation is to already consider oneself deserving of a certain kind of treatment, of a normative status that is denied. Such feelings, therefore, cannot themselves constitute the motivation for recognition, rather they are symptoms of the prior existence of a conviction that one must be treated in a better way.

If the motivation for recognition cannot be accounted for metaphysically (by the teleology of social existence), or empirically (by the facts of one's psychological nature), or emotionally (by the powerful feelings that signal the need for social change), then it must somehow be explained with reference to the ideas that together make up the theory of recognition. These ideas include specific understandings of individuality, self-realization, freedom, authenticity, social dependence, the need for social confirmation, in addition to notions of dignity, esteem, and distinction, among others. To be motivated to struggle for recognition is to already be shaped by a historical tradition where such notions have become part of how we relate to ourselves and others, and the normative expectations that structure such relations; as McBride (2013, p. 137) observes, "we are the inheritors of a long and complex history of ethical, religious, philosophical, and, more recently, social scientific thought about the stuff of recognition: pride, honour, dignity, respect, status, distinction, prestige." It is partly that we are within the space of these notions that we can see, as pointed out in section 3.5.2, that living a life of delusion and disregard for what others think, or a life of total absorption in social norms, is not to live a worthwhile life, for we would be giving up altogether either on social confirmation or on our individuality. We are motivated by these notions in so far as we are already constituted socially so as to be moved by them.

Putting the issue this way may raise concerns. By grounding the motivation for recognition in the subject's prior socialization, it becomes harder to establish whether that motivation is, ultimately, a means for the individual to broaden his or her social freedom, or a means for reproducing existing relations of domination. As McNay (2008, p. 10) says, "the desire for recognition might be far from a spontaneous and innate phenomenon but the effect of a certain ideological manipulation of individuals" (see also Markell 2003; McBride 2013, pp. 37–40). Honneth (2012, p. 77) provides several examples where recognition may be seen as contributing to the domination of individuals:

> The pride that "Uncle Tom" feels as a reaction to the constant praises of his submissive virtues makes him into a compliant servant in a slave-owning society. The emotional appeals to the "good" mother and housewife made by churches, parliaments or the mass media over the centuries caused women to remain trapped within a self-image that most effectively accommodated gender-specific division of labour.

Instead of constituting moral progress (in the sense of an expansion of individual freedom), recognition becomes a mechanism by which people endorse the very identities that limit their freedom. They seek recognition for these identities and in this way "voluntarily take on tasks or duties that serve society" (Honneth 2012, p. 75). There is a need, therefore, to see if we can distinguish ideological forms of recognition from those relations of recognition in which genuine moral progress can be said to have occurred, since what we are after are relations of the latter sort.

4.3.2 The problem of ideology

I first consider, and exclude, some ways in which the problem of ideology *cannot* be solved. It may seem attractive to find a solution by appeal to a Kantian notion of rational autonomy, where the subject withdraws from social life in order to know what it ought to do. If such withdrawal were possible, we would have had an instance of genuine recognition in the sense that an autonomous choice had been made. But as argued in section 3.2, withdrawing to pure reason can only produce the form that moral principles must take, without those principles thereby possessing sufficient content that can guide action. Moral principles acquire content, and hence can be action guiding, through the very social practices that Kant urged us to withdraw from in order to exercise our rational autonomy. Somehow then, the distinction between ideological and genuine recognition, if it can be made at all, will have to be drawn from within those social practices, as an appeal to a noumenal realm of freedom where we can rationally will what we ought to do cannot work. This is further complicated by the fact that both genuine and ideological recognition—being forms of *recognition*—must meet the approval of the subject in the sense that both must make the subject feel valued and be considered as positive developments conducive to individual growth. Hence, the *experience* of the subject cannot help us here either. Ideological recognition then consists in practices that are "intrinsically positive and affirmative" yet "bear the negative features of an act of willing subjection, even though these practices appear *prima facie* to lack all such discriminatory features" (Honneth 2012, p. 78). How can these acts of recognition be identified?

The key seems to lie in the notion of "willing subjection" and the possibility of identifying this *despite* subjects' pronouncements of their well-being. The judgment that particular practices of recognition are ideological in the sense that they constitute acts of willing subjection must therefore be made by an external observer. The observer needs to perceive subjection, while at the same time explaining away the person's acceptance of the situation as an indication that he has internalized his oppression in such a way that he willing subjects himself. The case of the "good mother" is a case in point; by voluntarily endorsing that role, she remains uncompensated for her work and many other opportunities in life would be foreclosed to her. Now the observer, in this kind of theoretical narrative, is no longer concerned with the quality of interpersonal relations or the subject's experience of freedom and well-being. What is at issue here seems to be that the observer *disagrees* with the values and beliefs that structure those relations, rather than the quality of those relations being relations of mutual recognition. A contemporary example can further clarify.

Consider the claim, often heard in certain public discourse, that Muslim women who cover their hair—who wear a *hijab*—are "oppressed." Frequently, the claims made do not require that the women in question report any oppression, and hence concepts such as "internalized oppression" are invoked to explain the lack of a negative experience. Of course, some women are coerced into wearing the *hijab*, and given the right context they would remove it and see it as an unnecessary imposition on them. For others the *hijab* is about modesty and has religious connotations. For them, it is not a symbol of their oppression and may even be regarded as a feature that can generate positive recognition as a pious and religiously observant person. An observer who claims that the desire for recognition in such cases is ideological—that women who cover their hair are willingly (and subconsciously) subjecting themselves to existing norms—is making a statement about his or her views on the cultural context: the problem the observer has is with the religious weight placed on clothing, or the fact that it is mainly women who have to observe such practices. Some women who wear a *hijab* reject this account since it bypasses their own understanding of what they are doing and the value they attach to it (in fact such an account can itself end up being a form of misrecognition). Not surprisingly, the exact claim is made in reverse by some Muslim women who argue that "Western" women who dress "immodestly" are oppressed by a dominant, male culture that subtly forces them to show their bodies. Those who believe that dressing in this way is an expression of freedom and secularism have simply internalized the values by which they willingly subject themselves to existing norms.

The point of presenting this case from both sides is to show that once we bypass people's accounts of what they are doing, and put aside their reported experience of freedom and well-being, we can see that what is going on is an ideological conflict between two worldviews. This conflict can itself be described within the framework of misrecognition as a continued devaluing of agent's identities under the cover of an interest in their well-being. Of course, people are not always right about what they are doing, and our psychological depth is such that we can deceive ourselves and accept an abusive situation, even more not be able to see that it is abusive. We may convince ourselves that a particular role is exactly right for us, whereas others can see that it is obviously limiting our lives. But psychological depth and the possibility of self-deception go both ways; if that person over there is not transparent to himself then neither am I, even if transparency admits of degrees. Hence, if we are going to argue that a person is willingly subjecting herself, we also need to account for our motivations in making such an argument and what we are, in a sense, getting out of it in terms of validating our worldview, our take on what matters.

This perspective on the idea of "willing subjection" should not be interpreted as a call for inaction; what it is, is a call for *personalizing* and *contextualizing* our moral and political responses and analyses of the lives of others. This means that if we are inclined to persuade individuals to change their understanding of their situation, then we cannot simply bypass their experience of well-being and their specific circumstances. In other words, sweeping judgments that take the form "group x is oppressed" are not helpful; clearly there are all sorts of possibilities and the only way to sort these out is to be aware of this complexity, without losing sight of "structural" discrimination in a particular community. With this in mind we will find that the spectrum of oppression includes the following: some in group x are oppressed and are already fighting to change that; some do not consider themselves oppressed but change their take on the situation once they are presented with a different analysis of it; some do not consider themselves oppressed—despite clear evidence to the contrary—yet no amount of persuasion can get them to see this; some consider your interest in their freedom as an attempt to oppress them; others consider themselves perfectly free and empowered.

Returning to our original question—the distinction between ideological and genuine forms of recognition—it appeared, to begin with, that the idea of "willing subjection" held the key to that distinction. However, on having a closer look at this idea it emerged that what it communicates is a conflict of worldviews rather than a view on the quality of interpersonal relations as relations of recognition. As argued earlier, whether "ideological" or "genuine," if the relations in question are to be relations of recognition, then the individuals concerned must feel valued for who they are and be able to see existing relations as contributing to their personal growth and fulfillment. In this sense the distinction between ideological and genuine recognition cannot be drawn using the notion of "willing subjection." What this notion brings to light are the very real, and very deep, disagreements in beliefs, values, social roles, and life goals that exist across contexts and ideologies. And while it certainly is of importance to debate and negotiate these differences, in order for such disagreements not to end up themselves generating conditions for misrecognition, it is necessary not to lose sight of the individuals involved, including their take on what they are doing and their experience of freedom and well-being.

4.4 **Psychological consequences of recognition**

The reconstruction of the Hegelian concept of recognition in Chapter 3 demonstrated that Hegel was not after some basic fact of human psychology, rather, he was developing a conception of freedom for which recognition is a necessary condition. To be a free agent is to have my self-conceptions, beliefs, and reasons for action recognized as valid, and for this recognition to issue from those whom I consider capable of offering it. It is for what I take to be authoritative (my subjective certainties) to be really authoritative not just for me but in general (and in this way to attain an objective validity) (Pinkard 1994, pp. 52–4).[11] As Pippin (2008b, p. 62) writes, this argument "is not based on a claim about human need, or derived from evidence in developmental

----

[11] See sections 3.3.2, 3.3.3, and 3.4.2 for further elucidation of this point, and for an understanding

or social psychology. It involves a distinctly philosophical claim, a shift in our under-standing of individuality." Indeed, in section 3.5.2, I made a point of distinguishing this claim—and its normative content and implications—from empirical consider-ations pertaining to how people actually form identities. On the one hand, we have recognition as a normative status involving affirmation of an individual's success as an agent; on the other hand, we have the empirical conditions under which a person is able to attain this normative status. Even though these two determinations have to be distinguished from each other, they do interact: to the extent that a person is related to as a successful agent, we can expect his identity to develop in a positive direction; and to the extent that his identity develops in a positive direction, we can expect that he is more likely to be related to as a successful agent. This is to be expected of course; we are psychological beings, and the attitudes that we are subject to are bound to impact on how we regard ourselves. Important strands in the literature on recognition develop this latter point and ask: What are the psychological consequences of recognition? By far, Axel Honneth has done the most to advance an answer to this question, and this section focuses primarily on his work. I begin by outlining Honneth's argument for the connection between recognition and self-relations, followed by an account of the forms of recognition that correspond to these self-relations, and concluding with a discussion of some problems and implications of Honneth's account.

4.4.1 **Recognition and self-relations**

In the introduction to Axel Honneth's landmark study, *The Struggle for Recognition* (1996), the translator Joel Anderson summarizes the approach as follows:[12]

> The possibility for sensing, interpreting, and realizing one's needs and desires as a fully autonomous and individuated person—in short, the very possibility of identity-formation—depends crucially on the development of self-confidence, self-respect, and self-esteem. These three modes of relating practically to oneself can only be acquired and maintained intersubjectively, through being granted recognition by others whom one also recognises. As a result, the conditions for self-realisation turn out to be dependent on the establishment of relationships of mutual recognition. (Honneth 1996, p. xi)

What is the nature of the connection between recognition and the development of positive self-relations? Honneth and Anderson describe this connection in particularly strong terms: positive self-relations *can only* be acquired through mutual recognition. Elsewhere, Ikaheimo (2009, p. 32), in a commentary on Honneth, writes that it would be "very difficult, if not impossible" for positive attitudes toward oneself to arise without "the experience of being an object of [corresponding] attitudes of recognition."

These strong formulations of the connection between recognition and the develop-ment of positive self-relations need to be weakened. What we are talking about here are the *empirical* conditions under which a person can develop a positive identity, and being empirical in nature they cannot be described as necessary. To be sure, if a

---

of the specific meaning of the terms "certainty" and "truth," "subjective" and "objective."

[12] Axel Honneth described his theory of recognition in several works, most notably *The Struggle for Recognition* (1996) and *Redistribution or Recognition* (Fraser and Honneth 2003).

person is consistently met in every wake of life with negative attitudes toward his or her attributes or achievements—such as with certain instances of racism—then that person may struggle to develop a positive identity since he or she would not have received the encouragement and endorsement required to constitute and maintain the positive self-relation in question. But we can't account for the potential of the human mind in this way: in section 3.5.2 I described the hypothetical case of Nadia who believes she is Queen Nefertiti and carries the self-esteem coterminous with her assumed status, and this despite receiving no recognition whatsoever for what is a false identity. Similarly, an inspired individual may persist in absolute conviction of her identities and beliefs, and only later is able to convince people of her point of view. It would be more accurate, then, to state that many of us need feedback in order to develop positive attitudes toward ourselves, and to have sufficient confidence and esteem in our attributes and abilities. The absence of such feedback can impair this, and in this sense can constitute a psychological harm (a point I return to shortly). With these caveats in mind we can return to Honneth's account of recognition and self-relations.

The core of Honneth's account is the following thesis: in order for identity to develop properly, the subject needs to engage in processes of mutual recognition that provide for the possibility of acquiring self-confidence, self-respect, and self-esteem. What are the forms of recognition that correspond to these modes of relating to oneself?

4.4.2 **Forms of recognition**

In his widely cited essay *The Politics of Recognition*, Taylor (1994a) distinguishes three forms of recognition identifiable in modern society. The first exists in the "intimate sphere" where our identity and sense of self are forged in "dialogue and struggle with significant others" (1994a, p. 37). Here, recognition, or its absence, can have crucial and lasting impact on the development of identity. The second and the third forms of recognition exist in the "public sphere" under the rubric of the "politics of equal recognition." These manifest as a politics of universalism and a politics of difference. The politics of universalism is familiar to us as an emphasis on the equal dignity of all citizens, and their entitlement to respect by virtue of having the universal human potential for rational agency. As Taylor (1994a, p. 41) points out, it is "this potential, rather than anything a person may have made of it [which] ensures that each person deserves respect." By contrast, the politics of difference demands recognition of precisely that which the politics of universalism insists on eliding: the uniqueness and distinctiveness of identities and "cultures." This three-part division of forms of recognition is also found in the work of Honneth. Roughly corresponding to Taylor's distinction, Honneth (1996, p. 129) identifies *love* in primary relationships, *rights* in civil society, and *solidarity* in communities of value as three forms of recognition relating, respectively, to our needs and emotions, our moral agency, and our traits and abilities.

The recurring tripartite distinction among forms of recognition has led some commentators to suggest that there is something systematic and formal underlying it. The idea is that each form of recognition corresponds to one of three logically available ways in which a human subject can be related to, viz. as a person (universality), as a certain kind of person (particularity), and as a certain person (singularity) (Ikaheimo

2002, pp. 450–2; also Laitinen 2002, pp. 470–3). To relate to someone *as a person* is to recognize in her a universal capacity to which both her particular features and her singular, unique nature are irrelevant. To relate to someone *as a particular kind of person* is to recognize in her specific features which she instantiates, but which she may also share with others, for example being of a specific identity or profession. To relate to someone *as a certain person* is to respond to her as a unique and irreplaceable individual, as we do in love and friendship. These three possible categories of relating correspond to Taylor's and Honneth's three forms of recognition, respectively: *universality* (politics of universalism/rights in civil society); *particularity* (politics of difference/ solidarity in communities of value); *singularity* (the intimate sphere/ love in primary relationships).

While this is a helpful way of grounding forms of recognition, Taylor and Honneth remind us that the dimensions of personhood in question, and the forms of recognition that correspond to them, are not ahistorical, socio-ontological givens but historical developments (Taylor 1994a; Honneth 2002, pp. 511–12). For example, the politics of difference is made possible by a modern understanding of identity. And, to anticipate what follows, legal rights in premodern times were not conceived of universalistically and were tied to social esteem. Nor is there a reason to suppose that our current conception of the dimensions of personhood and their significance will not change with the perpetual "cultural transformations of our lifeworld" (Honneth 2002, p. 512).[13] The three forms of recognition are historical achievements rather than derivations from the three logically available ways in which a person can be related to.

Honneth's innovation, which he partially supports with empirical evidence from social psychology and psychoanalytic theory, is to map the three forms of relations of recognition onto the three modes of relating to oneself (self-relations)—the former being conditions for the latter. When these forms of recognitive relations are withdrawn, the development of one's identity may be undermined. In Honneth's account (detailed in what follows), self-confidence develops and is maintained through relationships of *love* and friendship that recognize the individual's needs and emotions; self-respect arises out of legal relations that guarantee equal *rights* and recognize the status of each individual as a responsible agent (motivating a politics of equality); and self-esteem arises out of *solidarity* in communities of value by which are recognized the unique traits and abilities of the individual and his or her particular contribution to society (motivating a politics of difference).

Love: Love is a form of reciprocal recognition where two people mutually acknowledge the other's unique individuality while recognizing their dependence on each other for the satisfaction of their desires and needs (see Honneth 1996, pp. 95–107). Honneth (1996, p. 96) follows Hegel in seeing love as "being oneself in another,"

---

[13] It was Hegel in his early Jena lectures who first explicitly differentiated love, rights, and social esteem as progressively complex forms of recognition that reflected the ethical progress of society (Hegel 1983; this point is repeatedly noted by Honneth 1996, 1997, 2001b). It was also Hegel who, in his later work the *Philosophy of Right* (1991), proposed the family, civil society, and the state as the respective spheres of action in which these forms of recognition can be realized.

which is to be understood as referring to the capacity to balance independence and attachment. This is something we first learn in our primary relationship with a caregiver and continues in adult intimate relationships and friendships. In these relationships, there is affirmation of the emotional and physical needs of the individual in a manner that does not prioritize considerations of utility or value.[14] Basic self-confidence is the self-relation acquired through this form of recognition: if one is secure through the love of others in the knowledge that care and concern will be forthcoming unconditionally, then one can develop the self-confidence required to "engage with one's deepest feelings both openly and critically" (Anderson and Honneth 2005, pp. 133–5). A person who is able to do that, is also able to articulate with confidence what his wants and desires are, and hence is able to relate to himself, in more complex ways, as a respected person in society (Anderson and Honneth 2005). In this sense, basic self-confidence is a "psychological precondition" for the development of the other two relations to self (Honneth 1996, p. 107).

Rights: Whereas self-confidence arises from relationships of love and friendship, self-respect arises from legal relations by which the individual is recognized as a bearer of rights. How does this relation-to-self come about? In order to understand oneself as a bearer of rights, the individual must internalize the perspective of the "generalized other" and hence understand that others too are bearers of rights whose claims, like one's own, are to be met (Honneth 1996, p. 108). By recognizing that I have obligations toward others, and by being recognized in turn as a bearer of rights, legal relations become a form of reciprocal recognition. But such a general conception does not fully capture what it is about the person that legal relations recognize. For instance, in a tradition-bound society, as Honneth (1996, p. 109) points out, this conception is consistent with a legal order in which rights and obligations are asymmetrically ascribed, say on the basis of social status. But with the modern social order, what is recognized in the person is not his or her social status but a universal capacity as a free, rational agent (1996, p. 120). This transition required that legal relations are conceived of independently of social esteem; that the hierarchical arrangement of individuals on the basis of their social location—an arrangement by which rights and obligations are distributed—is replaced with "universal respect for the 'freedom of the will of the person'" (1996, p. 112). To the extent that this recognition is forthcoming, the person is increasingly able to relate to him- or herself with respect, since in deserving the respect of everyone else as evident in being recognized as a legal person, one is able to respect oneself (1996, pp. 118–19). Conversely, denial of rights and exclusion can undermine "the opportunity for individual self-respect," and has been a primary motivation for resistance and protest movements over the past sixty years (1996, pp. 120–1).

---

[14] The conception of love as a human relation that should not be governed by utility has a historical basis; Honneth (2002, p. 511) writes that "love was not uncoupled from expectations of utility until the modern period" (see also Fraser and Honneth 2003, p. 139). This point, however, may apply to adult relationships and not to parent–infant relationships, as the latter are likely to have always been ideally driven by unconditional interest in the well-being of the infant.

Solidarity: The last form of recognition to be discussed is not concerned with one's status as a universal moral agent—which legal relations respond to—but with a person's concrete traits and abilities (Honneth 1996, p. 121, 125). In order to be able to relate positively to one's traits and abilities, and hence to develop a sense of self-esteem, it is likely that one requires confirmation from others of their value. Just as the ability to understand oneself as a bearer of rights requires that one internalizes the normative expectations of the generalized other, in order to experience the value of one's way of life:

> every individual must learn to generalise the value-convictions of all of his or her interaction partners sufficiently to get an abstract idea of the collective goals of the community. For it is only within the horizon of these commonly shared values that one can conceive oneself as a person who is distinguished from all others in virtue of a contribution to society's life-process that is recognised as unique. (Honneth 1996, p. 87)

Such a perspective on esteem has become possible over the course of historical developments akin to those that made possible modern conceptions of legal relations. In traditional societies, self-esteem—then understood as "honor"—was something a person acquired by realizing the moral and practical expectations internal to the social group to which he belonged. But social groups themselves, based on, say, class or caste or vocation, were ordered on a scale of value arising "from the socially determined degree of their collective contribution to the realisation of societal goals" (Honneth 1996, p. 123). Hence, what is being recognized is not "a biographically situated subject" but the relative value of a specific group. In earlier societies, recognition could not yet arise as a problem as it was "built into the socially derived identity from the very fact that it was based on social categories everyone took for granted" (Taylor 1991, p. 48).

By contrast to traditional relations of recognition, modern relations aspire to recognize individuals *qua* individuals and, as far as possible, on a symmetrical basis. For this to be possible, the basis of the value-hierarchies by which social groups were ordered had to be questioned as they lost their religious and metaphysical grounding and became less convincing (Honneth 1996, p. 124). Further, the target of recognition had to change from a social group to an individual with a unique life-history and identity. A value came to be placed on self-realization, and identity came to be seen as something whose development can proceed well or badly (as discussed in section 4.2). In order for relations of recognition to respond to the diversity of individual ways of life, the intersubjectively shared horizon of social values and goals must be sufficiently broad and pluralized. Further, it must be sufficiently horizontal, as opposed to hierarchical, in order to allow for *symmetrical* relations of recognition. Of course, these requirements are often lacking, and individuals are frequently unable to interpret their traits and contributions as valuable. From this we can reflect back on the many struggles for recognition prevalent today as attempting, in one way or another, to transform the intersubjective horizon of social beliefs and values—society's "cultural self-understanding"—and make it more accommodating and symmetrical.

To illustrate the different forms of recognition in relation to activism, consider mental health activism and the many initiatives that can be identified (Chapter 1): some reform-minded activists do not reject the medical model or psychiatric concepts and campaign for equal rights and against coercive treatment. They are, therefore, primarily concerned with the second form of recognition: rights and self-respect. Mad activism—while also concerned with rights in this sense—takes on a broader challenge that aims at transforming the total symbolic and cultural space within which madness is apprehended. Such activism seeks to redefine society's cultural understanding of the meaning and value of madness. In this sense, Mad activism is primarily concerned with the third form of recognition: solidarity and self-esteem. What about the first form of recognition, love and self-confidence?

Recall that Honneth regards self-confidence as a prerequisite for self-respect and self-esteem. Let us assume, for the sake of argument, that that is the case. If so, then individuals who have not had the chance to develop basic self-confidence would struggle with accessing more developed self-relations. In such cases, the argument can continue, it would be premature to engage in the kind of social and political action that aims at repairing social relations in a way that would provide individuals with the possibility of acquiring self-respect and self-esteem, since the obstacle lies at a more basic level, viz. self-confidence. Indeed, it is frequently pointed out that some individuals diagnosed with a serious mental health condition as adults may not have experienced positive and sustaining care-giving relationships in their formative years. The development of identity, in their case, may be impaired at a more basic level than can be addressed through social and political action. This suggests that what they need is support and therapy to author an identity, and not (not yet) social and political recognition. This is an important argument and one that I examine in considerable detail in Chapters 7 to 9 where the viability of the notion of Mad identity as a route to recognition is assessed.

4.4.3 Problems and implications of Axel Honneth's account

Honneth's account seeks some empirical support in social psychology and psychoanalytic theory but falls short of being an empirical theory. While it derives some ideas from the empirical literature, it relies heavily on the necessity of mediation for the possibility of self-relation: my relation to myself must be mediated via my relation to an other in order for it to be more than a tautology (see section 3.3.2). The latter claim is not an *empirical* theory about the formation of self-relations, but a *normative* standard by which we can judge the *right* kind of self-relations. Hence, it is not a claim that Honneth can help himself to in constructing his empirical account, and he requires more empirical evidence in order for it be compelling. That is why I had to refer to his claims about the importance of recognition for the development of positive self-relations as a matter of likelihood and nothing stronger than that. In this weaker sense, we can provisionally accept his account while noting its limitations.

Another problem is the paradox of misrecognition, for example, of a subject who has been unable to develop self-confidence, self-respect, and self-esteem, yet is able to find the resources to struggle for recognition: From where could he derive these resources? If I have no confidence in my reasons for action, and if I am unable to command respect from others, and if I can see no value in my traits and abilities, it is unlikely that I can engage in political action whose main aim is to reverse people's views about me in these dimensions. To address this point, we need to return to the account of the motivation for recognition presented in section 4.3.1. I argued that we demand recognition in so far as we perceive ourselves to be denied a normative status we are worthy of. This perception arises from our exposure to the ideas and the moral concepts that make up the modern discourse of recognition. Our emotional experiences of disrespect, I argued, do not in themselves constitute the motivation for recognition; rather they indicate the prior conviction that one must receive better treatment from others (cf. Honneth 2007). In the absence of this conviction, a person's response to his treatment by others might manifest in the experience of shame for *who he is*. The key point then becomes, how can this person transition from drowning in a sense of shame to demanding that you accept him for who he is? A possible answer is that he needs to reinterpret his situation in terms of the discourse of recognition or, more broadly, the discourse of civil rights. Achieving this kind of transition is a fundamental aspect of grass-roots activism; we have already encountered it in Chapter 1 in the concept of "consciousness-raising," which is a group activity where individuals share experiences and reinterpret their situation in terms of ideas such as misrecognition, systematic oppression, and others (see section 1.2.4). An outcome of this process is that individuals may be able to regain some confidence in their abilities, to shed a previously ingrained sense of inability, and to demand social change. Returning to the paradox of misrecognition with which we started, we can now see the importance of the group for generating sufficient confidence, self-respect, and self-esteem in its members such that they can demand change from the wider society.

Finally, there is an important normative implication to Honneth's account. Implicit in his account is the idea that being loved, being respected, and being esteemed are desirable states. We can argue that any reasonable conception of psychological health must include an adequate realization of these three states. If so, then recognition plays a key role in our psychological health as one key empirical condition. From there it is only a short step to its converse: misrecognition can impair our psychological health. Given that the latter is a desirable state for the individual, and the former a threat to its realization at the level of social relations, we can see one way in which this can pan out: Honneth (e.g., 1996) describes the situations where social relations result in psychological harms of this kind as social pathologies that we ought, in some way, to socially or politically address. This issue is examined in Chapter 5.

4.5 **Conclusion**

This chapter continued the overall aim of Part II which is to construct a theory and politics of identity and recognition that can enable us to respond to Mad activism's demand for recognition. Informed by the conclusions of Chapter 3, the focus in this chapter had been on the nature of identity, the motivation for recognition, and the psychological consequences of recognition.

Section 4.2 developed the notion of identity and made the following key points: identity is a person's self-understanding expressed in terms of the beliefs and values that orientate a person in making choices and, more broadly, in deciding what would be a worthwhile life to pursue. Social categories play a key role in constituting this self-understanding. Modern ideals emphasize the individual nature of identity, and the importance of deciding for oneself the extent to which—and the way in which—certain social categories figure in a person's understanding of him- or herself. Identity is contested, and the social categories that constitute its sources are subject to constant challenges, attempts at redefinition, and struggles for recognition. The motivation for these struggles cannot be accounted for teleologically (as a forward-driven resolution of the tension between an agent's certainty of what it is and the social truth of that certainty), or by our psychological nature: we demand recognition in so far as we perceive ourselves to be denied a normative status we are worthy of. And we perceive ourselves in this way owing to our prior exposure to the historical and contemporary ideas and concepts that make up the discourse of recognition (section 4.3).

Section 4.4 explored the psychological consequences of (mis)recognition through the work of Axel Honneth. There are four main points to take with us to the next chapter. First, recognition as a normative status (as affirmation of agential success) must be distinguished from the empirical (psychological) consequences of being related to as a successful agent. Second, these consequences include the development of positive self-relations in the dimensions of confidence, respect, and esteem. Third, misrecognition can result in impaired identity development and hence in psychological harms. Fourth, it is a possibility that this harm is one that we ought to correct through social and political action.

Given the theoretical account of identity and recognition developed over Chapters 3 and 4, the following chapter offers a framework for thinking about, justifying, and responding to demands for recognition.

Chapter 5

Misrecognition: Political reform or reconciliation?

5.1 **Introduction**

In contemporary society it is common to encounter various groups claiming that features central to their identity are portrayed in demeaning and disrespectful ways. These portrayals, it is argued, are harmful to the well-being of the individuals involved. Claims of misrecognition are usually accompanied by demands for cultural transformations in society in order to address the problem. Drawing on Chapters 3 and 4, this chapter seeks an outline of an approach that would enable us to justify and address these demands.

In Chapter 3, the reconstruction of the concept of recognition in light of the problem of freedom led us to a distinctive view of freedom: to be a free agent is to have my self-conceptions, beliefs, and reasons for action recognized as valid, and for this recognition to issue from those whom I consider capable of offering it; that is, whom I recognize, in turn, as free agents. It is for the person that I take myself to be and for what I take myself to be doing (my subjective certainties) to correspond to how people take me to be and what they consider me to be doing. In the terms argued in Chapter 3, the concept of recognition completes the conditions under which an autonomous subject can become a free subject. In the absence of recognition, my attempts at self-determination are provisional, unrealized or, in the worst case, delusional. In so far as we accept the arguments underpinning this view, mutual recognition is a philosophical concept that implies how we ought to think about freedom and social relations (see section 3.5). Beyond this implicit normativity, it is not clear what role the concept can actually have in social and political life; as Ludwig Siep (2011, p. 136) asked, "what is the importance of the concept of recognition for contemporary ethics, social and political philosophy?".

We can approach this question in two ways: a broad and ambitious attempt to demonstrate how the concept of recognition can be a sufficient (or, at least, a primary) concept in normative political theory; and a more limited and modest attempt to employ the concept of recognition to those cases in which a demand for recognition (a claim of misrecognition) is actually made, as a way of justifying those claims and considering possible responses to them. Demonstrating that the concept of recognition can be a sufficient principle for social and political analysis and action is much more difficult and controversial than it is to show that it can play an important role in justifying and addressing certain social harms.[1] The latter attempt is sufficient for Part II, where the main aim is to develop a resource for responding to claims of misrecognition.

This chapter proceeds as follows: section 5.2 outlines the harms of misrecognition and the way in which they are social harms (i.e., collectively generated). The guiding question is: What follows if a person is consistently related to as an unsuccessful agent? Having identified some possible harms, we can ask whether misrecognition should be addressed through political reforms (bringing in considerations of human flourishing and social justice) or through cultivation of interpersonal reconciliation (bringing in attitudes and practices aimed at mutual acceptance). Sections 5.3 and 5.4 explore these two possibilities, respectively. Finally, section 5.5 concludes with an argument for a dual perspective in which both institutional responses and the attempt to seek interpersonal reconciliation are required for addressing demands for recognition.

5.2 **Misrecognition as a social harm**

The harms of misrecognition are the consequences of being consistently related to as an unsuccessful agent, that is, as a person whose self-conceptions, reasons for action, and beliefs are in some way invalid (invalidity may concern a category error—thinking oneself x where one is y—or it may concern a disagreement on interpretation—thinking of one's attributes positively while others think of them as deficiencies).[2] To say that these harms are *social* harms is to say that they are collectively, rather than individually, generated and maintained. The problem is not of a single individual misrecognizing another (though that is how it can play out in practice), but of social patterns of representation and value that undermines peoples' identities (and which allow interpersonal interactions to play out in practice the way they do). So what are the harms of misrecognition?

To deny people recognition is to deny that they are successful agents in the meaning of successful agency deployed here and in Chapter 3. It is to be disqualified as an authority on yourself and on the world: in the domain of identity, it is to be told that you are wrong about who you think you are. Of course, you might be genuinely wrong about who you think you are, and the claim that you are wrong would be, in that case, justified. But this is to go too far ahead of what we are considering here (see Chapter 7 for the distinction among various sorts of mistakes an agent can make); the

---

[1] For a laudable attempt to construct a comprehensive political theory underpinned by the concept of recognition, see Axel Honneth's arguments in the debate with Nancy Fraser, and Fraser's rebuttals (Fraser and Honneth 2003).

[2] We can conceive of misrecognition per se as a harm irrespective of its consequences. Here, something like Kantian respect for the dignity of human subjects is at play. As I pointed out in Chapter 3, footnote 13, it has been noted that Hegel's account of the paradigm case of misrecognition—the master/slave relation—contains the moral insight that one must always treat others as an end, never as a means. One can certainly draw this insight from that relation, but this would be to put the cart (the dignity of human subjects) before the horse (relations of recognition). Meaning: whether or not subjects have absolute dignity is itself an outcome of relations of recognition, a positive outcome no doubt, but one that cannot be imposed from without.

main point to highlight at this stage is that the denial of recognition—whether justified or not—can amount to a social harm: to disqualification. There are many entry points to social disqualification; the one we are considering here has to do with the implications of not being regarded as an authority on yourself, with the likelihood that you are thereby not regarded as an authority on others or on the world. You can become epistemically marginalized in the sense that your point of view on the world is not heard or, if heard, is not taken seriously. Unable to have significant epistemic input in the world you become socially marginalized, and your ability to become an effective agent diminished. The effects of such disqualification are no more apparent as they are for individuals considered to be mad or mentally ill. As we have seen in Chapter 1, the struggle to have one's voice heard is at the heart of mental health activism, and the social representations of madness as deficit and disorder (with not much to say) are a fundamental obstacle to this.

Aside from social disqualification, the other harm I want to mention here is psychological. In section 4.4 I presented an outline of Axel Honneth's account of the psychological consequences of recognition. According to Honneth, to be related to (recognized) as a successful agent is one key empirical condition in the development of a positive identity. Recognitive relations in the form of *love* in primary relationships, *rights* in civil society, and *solidarity* in communities of value, turn out to facilitate the development of corresponding self-relations characterized by, respectively, self-confidence, self-respect, and self-esteem. To be denied an adequate realization of these forms of recognition is likely to impair the development of a positive identity. Further, this may instate a vicious cycle of misrecognition in which the absence of positive self-relations makes it less likely for the person to be related to as a successful agent, since in lacking self-confidence, self-respect, and self-esteem that person would not be in a position conducive to a meaningful and convincing presentation of his or her identity and beliefs. With a range of caveats in place—including crucially that this is an empirical account for which more empirical support is required (see section 4.4.3)—we can, for the purpose of this argument, accept that misrecognition can result in psychological harms of the kind just described, and that these are social harms in the sense defined earlier.

If we accept that misrecognition can lead to social disqualification and impaired identity, and if we accept that repairing social relations can play a role in addressing these harms, what would be the right kind of response? Are we within the scope of a political institutional response or are we within the scope of cultivating reconciliation in social relationships? Robert Pippin (2008b, p. 76) notes these possibilities when he writes:

> we may have demonstrated the centrality, essentiality even, of forms of mutual recognition for a satisfying human life, but these are largely ethical matters that are not proper subjects for political remedy, that they lead us closer to moral and religious practices than to any program for social reform.

Political remedy is a common way of addressing claims that are judged to be within the scope of social justice. One way to change negative social scripts pertaining to specific identities is to initiate a program of reform, of education for instance, to bring about the necessary change. We are familiar with this in campaigns that discourage—and in some cases criminalize—certain patterns of discrimination. On the other hand, reconciliation seeks a more profound and demanding change in attitudes, yet it is a change that cannot be legally binding in the way political remedies may be. Reconciliation aims at a genuine state of mutual acceptance that does indeed bring to mind, as Pippin phrases it, "moral and religious practices." Which approach is more appropriate, or do we need both? In the following two sections I explore, in turn, political reform and reconciliation, and in section 5.5 I compare the two approaches.

5.3 **Misrecognition and political reform**

If we go down the route of a political response to the harms of misrecognition, then we have to justify the case for political institutions to use incentive or coercion to bring about a change in the social conditions that generate and propagate these harms. Misrecognition would be similar to, say, denial of employment rights to a certain group in so far as both are social problems that require political institutional intervention and possible sanctions to the offending parties. I am doubtful that such a case can be made, not because misrecognition cannot be a serious harm, nor because these harms cannot be understood as social injustices, but because it is not the kind of harm that can be adequately corrected by political responses that involve incentive and coercion. I will get to this point shortly (in section 5.3.3), but first let us see in broad outline what such a case would look like and what problems it would raise.

5.3.1 **The theory of recognition as an ethical conception of the good**

The case for a political response to misrecognition can argue that the harms of misrecognition are impediments to human flourishing, and that denying people the conditions to flourish can amount to a social injustice.[3] Axel Honneth (1996), for example, regards social relations that result in such harms as social pathologies that ought to be addressed. The first point seems plausible enough; it is hard to imagine a life going well where one is not considered an authority on oneself or the world, is unable to be an effective agent in ways that matter, and is unable to adopt positive attitudes toward

-----

[3] True Hegelians would balk at this way of proceeding. They may see it as an inappropriate "analytic" approach to Hegel's dialectical and holistic philosophy. They could argue that to put the issue in this way—that misrecognition can amount to a social injustice—is not yet to have grasped the meaning and the structure of recognition: "I am only truly free when the other is also free and is recognised by me as free" (Hegel 1971, p. 171). The issue, for them, is not a matter of social justice, but of a deep and mutual dependency that is a condition for freedom. If one grasps the meaning and structure of recognition, then one would immediately see that misrecognition is a "social pathology." However, the "true Hegelian" approach is not going to be sufficient for contemporary political reflection, where some sort of independent normative justification is usually required. Even though the concept of recognition is one that ought to inform our thinking about freedom and social relations (as I argued in section 3.5), the political implications of this have to be worked out separately, and running the issue in terms of social justice is one way of doing so.

oneself. Or is it? An immediate worry at this point are the innumerable examples where people have imagined for others how their life must go if it is going to go well, or that it would go better if they would adopt this or that set of values. In other words, is the theory of recognition an ethical conception of the good, a parochial view on how we should live grounded in a certain view of human flourishing? If it is, then it cannot presume to offer a standard with which to judge social relations and prescribe how they ought to be corrected; it cannot, that is, function as an aim for social justice. On the other hand, if it is not—if it does not possess substantive ethical content—then it cannot inform social and political life beyond a very general sort of recommendation; it becomes an indeterminate theory. The theory of recognition, according to these criticisms, is damned if it is a theory of the good life and damned if it is not.

The first point to note in response to these criticisms is this: "a theory of the good life" as opposed to what? A possible answer: as opposed to a perspective that remains neutral with respect to ethical conceptions, busying itself only with providing the conditions under which persons can realize their own idea of the good. This would be a version of procedural liberalism where the aim is to advance a moral and political perspective that withdraws from specific ends in order to establish a neutral ground from where all can receive equal and just treatment.[4] The problems of procedural liberalism have long been debated, most famously in the exchange with the "communitarians."[5] In so far as it is grounded in the Kantian tradition, among the pitfalls of procedural liberalism is that it fails to take account of the conceptions of the good on which moral principles are dependent. We do not need to get into the details of this debate or to critique procedural liberalism at the level of political theory, for we have already addressed it at the conceptual level in section 3.2. Briefly, by contrasting Kant's moral theory with Hegel's ethical life, it emerged that the attempt to provide principles of morality that can be action-guiding presupposes prior social practices and traditions.

----

[4] Liberal political morality is underpinned by the idea that human dignity finds its source in our capacity for self-governance (autonomy). As autonomous agents we have the capacity to determine each for him- and herself a conception of the good, of what is valuable and worth pursuing. This power—and not what is made of it—is to be respected equally in all subjects, hence in order for government to treat its citizens with equal dignity it must remain neutral and not espouse a particular conception of what gives value to life (Dworkin 1978; see also Kymlicka 1991).

[5] Communitarians took issue with several facets of the liberal project. One of the points of contention was the assumed relation between self and community. In its focus on and prioritization of individual autonomy over community, liberalism exaggerated our capacity for choice by relying on an incoherent conception of self. The liberal self appeared to stand outside of society, capable of detaching itself from all commitments, perusing its options and choosing what is valuable. Liberals, according to this criticism, failed to appreciate the ways in which our identities are constituted through the communities and roles in which we are embedded. (For representative readings on the liberalism/communitarianism debate consult, Sandel (1982), MacIntyre (1984), Caney (1992), Taylor (1994b), and Shapiro (2003).) Another way of putting this is to say that procedural liberalism presupposes that participants in the democratic order *already* have a voice (i.e., they already are recognized as successful agents). That, of course, is not always the case, an issue emphasized in the theory of recognition.

Purely formal principles cannot guide action since they are lacking in content, and content can only be acquired from existing practices and other contingencies. We cannot do without ethical life—we cannot withdraw fully from some kind of orientating value or end in moral or political deliberation. The question then becomes whether or not we can put forward a view of ethical life—a conception of the good—that is formal enough to permit multiple concrete realizations, but substantive enough to function as an aim for social justice. In his work on recognition, Axel Honneth tries to provide such a balancing act.

Honneth argues that the theory of recognition offers a *weak* ethical conception of the good that provides a formal view on the general structures of a good life, while leaving room for these structures to be populated with a diversity of concrete conceptions (Honneth 2001b, p. 51; Fraser and Honneth 2003, p. 259). For example, referring to the three patterns of recognition—love, rights, and solidarity—he writes (see section 4.4.2):

> On the one hand, the three patterns of recognition—which now can count as just as many preconditions for successful self-realisation—are defined in a sufficiently abstract, formal manner to avoid raising the suspicion that they embody particular visions of the good life. On the other hand, from the perspective of their content, the explication of these three conditions is detailed enough to say more about the general structures of a successful life than is entailed by general references to individual self-determination. (Honneth 1996, p. 174)

In being "detailed enough," this formal conception of ethical life can function as an aim for social justice which, in this context, would consist in securing the conditions for relations of reciprocal recognition under which "personal identity-formation, hence individual self-realization, can proceed adequately" (Fraser and Honneth 2003, p. 174). Elsewhere, he clarifies:

> The various attitudes that, taken together, make up the moral point of view are introduced with reference to a [teleological] state that is considered desirable because it serves human well-being. Thus in contrast to the Kantian requirement, it is an ethical conception of the good according to which the meaning and scope of what is morally right can be measured. (Honneth 2007, pp. 137–8).

In his defense of the theory of recognition, Honneth treads a thin line between the right and the good, between morality and ethics, between deontological moral principles underpinning justice and an ethical theory underpinning a conception of the good life (Fraser 2001, pp. 22–3). He is driven to do so because he wants the theory to lie midway between the formalism of deontological principles (which found its way to procedural liberalism) and communitarian ethical particularism, while at the same time avoiding the pitfalls of both. Has he succeeded in this balancing act?

5.3.2 Two criticisms

According to Nancy Fraser and Christopher Zurn, Honneth fails at realizing a theory of recognition that has determinate moral content without being sectarian. But whereas for Fraser, Honneth's failure leaves him with a morally vacuous theory, for

Zurn it leaves him with a sectarian theory: two contrasting criticisms; I begin with Fraser's.

Nancy Fraser (2001, 2008, and with Honneth 2003) doubts the ability of the theory of recognition to justify and judge claims for recognition. For a theory of justice to be able to adjudicate it must meet two requirements: it must be nonsectarian while being sufficiently determinate in order to offer a foothold from where to judge such claims. Nonsectarianism is required since societies are composed of multiple value horizons and a theory of justice cannot advance one account of the good over another without thereby losing its normative force vis-a-vis other groups. On the other hand, not all claims for recognition are straightforward and in some cases judgments will have to be made, for example in cases where the recognition of cultural identities would violate gender equality (Fraser and Honneth 2003, p. 223). The challenge is to adjudicate such claims without falling into sectarianism, a double-requirement with which Honneth would agree. Yet, according to Fraser, it is a challenge that the theory of recognition cannot meet.

Fraser's contention is that the theory fails to offer a useful theory of justice because it tries too hard to avoid sectarianism and ends up being empty of determinate moral content. Thus, while the theory highlights the importance of recognition for being an effective agent, it cannot specify the parameters of effective agency; similarly, while it highlights the importance of recognition for developing positive self-relations in the dimensions of self-confidence, self-respect, and self-esteem, it cannot supply content to these categories by specifying what would constitute adequate care, justified respect, and valuable achievement. To do so would be to advance a specific horizon of values and hence to fail to abide by the requirement for nonsectarianism; we would be back with communitarianism and its problems. Yet without supplying such content, maintains Fraser, the theory would fail to adjudicate competing and potentially problematic claims for recognition:

> By grounding his account of justice in a theory of the good life, [Honneth] is forced to take extraordinary steps to avoid capitulating to ethical sectarianism. Constrained to construe his normative principles formally, he must drain them of substantive content—hence, of normative force. In seeking to resist teleology's built-in temptation to sectarianism, he ends up succumbing to indeterminacy. Ironically, then, an ethical starting point designed to overcome empty formalism itself descends into moral vacuity. (Fraser and Honneth 2003, p. 228)

In my view, Fraser's critique overlooks the normative potential of the theory of recognition in adjudicating claims. The theory contains internal tensions that generate constraints by which the validity of claims for recognition can be assessed. In addition to this, the process of adjudication is overseen by the aim of the theory as a whole, which is social justice.[6] Consider the following typical cases. With certain demands

---

[6] Another point of contention between Fraser and Honneth (2003) is the relation between the two dimensions of justice: redistribution and recognition. Fraser argues that even though these two dimensions influence each other, they are not *reducible* to each other. Status subordination (misrecognition) and class subordination (mal-distribution), on her account, interact in a variety of complex ways, and in order to not lose sight of the unique injustices of

for recognition, even though it may be possible to demonstrate that social relations impair agency and identity development, there may be other reasons to withhold recognition. An example that comes to mind are self-identified racist identities. Fraser rightly points out that if identity impairment is the whole story, then some racists may demand recognition by arguing that their self-esteem depends on it (Fraser and Honneth 2003, p. 38).[7] How can the theory respond to such demands? Another example offered by Fraser is when demands for cultural recognition—think of certain religious identities—conflict with gender equality (Fraser and Honneth 2003, p. 223). Again, it is not clear whether such claims are justified. Fraser argues that Hegelian theories of recognition cannot deal with such problems, for if effective agency and psychological health are at stake, any claim to the effect that one is impeded in either would seem justified, irrespective of whether or not such claims are considered racist or misogynist. All of which is to say that there are other intuitions at play aside from the concern with flourishing in this sense. The theory of recognition, however, can cope with these kind of demands.

On the question of the moral evaluation of struggles for recognition, Honneth writes:

> It is obvious that we cannot endorse every political revolt as such—that we cannot consider every demand for recognition as morally legitimate or acceptable. Instead, we generally only judge the objectives of such struggles positively when they point in the direction of social development that we can understand as approximating our ideas of a good or just society. (Fraser and Honneth 2003, pp. 171–2)

A just society, as indicated earlier, is one in which the conditions exist for reciprocal relations of recognition such that individuals can flourish. Reciprocity is precisely that which racist identities fail to maintain, which renders recognition in such cases akin to the master/slave relation discussed in Hegel's *Phenomenology of Spirit*: it is not a relation between equals and, ultimately, the recognition that it affords the master is vacuous and unstable (see section 3.3.3). People who hold racist identities, by the very definition of their worldview, perpetrate on their targets an instance of misrecognition, and hence deny them the same conditions for flourishing that they are claiming for themselves. For this reason, their demand for recognition cannot be justified, irrespective of the positive case that they can make in terms of impaired agency and identity.

What about conflicts between gender equality and demands for recognition of certain religious identities? The key to responding to such conflicts is to recall the

---

each dimension, they must be kept analytically separate. Honneth, by contrast, holds that recognition provides a sufficient framework that can make sense of material as well as cultural injustices. Thus, problems of distributive justice can be understood as problems with the recognition of the achievements of specific groups in society. This debate, though important for social and political theory, exceeds the concerns of this book.

[7] As Fraser (2001, p. 32) writes elsewhere, if self-esteem was the sole consideration, then "racist identities would seem to merit some recognition, as they enable poor Europeans and Euroamericans to maintain their sense of self-worth by contrasting themselves with their supposed inferiors."

different dimensions of recognition described in section 4.4.2. The second dimension of recognition—rights and respect for autonomy of persons—places constraints on the third dimension of recognition—solidarity and self-esteem. The provision of the conditions for self-esteem cannot be at the expense of violating the autonomy of certain subjects. The concept of recognition, after all, is about *reconciling* individual autonomy with the social world and this for *all* subjects, ideally (see section 3.2). By this constraint, the values that play out in the dimension of solidarity and self-esteem "are subject to the normative restrictions set by the legally sanctioned autonomy of all subjects . . . and need to coexist with the two other patterns of recognition, that is, love and rights" (Honneth 1996, p. 178). The price for self-esteem cannot be the recognition of collective values and goals that deny others their chance to participate as equals in social life.

In summary, the theory of recognition possesses normative resources for adjudication: it operates with an ideal that functions as an aim for social justice and against which demands can be assessed, and it contains internal constraints that exclude morally objectionable identities and demands. In Chapter 10 I employ these and other resources in the process of responding to the demand for recognition of Mad identity.

The second criticism of Honneth's approach that I shall consider is by Christopher Zurn. Zurn (2000) objects that the theory of recognition embodies a parochial view of human flourishing and hence cannot function as a universal standard with which to assess social relations. The problem here is not, as Fraser would have it, that the theory is devoid of moral content by virtue of offering a formal and empty conception of the good, but that it offers too much content. Zurn argues that the view of human flourishing advanced by the theory—and which he refers to as self-realization—emerges from an understanding of the good life that arose in "Western" thought (see section 4.2.2). Given this, he questions whether Honneth is able to defend the claim that "uncoerced, full self-realisation can serve as *the* critical yardstick for the social conditions of the good life" (Zurn 2000, p. 119). After considering, and finding unsatisfactory, three possible responses, he concludes by noting that "the question of how such [an ethical ideal] might serve as the normative grounds for a diagnostic social philosophy that could transcend the limits of our own particular social forms remains open" (2000, p. 122).

Zurn is correct in rejecting the sort of defense that tries to secure a universal basis for this ethical ideal by appeal to a philosophical anthropology where the drive to self-realization is the essence of human nature. He is also correct in reminding us of the skeptic's retort: why self-realization and not other conceptions of the good such as "virtuous subservience to communal ends, or righteous obedience to the moral law, or maximization of the pleasure of others"? (2000, p. 121). In order to respond to this objection, we can recall the point, made earlier, that we need an overall view of ethical life in order for moral and political deliberation to have something to aim for. The question then becomes whether the ideal of recognition can fulfill this role, and the answer rests on a key determination: Can the ideal accommodate within it a diversity of conceptions of the good? The reasoning here is that, if we are after an overarching aim for moral and political deliberation, then an ideal that can accommodate as many other ideals as possible is preferable to one that cannot; it will be more inclusive and will bring under its purview the well-being of a larger number of people.

To address this question, we can begin by agreeing with the skeptic that different groups have rather different ideas about what would constitute a fulfilling life. Certain religious traditions consider it most liberating to live in subservience to the common good in accordance with Divine dictates. For others, a key goal is to eschew worldly desires and possessions in order to liberate one's self and connect to a higher realm. What these traditions share is that they are all involved in self-making, in training the self such that it becomes an embodiment of the higher principle aspired to. While each of these ideals regards self-making to be of importance, it advances a specific vision of what this would entail. That vision is a detailed account of the values and beliefs by which a person must live. Accordingly, these ideals cannot accommodate—in fact positively and wholly exclude—other visions of self-making. On the other hand, the ideal of recognition is able to accommodate diverse visions of self-making *in so far as they do not force people to adopt a particular way of life.*

Our skeptic, however, is unlikely to be satisfied with this response. She could note that the qualification in italics in the previous paragraph is precisely the problem that prevents the ideal of recognition from being a critical yardstick for adequate social relations. Why, she might ask, should adopters of a religious ideal assent to the limit placed by the ideal of recognition on the coercive elements of their vision of self-making? At this point it is evident that there is a basic rift in starting assumptions. On the one hand we have religiously grounded assumptions pertaining to the nature of human beings, the relation of individual freedom to Divine and social authority, and the purpose of human activity; on the other hand we have a set of liberal, secular assumptions pertaining to the value of individual autonomy, and the importance of reconciling autonomy with the social world. These two perspectives appear incompatible, even if there are many important scholarly and cultural attempts to reconcile them with each other. That being said, an ideal that forces or coerces people to adopt a particular way of life falls short of the basic understanding of autonomy and freedom that unfolded over the past two chapters and in the modern rational, secular tradition. Within this tradition, the ideal of recognition—by virtue of having sufficient content for adjudication while, at the same time, being able to incorporate diverse visions of self-making (with the aforementioned provisos)—can function as a critical yardstick for assessing social relations.

5.3.3 Social justice and the limits of political reform

Assuming we have established that the harms of misrecognition are impediments to human flourishing, is it the case that denying people the conditions to flourish (in this sense) is a social injustice? Let us recap the consequences of misrecognition (section 5.2): to deny people recognition is to deny that they are successful agents. Such denial can have two possible consequences: the person is unable to become an effective agent (since their point of view is not considered or taken seriously—they are socially disqualified); the development of identity is impaired. Social disqualification owing to epistemic marginalization has been formulated as an injustice—an epistemic injustice—in some recent work.[8] Impaired identity owing to misrecognition can also be formulated as an injustice; social relations by which one can acquire self-respect and self-esteem would be, on this view—and in Rawls' (1973) term—"primary goods" akin to, for example, material resources, education, and freedom of expression (Rawls does, in fact, talk about the "social bases of self-respect").[9] We can engage with those particular views on their own terms and ask whether the harms in question *really* are injustices. However, I will not pursue that path, for there is a more fundamental issue at stake whereby even if these harms were injustices, they cannot be adequately addressed through political reform. The issue has to do with the nature of the problem that led to these harms, viz. misrecognition, and how it can be corrected.

The subject of misrecognition is an agent whose self-conceptions, beliefs, and reasons for action are socially regarded to be invalid (either factually or evaluatively). It follows that correcting for misrecognition (and for the harms that can arise from it) requires that we affirm the validity of the agent's self-conceptions, beliefs, and reasons for action. But such affirmation cannot be offered unconditionally (i.e., prior to actual engagement, adjudication, and evaluation of the claims in question). If it is offered on demand, then that affirmation would be nothing more than a forced lie, a condescending agreement, or a thoughtless nod to the zeitgeist—the latter being, in some circles, that *any* demand for recognition is *ipso facto* a valid demand, a position that, if it were to be applied across the board, would render meaningless the social struggles in question. For a key point of a struggle for recognition is to have one's success as an agent *genuinely* affirmed by others, and this inevitably comes with the risk that not all demands will be regarded as valid (more on this in section 5.5). If that is the case, then coercing or incentivizing people to affirm the validity of other people's identities is not an appropriate solution, for it might produce nothing but the appearance of agreement and none of the intended repair of social relations. So while we can formulate social disqualification owing to epistemic marginalization, and impaired identity owing to misrecognition, as social injustices, correcting for these injustices cannot be achieved by the coercive or incentivizing actions of political institutions. Where political action can be helpful, however, is in creating the right conditions under which people can meet, and in this way encourage what I consider to be a more adequate response to demands for recognition, its adequacy consisting in that it takes into account the nature of recognition: that response is the attempt to achieve *reconciliation*.

5.4 **Misrecognition and reconciliation**

We concluded section 5.2 by noting two kinds of response to demands for recognition, responses aimed at repairing social relations and affirming the status of the other

---

[8] See Fricker (2007) for an account of the concept of "epistemic injustice" that works out the nature and implications of the lack of epistemic authority. See Sanati and Kyratsous (2015) and Dübgen (2012) for applications of the concept to, respectively, the domains of mental health and international relations.

[9] See McBride (2013, Chapter 4) for a discussion of a range of views on recognition, self-relations, and justice.

as a successful agent: political reform and reconciliation. The notion of reconciliation operates in a different thought space to that of political reform. Whereas the latter, as we have seen, operates under considerations of social justice and the actions of incentivizing/coercive institutions, reconciliation brings to mind a certain kind of acceptance of the other that cannot be forced and is not in any direct way a matter of social justice.

5.4.1 The meaning of reconciliation

Reconciliation, as I understand it, requires mutual accommodation between self and other in the life contexts in which they interact. It involves "making one's peace" with a state of affairs; "instead of trying to resist or change the reality, the reconciled person accepts it and tries to integrate it with his own goals and way of life as much as possible" (Disley 2015, p. 13). *Integration* is a key word here, as it implies that the person has been changed in some way and is not merely tolerating the other; integration implies transformation. For example, in a long-standing partnership, integration can be said to have occurred to the extent that the other person's desires and goals now feature in *my* life-plan not as obstacles to be circumvented, but as further factors to be considered alongside my desires and goals in the process of constructing a plan that can then be described as *our* life-plan. For this to be possible, I need to make space for my partner's desires and goals alongside mine, and to accept that their satisfaction is to count as much as the satisfaction of my own. When integration occurs mutually, my individuality is reconciled with my partner's, which in the best cases results in the unity that we call a good partnership.

This structure should be familiar to us from the discussion of the concept of recognition in Chapter 3. The ideal of mutual recognition is a situation in which each partner in the interaction voluntarily restricts her autonomy, thereby recognizing the other's independence. To recognize the other's independence is to recognize her as a successful agent, which is for the identity, beliefs, and reasons for action that she attributes to herself to be affirmed as true (i.e., as corresponding to what she takes them to be). Recognition that is uncoerced, reciprocal, and equal achieves an ideal of unity where each agent's self-conception is mirrored by the other such that it can become its truth, and where both agents take it that this kind of satisfaction in the other depends on the other also receiving it. This is what Hegel (1977, p. 112) means when he refers to the final realization of the process as follows: "They *recognise* themselves as *mutually recognising* one another."

This final ideal is realized in the form of recognition that Hegel refers to as *love*, the exact opposite of which is the first form of recognition (or rather of misrecognition) that he raises, the master/slave relation. As discussed in section 3.3.3, Hegel (1977, p. 113) begins his account of determinate forms of recognition with the master/slave relation, a relation of absolute inequality in that one self is "being only *recognised*, the other only *recognising*." The interpersonal experience of recognition thus begins with an example where mutuality is absent: the master seeks to retain absolute independence and to receive the slave's recognition without having to accord any recognition to the slave, except for the minimal recognition required for the slave to be a being capable of affirming the master's status (i.e., the slave is not an object to be consumed as in "desire", but a being in its own right, albeit a being whose satisfaction does not count). That relation, as Bernstein rightly notes, "is the paradigmatic form of moral injury and misrecognition."[10] The mirror opposite of the master/slave relation—and the conceptual culmination of the process—is a state of reconciliation. It is a relation of equivalence where each partner in the interaction is able to find itself confirmed in the other, and where the other is no longer an alienating presence that needs to be dominated. While Hegel uses the term love (*liebe*) to refer to this state, I will refrain from doing so to avoid the impression that this term is limited to *romantic* love.[11] It is true that Hegel regards the latter to be a perfect example of mutual recognition, but it is just one possible example, the main point being the structure of recognition in question and which was described in the previous paragraph. I will therefore continue to refer to that structure using the term reconciliation, as it is broad enough to encompass close relationships ("love"), partnerships united by shared goals, and communities trying collectively to come to terms with and resolve past and present social harms, violence, and moral injuries.

Reconciliation is both an outcome and an attitude. As an outcome, it is to be actually reconciled with each other in the terms defined in this section; as an attitude, it is to approach others with the implicit acknowledgment that their satisfaction counts, that their ability to find themselves at home in the world matters as much as mine does (in the meaning of *satisfaction* and *finding oneself at home in the world* developed over the past two chapters: to find a place in the social world for one's identity and projects is to be able to enact them and to receive confirmation of their worth). We can therefore distinguish the *intention* of reconciliation as a basic attitude we hold toward others, from the *outcome* of reconciliation as the realization of an ideal. This distinction shows that while we can (and perhaps should) approach others with the intention of reconciliation, we cannot force it as an outcome as that would undermine the kind of change that is required. This change has to be genuine, voluntary, and mutual, a point elaborated on in section 5.5. But first there is an outstanding question.

5.4.2 Why *should* we approach others with an attitude of reconciliation?

At their best, friendships and partnerships embody an unconditional and mutual attitude of reconciliation. This means that each partner in the interaction regards the other as someone whose ability to find satisfaction in the social world matters as much as one's own. An attitude of reconciliation does not mean that people are bound to agree

---

[10] The Bernstein Tapes Project. Online: http://www.bernsteintapes.com/hegellist.html

[11] Hegel (1991, p. 199) saw love in those terms: "Love means in general the consciousness of my unity with another, so that I am not isolated on my own, but gain my self-consciousness only through the renunciation of my independent existence and through knowing myself as the unity of myself with another and of the other with me . . . The first moment in love is that I do not wish to be an independent person in my own right and that, if I were, I would feel deficient and incomplete. The second moment is that I find myself in another person, that I gain recognition in this person, who in turn gains recognition in me."

on everything, only that in their interactions there is a genuine attempt to consider what the other is saying and doing—to make room for the other—even if, ultimately, reconciliation cannot be arrived at in practice. Why *should* we approach our friends with such an attitude? Phrasing the question this way is not entirely appropriate, for we do not ordinarily think of our interactions with our closest friends and partners as dictated by an ought, by a sense of moral obligation; we simply care for the other's satisfaction, we don't need justifications of a moral nature.[12] Richard Rorty (1999, p. 78) makes a similar point when he asks:

> Do I have a moral obligation to my mother? My wife? My children? "Morality" and "obligation" here seem inapposite. For doing what one is obliged to do contrasts with doing what comes naturally, and for most people responding to the needs of family members is the most natural thing in the world.

This recalls the point I made earlier that in contrast to political reform, reconciliation does not evoke the language of moral obligation and social justice: I do not hold an attitude of unconditional concern for my friend's satisfaction because it would be unjust not to do so; I hold it because unconditional concern for him comes naturally out of concern for myself (but not necessarily in an instrumental way). Concern for my own satisfaction is not analyzable into further moral principles; it would be absurd to argue that the reason I should hold such concern toward myself is that I would be committing an injustice against myself not to do so.[13] My close friend, obviously, is not me, but our emotions and self-understandings are intertwined such that mutual concern can arise naturally (i.e., with no need for further justification, whether moral or instrumental). Words like "love" and "friendship" are all shorthand ways of referring to this, to relationships where I am acquainted with another person, and where we see key aspects of ourselves in each other.[14]

As I pointed out in section 5.4.1, reconciliation can encompass close relationships ("love" and "friendship") as well as communities going through social upheaval and violence. Yet so far when discussing the attitude of reconciliation, the discussion centered on close friendships and partnerships. Indeed, this attitude, as presented here, is beyond moral justification precisely because it involves individuals with whom a person's identity and emotions are intertwined. Can such an attitude be extended to strangers, to members of the community, to people a person hears about, might encounter in the street, but is unlikely to ever get to properly meet? Why should I care

---

[12] In fact, if I begin to wonder why I should treat my friend well, and seek justifications for this in the "great tradition of friendship," this may reflect that our relationship is not as close as it used to be.

[13] Whereas it is sometimes argued that I do have an obligation *toward others* to look after myself so that I do not impede their well-being through neglecting myself.

[14] Parent/child relationships may appear different in that they have an unequal sort of dependency at their core. Still, my daughter is a young person whose ability to find herself at home in the world matters to me crucially, even if she needs guidance and material and emotional care so that one day she can independently pursue her satisfaction.

about *their* ability to find themselves at home in the world; is there a moral obligation to do so?

For Rorty (1999, pp. 79–82), the language of moral obligation kicks in when we are no longer able, or willing, to identify with others in such a way that concern for them would come to us naturally. Some of us, out of the conviction that we ought to do what is right, what morality obliges us to do, may have a strong impulse to help others. But obligation—however presented (Kant's moral law or Allah's divine dictates) and however incentivized (pure reason or eternal reward/punishment)—is not going to be sufficient on its own to generate concern for others if we do not see them as like us, or as belonging to our group or tribe or community. In fact, for many people, the "moral law" is not at all relevant for them when it comes to deciding who is going to receive their care, help, and attention. Campaigns seeking to get people to donate money to a cause do not start by reminding us of our obligations under the moral law, or by appealing to our capacity for reason or even to our self-interest; they show us pictures of human suffering and tell us stories about the individuals who are suffering; they try to personalize and humanize those individuals as a way of generating concern for them; they try to show that, in a fundamental way, they are like us. For there is no doubt that for many people, the field of their concern for others is limited; for most, in fact, it stops at the boundary of the immediate family. And yet, as Rorty (1998, p. 177) argues, moral philosophy has always given more attention to the question "why should I be moral"—and hence to the "rare figure of the psychopath"—to the neglect of what is by far more common:

> the person whose treatment of a rather narrow range of featherless bipeds is morally impeccable, but who remains indifferent to the suffering of those outside this range, the ones he thinks of as pseudo-humans.

From this we can understand Rorty's (1999, p. 79) view that "moral development in the individual, and moral progress in the human species as a whole, is a matter of re-marking human selves so as to enlarge the variety of the relationships which constitute those selves." This requires that we "expand the reference of the terms 'our kind of people' and 'people like us'" to include more and more people (Rorty 1998, p. 176). It is for the question "why should we approach others with an attitude of reconciliation" to appear as inappropriate as it did when we asked it of close friends and partners.[15] How can this be achieved with people who are not, and will never be, our friends or partners?

There are many obstacles that prevent us from extending our concern to individuals beyond our close family and friends. To begin, we do not share an emotional bond with them, and this counts for a lot. Further, however we act toward them, it is unlikely that this will have repercussions on our life; we lack the element of self-interest. Not to mention a host of motivational and social-psychological impediments such as apathy,

---

[15] "The ideal limit of this process of enlargement," writes Rorty (1999, p. 79), "is the self envisaged by Christian and Buddhist accounts of sainthood—an ideal self to whom the hunger and suffering of *any* human being . . . is intensely painful." It is telling that we refer to people who attain this almost impossible ideal of universal concern for human life as *saints*.

denial ("this beggar is richer than you and me"), and the bystander effect ("someone else is going to help them"). These difficulties aside, a key factor in our lack of concern toward others is that we might not regard them as like us with respect to fundamental aspects; we dehumanize them. Dehumanizing narratives are rife in our communities and tend to apply to entire groups of people. The central premise of these narratives is that members of this group lack substantial psychological or moral depth, or that they are incapable of suffering in the way that "we" do (see Gaita 2000, pp. 57–72). I am sure many readers have encountered statements such as these: a person explaining to his listener that a particular ethnic group "do not value life as you and I do, that is why they don't care if their children die"; a person asking whether people of a particular race "can also feel so sad so as to be depressed like us"; another offering the view that "homeless people do not feel the cold like us, it's okay for them to sleep rough." In all these cases, there is no concrete knowledge as such of the individuals in question, just an imagined set of conceptions. But if it is about imagination, can't we also imagine the converse: that they, like us, have psychological and moral depth and are capable of suffering? If we begin to imagine that, then, at least, we might begin to adopt an attitude of reconciliation toward them, even if we do nothing else to work toward an outcome of reconciliation. In fact, humanizing others in this minimal sense is the very first step in addressing misrecognition, and is a prerequisite to more substantial engagement with the claims of those demanding recognition (for a similar point, see Ikaheimo 2012, pp. 22–3).

As we know all too well, even this basic step is hard to achieve socially. There are plenty of psychological, social, economic, political, and cultural reasons why this is so. A key observation that goes to the heart of the matter is that most people

> think of themselves as being a certain *good* sort of human being—a sort defined by explicit opposition to a particular bad sort. What is crucial for their sense of who they are is that they are *not* an infidel, *not* a queer, *not* a woman, *not* an untouchable. (Rorty 1998, p. 178)

As long as we continue to contrast "*us*, the *real* humans, with rudimentary or per-verted or deformed examples of humanity" (Rorty 1998, p. 179), and as long as this contrast remains fundamental to how we understand ourselves, the notion of human-izing others is bound to be threatening. Compounding this further is the common observation that economic and political instability make it much less likely for a per-son to be concerned about people with whom he or she does not normally identify (Rorty 1998, p. 180). If anything, as we see around us today in parts of Europe and North America, actual or perceived loss of security or privilege can once again delimit the category "people like us" to a certain racial or national boundary.[16] Humanizing others and adopting an attitude of reconciliation toward them is therefore a compli-cated task. In so far as a group of people find others to be a threat to their economic security or identity, they are unlikely to seek common ground with them. And in so far as they conceive of them as fundamentally different, they are unlikely to consider

---

[16] I am referring to the rise of nationalism and of far-right, White supremacist, and radical Christian groups in the aftermaths of the migrant and refugee crisis in Europe during 2015 and the global financial crisis of 2008.

them as part of the broader group and not as a threat. In order to break this cycle and create the possibility for reconciliation, political institutions have a role to play; for example, by getting people to meet and to know each other outside these exclusionary and often dehumanizing narratives. Reconciliation, therefore, while it constitutes the most adequate response to demands for recognition, can certainly be encouraged by specific kinds of political activity, as I discuss in what follows.

Returning to the question that we began this section with, "Why should we approach others with an attitude of reconciliation?", we can now see that this is not the right question to ask. Instead, we must ask, "what do we need to do in order for our field of concern to extend beyond our immediate family and friends?". And for this question the answers are going to be of a practical nature, though none of them are easy. It requires that we engage with the stories of other people, understand their point of view and, above all, resist the narratives by which we convince ourselves that they are less human than us.

5.5 Responding to misrecognition: A role for political reform and reconciliation

We have seen that an adequate response to demands for recognition requires both political reform and interpersonal reconciliation. The latter is the ultimate goal in that it focuses on the "internal" change that needs to occur by way of repairing social relationships. But the complexities in arriving there create room for the facilitating activities of political institutions. On the other hand, coercive political reforms in the absence of reconciliation can be counterproductive.

Let us begin by considering what a coercive political response to misrecognition might look like. We could have, for example, legislation that bans the use of words and narratives considered offensive to certain groups in society. This is already the case in relation to racial slurs and other expressions that fall under hate speech laws or similar legislation. The equivalent in the case of Mad activism (hypothetically) would be to criminalize or discourage the use of terms such as "psychotic" or "schizophrenic" (coterminous with this would be educational campaigns aimed at changing the terms of the public conversation). Coercive reforms can be considered a step forward in the same way that hate speech laws discourage some people from partaking in racist abuse of others. But there is also no doubt that coercive reforms of this kind are insufficient; on the one hand, they may breed resentment among those citizens who take such reforms as an attack on their right to free speech; on the other hand, they may create the illusion of a solution without actually having an effect on the contexts in which people interact, the contexts in which recognition and misrecognition are daily realities. It is difficult to force people to accept each other, and political reform without reconciliation is insufficient.

That being said, an attitude of reconciliation can be *encouraged* through political action. For example, the South African government passed the Promotion of National Unity and Reconciliation Act in 1995, upon which the Truth and Reconciliation Commission (TRC) of post-apartheid South Africa was able to commence its work.[17]

---

[17] I am not commenting on whether the TRC worked or not, only on its general approach to

Methodologically, a key approach of the TRC was to get people to hear each other's stories over thousands of encounters. In these encounters, people confronted each other, giving mutual testimonies and describing what they had done and what was done to them. It placed people in a context where they could meet with the explicit intention of reconciliation and forgiveness. In a more general sense, an attitude of societal reconciliation can be primed in a positive direction by prior work to address dehumanizing social narratives pertaining to specific groups in society. Further, the extension of certain rights to groups previously denied them can also increase the chances of reconciliation. We have seen this, to a certain extent, following same-sex marriage legalization in England. Political activity that gets people to share testimonies, or promotes equal rights, or advances positive views of devalued and despised identities, may foster a social attitude of reconciliation toward those individuals.

There is much that can be achieved through political action in terms of creating favorable cultural and practical conditions for people to adopt an *attitude* of reconciliation toward each other. Holding an attitude of reconciliation is only the first step; a full response to demands for recognition requires that we work toward achieving an *outcome* of reconciliation (see section 5.4.1). Such outcomes, as I noted at several points in this chapter, cannot be forced. For in demanding recognition—in demanding that their identities are registered by others in an adequate factual and evaluative manner—we can assume that people are seeking genuine and freely offered affirmation. While it is not impossible for some people to be satisfied by a positive yet insincere judgment—they may, for instance, consider it sufficient that they have been praised in front of their colleagues even though they know that this praise was dishonest—it is unlikely that people are going to be motivated to demand recognition with only the promise of disingenuous words to look forward to. They would want their value to be genuinely registered and experienced by others, even if they end up settling for less (see Taylor 1994a). A genuine judgment requires that identity claims are actually evaluated without any particular outcome preordained. To offer favorable judgments on demand is to forego, as Taylor (1994a) rightly argues, all standards of evaluation and hence to undermine the validity of those judgments. What we owe people, therefore, is not an a priori judgment of validity and worth, but to approach them with the kind of openness and humility that may lead to true appreciation (Taylor 1994a, p. 66), i.e. an attitude of reconciliation.

Honneth makes a similar point, noting that positive judgments of worth cannot be bestowed absolutely and can only arise from a process of evaluation that "escapes our control, just as sympathy or affection does" (Fraser and Honneth 2003, p. 168). Concurring with Taylor, he notes that what we owe other "cultures" and ways of life is to approach them with "well-meaning attention and consideration" and to judge them "according to an 'anticipation of completeness' (Gadamer) of their value" (Fraser and Honneth 2003, pp. 168–9). This attitude, proposed by Taylor and Honneth, includes the promise of registering the validity of a collective identity without the condescension and incoherence of offering positive judgments on demand. But as argued in this

societal trauma. The official TRC website can be found here: http://www.justice.gov.za/trc/index.html

chapter, the right attitude is just the first step, the ultimate goal being for the groups in question to achieve recognition, something that cannot be offered on demand and needs to be genuine and voluntary.

5.6 Conclusion

This chapter developed an approach for responding to demands for recognition (to claims of misrecognition). The starting point is the view that misrecognition can result in the social harms of disqualification and identity impairment, and that repairing social relations can play a role in addressing these harms. This places such demands within the space of society's normative concerns and calls for an inquiry into ways of responding to them. I explored two possible responses: political reform and reconciliation. We have seen that one way to justify a political response to misrecognition is to appeal to a notion of human flourishing for which adequate recognition is essential. If we then regard the denial of the conditions to flourish as a social injustice, we would have some justification for coercive or incentivizing political actions aimed at reversing misrecognition. Leaving aside the details of this case (aspects of which I explored in sections 5.3.1 and 5.3.2), I have argued that political activity that involves coercion or incentive cannot adequately address the problem of misrecognition; recognizing the other as a successful agent has to be a free judgment, and it has to arise from a genuine understanding and acceptance of the other. An adequate response to misrecognition is to seek interpersonal and societal reconciliation. As an attitude, reconciliation requires that we approach others with the acknowledgment that their ability to find themselves validated in the social world matters as much as our own. Political activity can play a role in facilitating this attitude. For example, political activity can create the conditions for people to meet on more equal terms, or could advance campaigns that seek to reverse dehumanizing narratives concerning others. Accordingly, even though seeking interpersonal and societal reconciliation is the adequate response to misrecognition, this can be encouraged through certain political activities. The framework developed in this chapter will be revisited in Chapter 10 in the process of responding to the demand for recognition of Mad identity.

Part III

Routes to recognition

Chapter 6

Mad culture

6.1 Introduction

Part II developed a theoretical and normative framework for recognition and outlined a range of responses to demands for recognition (political reform and interpersonal reconciliation). We are now in a position to raise the following question: What is the appropriate social response to Mad activism's demand for recognition? The answer to this question is the overarching point of this book, and even though we do now possess the framework to think about it, we are not in a position to answer it before certain major issues are addressed. If we recall the account of Mad activism presented in Chapter 1, we find that attempts to demedicalize madness do not merely reject bio-medical and clinical-psychological discourse: Mad activism presents alternatives to the language of illness and disorder. These alternatives—irrespective of their detailed content—are ultimately couched in terms of "culture" or "identity." Madness, so the claim goes, is grounds for culture or identity and not a disorder of the mind. The demand for recognition is, in part, a demand for society to acknowledge this. The aim of Part III is to examine this claim by asking: if Mad culture and Mad identity are two possible routes to recognition, do these routes lead us to a coherent demand, or do we meet, so to speak, insurmountable obstacles along the way? Mad culture is the topic of this chapter, while Mad identity is considered in Chapters 7 and 8.

"Culture" and "identity" are two routes by which social movements, in general, make the case for the value and importance of their way of life or shared self-understandings; we have seen this and continue to see it with Deaf culture, Deaf identity, Queer culture, Aboriginal culture, and various racial identities, to name a few examples. Claims couched in terms of "culture" may appear quite similar to those couched in terms of "identity"; in fact, in some discourses these two terms are used interchangeably. However, given the definition of culture with which I operate in this chapter (section 6.2), and the understanding of identity developed in Part II, the two concepts need to be kept distinct: they raise different issues and a consideration of how they interact yields important insights (section 6.4.3). Accordingly, this chapter proceeds by asking the following questions: What is culture? Can madness constitute a culture? What are the justifications for cultural rights?

6.2 What is culture?

Part of the difficulty in making sense of the notion of Mad culture is the meaning of culture as such. The term "culture" refers to a range of related concepts which are not always sufficiently distinguished from each other in various theoretical discussions. There are, at least, three concepts of culture (see Rashed 2013a, 2013b):

* *Culture as an activity*: the "tending of natural growth" (Williams 1958, p. xvi); "to inhabit a town or district, to cultivate, tend, or till the land, to keep and breed animals" (Jackson 1996, p. 16); to grow bacteria in a petri dish; to cultivate and refine one's artistic and intellectual capacities—to become cultured. This final meaning— culture as intellectual refinement—lives today in the Culture section of newspapers.

* *Culture as an analytic concept in the social sciences*: this is the concept of culture that we find, for example, in the academic discipline of anthropology. The academic concept of culture has evolved rapidly since its introduction by Edward Tylor in the late nineteenth century.[1] Today, "culture" is used to refer to socially acquired and shared symbols, meanings, and significances that structure experience, behavior, interpretation, and social interaction; culture "orients people in their ways of feeling, thinking, and being in the world" (Jenkins and Barrett 2004, p. 5; also see Rashed 2013a, p. 4). As an analytic concept it enables researchers and theoreticians to account for the specific nature of, and the differences among, social phenomena and peoples' subjective reports of their experiences. For example, a prolonged feeling of sadness can be explained by one person as the effect of a neurochemical imbalance, by another as the effect of malevolent spirits, and by another as a test of one's faith: these differences can be accounted for through the concept of culture. (See Risjord [2012] for an account of various models of culture in the social sciences.)

When we refer to "culture" in constructions such as Mad culture and Maori culture, we are not appealing to either of the two concepts just outlined. For what we intend is not an activity or an analytic concept but a *thing*. This brings us to the third concept of culture I want to outline and the one that features in political discussions on cultural rights.

* *Culture as a noun*: this is the societal concept of culture; Will Kymlicka (1995, p. 76) defines it as follows:

> a culture which provides its members with meaningful ways of life across the full range of human activities, including social, educational, religious, recreational, and economic life, encompassing both public and private spheres. These cultures tend to be territorially concentrated and based on a shared language.

Similarly, Margalit and Halbertal (1994, pp. 497–8) understand the societal concept of culture as "a comprehensive way of life," comprehensive in the sense that it covers crucial aspects of individuals' lives such as occupations, the nature of relationships, a common language, traditions, history, and so on. Typical examples of societal cultures include Maori, French-Canadian, Ultra-Orthodox Jewish, Nubian, and Aboriginal Canadian cultures. All these groups have previously campaigned for cultural rights

---

[1] In *Primitive Culture*, Edward Tylor (1891, p. 1) provides the following definition: "culture or civilisation . . . is that complex whole which includes knowledge, belief, art, morals, law, custom, and any other capabilities and habits acquired by man as a member of a society."

within the majorities in which they exist, such as the right to engage in certain practices or to ensure the propagation of their language or to protect their way of life.

To stave off the obvious objections to this final concept of culture, I point out that there is no necessary implication here that a given societal culture is fixed in time— Nubian culture can change while remaining "Nubian." Neither is there an implication that all members of the community agree on what is necessary and what is contingent in the definition of their culture, or on the extent of the importance of this belief or that practice. And neither is a societal culture hermetically sealed from the outside world: "there is no watertight boundary around a culture" is the way Mary Midgley (1991, p. 83) put it. Indeed, it is because there is no hermetic seal around a societal culture that it can change, thrive, or disintegrate through its contact with other communities. In proceeding, then, I consider the key aspects of a societal culture to be that it is enduring (it existed long before me), shared (there are many others who belong to it), and comprehensive (it provides for fundamental aspects of social life). In light of a societal culture's appearance of independence, it can be looked upon as a "thing" that one can relate to in various ways, such as being part of it, alienated from it, rejected by it, or rejecting it. Can madness constitute a culture in accordance with this concept?

6.3 **Can madness constitute a culture?**

In the activist literature we find descriptions of elements of Mad culture, as the following excerpts indicate:

> Is there such a thing as a Mad Culture? . . . Historically there has been a dependence on identifying Mad people only with psychiatric diagnosis, which assumes that all Mad experiences are about biology as if there wasn't a whole wide world out there of Mad people with a wide range of *experiences, stories, history, meanings, codes and ways of being with each other.* Consider some of these basics when thinking about Madness and Mad experiences: We have all kinds of *organized groups* (political or peer) both provincially and nationally. We have produced tons and tons of *stories* and first person accounts of our experiences. We have courses about our *Mad History.* We have all kinds of *art* which expresses meaning—sometimes about our madness. We have our own special brand of *jokes and humour.* We have *films* produced about our experiences and interests. We have *rights* under law both Nationally and internationally. We have had many many parades and *Mad Pride celebrations* for decades now. (Costa 2015, p. 4, abridged, italics added)

As the italicized words indicate, this description of Mad culture recalls key aspects of culture: shared experiences, shared histories, codes of interaction, and mutual understanding; social organization, creative productions, and cultural events. Many of these notions can be subsumed under the idea that Mad people have unique ways of looking at and experiencing the world:

> Mad Culture is a celebration of the *creativity* of mad people, and pride in our *unique way of looking at life,* our internal world externalised and shared with others without shame, as *a valid way of life.* (Sen 2011, p. 5)

> When we talk about cultures, we are talking about Mad people as a people and equity-seeking group, not as an illness . . . As Mad people, we have *unique ways of experiencing the world, making meaning, knowing and learning, developing communities,* and creating

cultures. These cultures are *showcased and celebrated* during Mad Pride. (Mad Pride Hamilton)

A key component of culture is a shared language, and cultural communities are frequently identified as linguistic communities (e.g., the French-Canadians or the Inuit). A similar emphasis on language and shared understanding can also be found in accounts of Mad culture:

> As Mad people we develop *unique cultural practices*: We *use language in particular ways* to identify ourselves (including the reclamation of words like crazy, mad, and nuts). We form *new understandings of our experiences* that differ from those of biomedical psychiatry. (deBie 2013, p. 8)

> The *experience of Madness* produces unique *behaviour* and *language* that many Normals don't understand but which make complete sense to many of us. (Costa 2015, p. 4)

> We can find a community in our *shared experiences*. We can find a culture in our *shared creativity*, our comedy and compassion. Sit in a room full of Nutters and one Normal, see how quickly the Normal is either controlling the conversation or outside of it. They do not share *our understanding of the world*, and here you can see evidence of our Culture, our Community. (Clare 2011, p. 16)

So, can madness constitute a culture? In the foregoing excerpts, activists certainly want to affirm this possibility. But the idea of Mad culture does not fit neatly with communities typically considered to be *cultural* communities. A typical cultural community, as outlined in section 6.2, tends to have shared language and practices, a geographic location or locations, a commitment to shared historical narrative(s), and offers for its members a comprehensive way of life. Compared to this, Mad culture appears quite atypical; for example, there is no shared language as such—references to "language" in the previous quotes refer to the kind of private codes that tend to develop between friends who have known each other for many years, and not to a systematic medium of communication. People who identify as Mad, or who are diagnosed with "schizophrenia" or "bipolar disorder," come from all over the world and have no geographic location, no single language, or a single shared history (the history of mental health activism in the English-speaking world is bound to be different to that in South America). Further, Mad culture does not offer a comprehensive way of life in the same way that Aboriginal Canadian culture may. Mad people can and do form communities of course—Mad Pride and similar associations are a case in point—the question here, however, is whether these can be considered *cultural* communities.

Perhaps Quebeckers and Maoris are not suitable comparisons to Mad culture. Another community to examine, and which may be more analogous in so far as it also continues to fight medicalization and disqualification, is Deaf culture. On visiting Gallaudet University in 1986—a university for the education of Deaf students—Oliver Sacks (1989, p. 127) remarked upon "an astonishing and moving experience":

> I had never before seen an entire community of the deaf, nor had I quite realized (even though I knew this theoretically) that Sign might indeed be a complete language—a language equally suitable for making love or speeches, for flirtation or mathematics. I had to see philosophy and chemistry classes in Sign; I had to see the absolutely silent mathematics department at work; to see deaf bards, Sign poetry, on the campus, and the range and

depth of the Gallaudet theatre; I had to see the wonderful social scene in the student bar, with hands flying in all directions as a hundred separate conversations proceeded—I had to see all this for myself before I could be moved from my previous "medical" view of deafness (as a "condition," a deficit, that had to be treated) to a "cultural" view of the deaf as forming a community with a complete language and culture of its own.

In Sacks' account, sign language appears as a central component of Deaf culture—the core from which other cultural practices and attitudes arise. The centrality of sign language to the Deaf community is confirmed through a perusal of writings on Deaf culture: the World Federation of the Deaf describes Deaf people as "a linguistic minority" who have "a common experience of life" manifesting in "Deaf culture."[2] Acceptance of a Deaf person into the Deaf community, they continue, "is strongly linked to competence in a signed language." In *Inside Deaf Culture*, Padden and Humphries (2005, p. 1) note that even though the Deaf community does not possess typical markers of culture—religion, geographical space, clothing, diet—they do possess sign language(s), which play a "central role . . . in the everyday lives of the community." The British Deaf Association remarks upon Deaf people as a linguistic minority who have a "unique culture" evident in their history, tradition of visual story-telling, and the "flourishing of BSL in a range of art forms including drama, poetry, comedy and satire."[3] Similarly, the Canadian Cultural Society of the Deaf and the American nonprofit organization Hands & Voices both describe sign language as the core of Deaf cultural communities.[4] Sign language is central to Deaf culture and is the crux around which a sense of community can arise. This community fosters awareness of deafness as a positive state, not a deficit; the Deaf person is frequently described as the Seeing person (distinct from the Hearing person), emphasizing the visual nature of sign language and Deaf communication.[5] Deaf culture is also supported by the existence of institutions dedicated for Deaf people such as schools, clubs, and churches. Finally, as a consequence of living in a world not always designed for them, and in the process of campaigning for their rights and the protection of their culture, Deaf people develop a sense of community and solidarity.

Even though Deaf culture differs from typical cultural communities, in its most developed form it does approach the ideal of offering its members "meaningful ways of life" across key human activities (Kymlicka 1995, p. 76). It may not be a comprehensive culture in the way that Ultra-Orthodox Jewish culture is, but its central importance to the life of some Deaf people—arising in particular from learning and expressing oneself in sign language—suggests that it can be viewed as a cultural community.

If we compare Mad culture to Deaf culture, we find many points of similarity. For example, like Deaf people, people who identify as Mad—at least in the English-speaking world—are united by a set of connected historical narratives, by opposition

---

[2] Online: http://wfdeaf.org/our-work/human-rights-of-the-deaf/

[3] British Sign Language (BSL). Online: https://www.bda.org.uk/what-is-deaf-culture

[4] Online: https://deafculturecentre.ca/canadian-cultural-society-of-the-deaf/ and http://www.handsandvoices.org/comcon/articles/deafculture.htm

[5] Online: http://www.handsandvoices.org/comcon/articles/deafculture.htm

to "sanism" and psychiatric coercion, and by phenomenologically related experiences (such as voices, unusual beliefs, and extremes of mood).[6] In addition, they share a tradition of producing distinctive art and literature and a concern with transforming negative perceptions in society surrounding mental health. But Mad people, unlike Deaf people, are not a linguistic community, and this does weaken the coherence of the idea that madness can constitute a culture. An alternative is to regard Mad people as forming associations within the broader cultural context in which they live, the very context they are trying to transform in such a way that allows them a better chance to thrive.

The comparisons drawn in this section cannot be the final word, as it is conceivable for different conceptions of societal culture and Mad culture to yield different conclusions. However, in what follows I shall argue that even if madness can constitute a culture, a consideration of the general justification for cultural rights leads us to social identity and not directly to culture as the key issue at stake.

6.4 **Routes to cultural rights**

Civil rights are the basic rights considered essential for equal citizenship. Traditionally, they are divided into three generations:[7] first-generation rights are legal and political and include the right to vote, the right to liberty, freedom of speech and association, and due process. Second-generation rights are socioeconomic and include access to employment, healthcare, education, and shelter. Third-generation rights are cultural rights and include the self-determination of ethnic and linguistic minorities, their right to practice their culture, language, and to protect their institutions against erosion by the majority culture.[8]

Third generation rights have featured in a range of social movements and underpin the struggles of groups as diverse as Native American tribes, New Zealand Māoris, Aboriginal peoples in Canada, French-Canadians in Quebec, and the Basque in Spain. In practice, the groups in question demand land rights and self-government, the right to have their language taught at schools, and to have special sites protected from development (see Kymlicka 2010, p. 101). It is important to note that third generation rights are rights that a group can claim in virtue of being a *cultural* community. Arguably, it is for the reason that a group is united by a language, history, traditions, and practices that the question of self-governance and protection can arise. It arises especially in the context of threats from the larger society to the "cultural integrity and durability of ethnic minorities" (Kukathas 1992, p. 105). These threats are, partly, a consequence of

---

[6] Sanism: discrimination and prejudice against people perceived to have, or labelled as having, a mental disorder. The equivalent term in disability activism is ableism.

[7] For a short history of the development of human (civil) rights, see the following United Nations article: https://unchronicle.un.org/article/international-human-rights-law-short-history

[8] The International Covenant on Civil and Political Rights (article 27) states that: "In those States in which ethnic, religious or linguistic minorities exist, persons belonging to such minorities shall not be denied the right, in community with the other members of their group, to enjoy their own culture, to profess and practise their own religion, or to use their own language." Online: http://www.ohchr.org/en/professionalinterest/pages/ccpr.aspx

the liberal-democratic state's impulse toward nation-building: at bringing all citizens under the same set of institutions, including language, education, and so forth (see Kymlicka 2001, p. 1). Why do these threats matter; what is the philosophical justification for cultural rights?

6.4.1 Culture as a context of choice

A key argument in support of cultural rights has been put forward by Will Kymlicka (1991, 1995, 2001). Locating himself within the liberal tradition, Kymlicka argues that cultural membership is a "primary good" in the sense articulated by Rawls (1973). These are things that would "normally have a use whatever a person's rational plan of life" and include "rights and liberties, powers and opportunities, income and wealth" (Rawls 1973, p. 62). Primary goods are basic requirements that enable subjects to develop and exercise their autonomy, to form and revise their choices, to live noncoercively in accordance with their chosen values and, most generally, to determine for themselves their idea of a life worth living.[9] Kymlicka supports the idea that cultural membership is a primary good by noting that the capacity for autonomy cannot be exercised in the absence of a secure cultural context from where individuals can form and revise their choices. Our cultural heritage, he continues, provides us with a context of choice, a range of options from where we can select what we deem valuable and worth pursuing. But the context itself we do not ordinarily choose: we grow up in a particular community with a distinctive language and historical tradition, and through them we come to awareness of a variety of roles and practices, some of which we already find ourselves in—and may choose to embrace—and others that present themselves as possible ways of life (Kymlicka 1991, pp. 164–5). "Liberals should be concerned with the fate of cultural structures," he concludes,

> not because they have some moral status of their own, but because it's only through having a rich and secure cultural structure that people can become aware, in a vivid way, of the options available to them, and intelligently examine their value. (Kymlicka 1991, p. 165)

Central to Kymlicka's (1991, p. 167) account—central to making it consistent with liberalism—is the distinction between the cultural structure and the specific character of a culture at any point in time. The cultural structure refers to the context of choice itself *irrespective* of the content of this context; irrespective, that is, of the specific language, beliefs, or practices of a particular community.[10] What Kymlicka was keen to establish is that the cultural *structure* is a primary good, a basic requirement for a flourishing human life much like income and shelter. Its absence—if such a state can

---

[9] Subjects in liberal political morality are defined as having an essential interest in determining for themselves their idea of a good life. Yet this is not, as Kymlicka (1991, p. 10) points out, the same as the "life we *currently believe* to be good"; we may find that we were mistaken about our chosen projects and our beliefs about what matters. Thus, we have an essential interest in being able to question and revise our views, and to lead our lives noncoercively according to our chosen values. In order to be able to do so, we require the facilitation and protection typical of liberal societies—the so-called *primary goods*.

[10] This is an important distinction as the idea is to recognize the right to cultural membership for individuals and not the specific norms and practices that make up a tradition and which an individual should be free to accept or reject. This position—known as liberal

be imagined—is a state of total alienation: a person with no community, history, or tradition, and hence with no orientation as to what would be a valuable life. Cultural rights, on this account, concern the right to *a* cultural context and not to a *specific* cultural context. This is an unusual way of thinking about cultural membership, but let us pursue it further.

If cultural membership is a primary good, then it is a good which the majority, typically, does not have to worry about securing. Minority groups, however, cannot take this right for granted and may have to claim it, subject as they are to the always present risk of losing their heritage and distinctive way of life if they are not protected from assimilative pressures arising from the majority culture. For example, by virtue of being a minority, Aboriginal Canadians can be politically outvoted in every possible matter that concerns their survival and well-being as a cultural community. On the other hand, English-speaking white Canadians do not have to worry about, say, losing the English language. Demands by cultural minorities for recognition and protection are therefore, in this sense, demands to correct for basic inequalities so that no group in society is disadvantaged before people begin to make their choices (Kymlicka 1991, pp. 182–9).

Consider, for example, threats to the integrity of Aboriginal Canadian culture. Individuals in this cultural minority who would be most obviously harmed by its loss are those who are unable to partake in the broader cultural context, in the institutions, language, and ways of life of the society in which they live. For an elder Aboriginal person in Canada it may not be possible to become adequately acculturated in majority culture. Disintegration of their culture would then be experienced as a loss of opportunities to practice their way of life. This could arise from the loss of ritual sites due to land development, and from the paucity of individuals with whom they could communicate due to the acculturation of the younger generation. For younger individuals the issues are somewhat different, but harms may also arise. Typically, they would have more access to the broader cultural context; they may be educated in the English language at school and would have more opportunities to interact with a different way of life. Yet they may still find themselves trapped between two worlds; one that is, as it were, falling apart and another that is taking more hold. In the worst-case scenario this struggle may result in breakdown in communication and loss of harmony between the generations. There is no question, therefore, that Aboriginal culture can be described as a context of choice and that its disintegration can be harmful.[11] What exactly would follow from that?

....

neutrality—requires that a liberal society remain neutral in relation to substantive ways of life; in order for government to treat its citizens with equal dignity, it must not espouse a particular conception of what gives value to life (Dworkin 1978; Taylor 1994a).

[11] If we apply this approach to Deaf culture we can describe it as a context of choice in so far as it provides Deaf individuals with a community in which they can learn and practice Sign, partake in Deaf institutions, and develop a sense of identity through narratives of Deaf history and solidarity. In the absence of this context of choice, Deaf individuals may be consigned to impoverished lives—they would not be individuals with a positive culture and a distinctive

6.4.2 **The right to *a* culture or to *my* culture?**

If we stay with Kymlicka's key idea that individuals have a right to *a* cultural context, then faced with a disintegrating cultural minority we would have at least two solutions: protect and support the existing culture, or assist those individuals with integration into majority culture. Thus, it may be the case that the appropriate response to cultural disintegration is not cultural protection but the provision of sufficient resources such that individuals of the minority culture can become perfectly acculturated, say through intensive language lessons and "cultural re-education." This solution may appear rather unattractive—and as I will argue in what follows, is insufficient—but it clearly is implied by the context of choice argument: If what matters is that individuals have a secure cultural context from where to examine their choices and form a view on how they wish to lead their lives, why can't this be any context? Is it not sufficient that they have full and supported access to the majority culture?

To demonstrate why it is not sufficient, recall the situations in which the question of cultural rights arises. These are situations where a culture's integrity and existence are threatened. In the case of an ethnic minority, as indicated in the previous section, this could be a result of the gradual erosion of its institutions by the majority. In the case of Deaf culture this could be through the increased prevalence of cochlear implants and the accompanying loss of education in sign languages.[12] In the case of Mad culture this could be through the continued medicalization and treatment of madness such that whatever coherence and unity Mad culture may have possessed would be lost. If we accept that this cultural loss can be harmful to the individuals involved—in the sense of restricting their autonomy, their choices—then, as argued earlier, we have two options before us: *protection* of the minority culture or *integration* into the majority culture. The latter solution is not satisfactory, and the reason why this is so can be brought to light with a simple thought experiment.

Imagine a hypothetical situation in which the harms experienced by members of a disintegrating cultural structure can be instantly eliminated. This is where all members of an ethnic minority are offered the option of acculturation in majority culture; all Deaf individuals are offered the possibility of bionic ear implants and instant cultural reintegration that can make them adapt perfectly to the hearing world; all Mad individuals are offered the possibility of fully efficient treatments that would reinstate them to the "standards" of normality they have been previously judged by. If such perfect solutions exist then for the purpose of this thought experiment there would

---

language, but people who cannot hear in a hearing world; they would be deprived of opportunities to thrive and their autonomy would be constrained.

[12] Cochlear implants are electronic devices that enable those with deafness and the hard-of-hearing a degree of hearing ability. They may enable children who are born deaf to learn to speak from a young age. The ethics of cochlear implants are subject to debate, and one of the issues frequently discussed is the one raised here: that deafness is similar to an ethnic minority, and that the use of cochlear implants—owing to the fact that it will diminish sign language and Deaf culture—is equivalent to the intentional destruction of the language and cultural institutions of an ethnic minority (see Sparrow 2005).

be no harms to speak of, that is, no constraints on the autonomy of those individuals whose culture is being lost. But even in this situation, some of the individuals offered those perfect solutions could reject them, precisely because for them there is something valuable about their culture that calls for protection notwithstanding the possibility of eliminating harms. When people demand cultural rights, they are demanding much more than the right to a cultural structure: they are demanding recognition of the particularity and value of their own Aboriginal, Deaf, or Mad way of life.

Kymlicka's critics have made this point. Taylor (1994b, pp. 259–60) writes that "for the people concerned, their way of life is a good worth preserving; indeed, it is something invaluable and irreplaceable, not just in the absence of an alternative, but even if alternatives are available." For Taylor this is evident in the case of people who live in French Canada and for whom the issue is not just the current existence of French-Canadian culture but its continued existence—its *survival* for future generations. Margalit and Halbertal (1994, p. 503) also take issue with Kymlicka's formulation, noting that "an individual has a right to *his* or *her* culture" and not just to any culture. They argue that this right derives from the interest individuals have in preserving the sources of their *identity*, the things that give meaning to their life. Tamir (1998, p. 282) makes the point that individual self-esteem is bound up to the group with which one identifies, and that humiliation of the group is at the same time a personal injury; hence, individuals "take pride and satisfaction in [the group's] success and prosperity." Gans (1998, p. 164) meanwhile distinguishes two kinds of justification for cultural rights: a freedom-based argument (of the sort advanced by Kymlicka and which supports the right to a cultural community), and an identity-based argument. According to the latter, people have an interest in their culture because it is a "component of their identity":

> They have an interest in adhering to it as it is the interest of people to adhere to every component of their identity they wish to adhere to (their sex, sexual orientation, religion), even though it may not serve other interests they have. (Gans 1998, p. 164)

In later works, Kymlicka (1995, 2001) partly concedes to these criticisms, now writing that people need access to their *own* culture owing to the strong bonds that they have toward their language and traditions. He explains these bonds by noting the importance of cultural membership to people's identity (Kymlicka 1995, p. 87). Elsewhere, in a summary of justifications for cultural rights, he writes:

> Some theorists emphasize the importance of respect for *identity*. On this view, there is a deep human need to have one's identity recognized and respected by others. To have one's identity ignored or misrecognized by society is a profound harm to one's sense of self-respect. Minority rights satisfy the need for recognition. (Kymlicka 2001, p. 47)

What emerges from these criticisms and from Kymlicka's restatement of his position is that people demand recognition and protection of their way of life because it enters deeply into their sense of who they are: their identity. An abstract right to a cultural community falls short of what is required, even if it satisfies the liberal commitment to neutrality with respect to ways of life. If we reconsider the question posed in the title of this section, we can answer it by saying that what the individual (may have) a right to is his or her culture—and not just any cultural structure—and that this right derives from the importance of cultural affiliation to identity.

6.4.3 From culture to identity

Consideration of the right to culture led to rejection of cultural integration as a satisfactory solution for the reason that what people wish to preserve are the sources of their identity and not just any random context of choice. Putting the issue this way, however, is expected to change the manner in which the right to culture can be justified. Recall that Kymlicka's initial formulation of the justification centered on the importance for individual autonomy of having a context of choice. Given that what matters now is not just any context but a specific one, the argument needs to be modified. Margalit and Halbertal (1994, p. 506) make a similar point when they argue that the right to culture is "justified by the right to identity" and not by the "right to freedom." I take this to mean that people have a right to identity *prior to* the right to culture, and that the latter is justified because culture is a key component of identity: culture, therefore, trades on the importance of identity.

There is no doubt that people care about their cultural affiliation and that it can enter into their understanding of who they are, but so do many other categories: culture is only one aspect of identity, others include professional, gender, racial, religious, and sexual identity. In some cases, cultural identity may not even be the most important identification in a person's life. Does it follow from this that a group or community that plays a fundamental role in people's identification requires protection or promotion? The answer to this question turns on how we understand the *right to identity*. The phrase *right to identity* is problematic for it either states a trivial point (that everyone has a right to form a self-conception) or a contentious one (that everyone has a right to have their identity accepted for what it is). I would rephrase this and say that individuals should endeavor to encounter each other through a reconciliatory attitude by which it may become possible, though not guaranteed, that they mutually recognize the validity and value of their respective identities (a point argued for in Chapter 5). And given that individual identity always appeals to various collective categories, recognition of individual identity cannot be sharply separated from recognition of the collective category in question (see section 4.2.4). In some cases, this may require protecting and promoting a minority culture. For example, to attempt to recognize the validity and value of Aboriginal Canadian cultural identity while, at the same time, the societal culture is stripped of land rights, its language is not taught at schools, and the community's way of life is engulfed by majority culture, is an empty gesture. In such a case the question of protection and promotion looms large, though deciding on how to manage it is not straightforward and is the subject of many debates in political philosophy (e.g., Kymlicka 2010; Mende 2016). Even though protection and promotion of a societal culture may be, in some cases, necessary for recognition, it is not thereby sufficient: one can imagine a cultural minority encouraged to thrive as a tourist attraction without receiving validation or respect on its own terms.[13] In other cases, protection and promotion are not the issue; what is at stake is not the health of a group in the sense of its continued existence, but rather the negative attitudes people who identify with the group face in society.

In summary, cultural rights can be justified on the basis of the "right to identity" and the importance of cultural affiliation to people's understanding of who they are. In some cases, adequate recognition of individuals' social identity requires protection and promotion of a societal culture, and while this in such cases may be necessary, it is not sufficient. Further, identity is broader than cultural affiliation and appeals to many other collective categories. For these two reasons—moral priority and broader reach—the question of cultural rights leads us to identity as the key issue and category at stake.

6.5 **Conclusion**

This chapter explored the viability of Mad culture as a route to recognition. We can now draw some conclusions: first, there are difficulties with the notion of Mad culture since it does not satisfy the typical understanding of a societal culture. Second, even if we think of Mad culture as a cultural community, the analysis of cultural rights conducted here led us to the consideration of identity (and not directly culture) as the key issue at stake. As I noted in the introduction, madness as identity is the second alternative to the view that madness is a disorder of the mind. The question of the right social response to the demand for recognition of Mad identity will occupy Part IV. Before that discussion can begin, there are complications pertaining to the possibility of Mad identity that need to be addressed, specifically: Can madness constitute the grounds for identity, or do the phenomena associated with "mental disorder" such as delusions, extremes of mood, and passivity experiences undermine the requirements for identity formation?

---

[13] Arguments for protection of, say, an indigenous language that is at risk of dying, or of a set of ancient rituals that are at risk of being forgotten, can be esthetic, intellectual, or even financial, none of which need to touch on questions of recognition or respect.

Chapter 7

Mad identity I: Controversial and failed identities

7.1 Introduction

In exploring routes to recognition in Part III, we began by considering Mad culture as one of two possible candidates (Chapter 6). A consideration of the moral basis for cultural rights led us to identity, and not societal culture, as the key issue at stake. We can now directly consider the second route to recognition: Mad identity. The expression "Mad identity" refers to a range of nonpathologizing counternarratives of madness that form key elements of people's self-understanding. Whether or not individuals refer to themselves as "Mad" is not the crux of the issue—while some identify with this term, others do not. The key point is for individuals to regard madness as one possible basis for identity; Triest (2012, pp. 20–1) expresses this well when he writes: "madness is an aspect of my identity—who I am and how_I experience the world—not an 'illness' that is separate from me or a collection of 'symptoms' I want cured." This raises a question: can madness be grounds for identity?

On the face of it, the question of whether madness can be grounds for identity appears misguided, for cannot anything be grounds for identity? As we have seen over the past many decades, people can elevate any features of their experience, or any traits that they share with others, to center-stage in their understanding of themselves. People can choose to strongly identify on the basis of sexual orientation, gender, race, ethnicity, religious affiliation, profession, to name some examples. Why would madness be any different; why cannot people identify on the basis of the kind of phenomena associated with madness? To answer this question, we need to modify the initial claim: anything can be grounds for identity *on the condition* that it does not impair the capacities for identity formation. Madness, as is commonly acknowledged, does exactly that, and hence the notion of Mad identity is incoherent: it claims a basis in the very same grounds that subvert its possibility. If this is true, serious implications follow for the demand for recognition of Mad identity.

Consider a group of individuals demanding that society recognizes Gay identity as a valid way of life. In many social and political contexts today, the demand they are making will be seen as one that requires consideration within the scope of recognition and misrecognition. Different societies will respond to this demand in different ways: from positive acknowledgment to toleration all the way to criminalization. Whatever the outcomes, it is clear that sexual orientation poses no obstacles to a person's ability to identify as such. There is no reason to suppose that these individuals' identity-forming capacities are impaired: the demand is regarded as one meriting a social and a political response. In the case of Mad activism, if phenomena such as delusions, passivity phenomena, hallucinations, and extremes of mood impair a person's capacities for identity formation, then identifying on the basis of madness places one outside the scope of recognition: the paradox lies in claiming an identity on the basis of phenomena that undermine it. If so, then responses to madness should be, perhaps, in the realm of therapy and care, and not recognition. On the other hand, if madness can be grounds for identity, then we are within the scope of recognition, and the demands of Mad activism can be addressed in those terms. A careful consideration of this issue is therefore required, a task to which this chapter and the following one are devoted. Two questions are raised by the problem before us: (1) What are the requirements for identity formation? (2) In what way does madness/mental disorder undermine those requirements?

In so far as identity formation is concerned, the theory of recognition presupposes that the subject of recognition is an agent, with a sense of herself as agent, and with the ability to participate in a shared medium of expression, such as a language (see section 4.2). These capacities enable an organism to express a self-conception and to be aware of oneself as an individual with that self-conception. They distinguish human beings from most life-forms and certainly from all inanimate objects: a rock cannot form a self-conception. In terms of the theory of recognition, having these abilities is only an entry point: the theory operates with a rich sense of identity to which being a self-aware agent and a language user are the barest requirements. Beyond the ability to hold self-conceptions, the subject of recognition must satisfy a range of requirements: (1) The self-conception for which recognition is demanded has to be of an epistemic status that can, in principle, be addressed through social and political action: in terms that are explored in this chapter, it needs to be a *controversial* and not a *failed* identity. (2) The self-conception must be an expression of a unified, and not a fragmented or disowned, mental life. (3) The self-conception must persist over a sufficient period of time. By satisfying these requirements, a person enters the scope of recognition, where the claim that one's identity is not being accorded the appropriate normative status can merit attention and be a potential candidate for a social or a political response.

As the literature recognizes, mental disorder undermines these three requirements. Jeanette Kennett (2009, p. 92) writes that in a subset of cases of mental illness "the central project we all have of constructing and maintaining our identity is profoundly undermined." Psychopathological phenomena such as delusions, hallucinations, and disordered thinking, Kennett (2009, pp. 94–5) argues, "may reduce or remove [the] capacity to recognize, or to weigh appropriately, relevant moral considerations and to judge accordingly." George Graham (2015, p. 372) writes that mental health patients "may be compromised or impaired not only in their capacity for self-responsible action or deliberate or reflective agency, but in their experiential appreciation of their identity as persons and agents." Mental illness can undermine the ability of the person to conceive of herself as a unified self over time, which in turn could hinder the ability to live out fulfilling life projects and plans (Kennett 2009, p. 97). Jennifer Radden (2004, p. 133) makes a similar point when she notes that "mental disorder inevitably challenges traditional ideas about personal identity" and can "profoundly alter and transform its sufferer, disrupting the smooth continuity uniting earlier and later parts of subjectivity and, viewed from the outside, of persons and lives."

A comprehensive examination of the claim that mental disorder undermines the basic requirements for identity formation is a major undertaking that cannot be done justice to in two chapters. Accordingly, what follows here and in Chapter 8 is not, indeed cannot be, comprehensive; the aim is to take certain key phenomena and demonstrate in each case the complexity of the claim that a particular phenomenon undermines the requirement in question. The further aim is to try and carve out a space where madness, despite these problems, can be grounds for identity (this is taken further in Chapter 9). In terms of the three requirements for identity formation noted here earlier, the phenomena/conditions are as follows: (1) Identities that are based on delusional beliefs are likely to be failed identities. (2) Passivity phenomena undermine unity of self. (3) The conditions known as schizophrenia and bipolar disorder manifest in discontinuity of self. These problems, of course, need not co-occur; a person may have one and not the other. But they are the kind of problems that could remove a person from the scope of recognition by undermining their ability to coherently form and maintain an identity.[1] This chapter focuses on the first requirement: controversial and failed identities in light of delusions. Chapter 8 addresses the second and the third.

7.2 The distinction between failed and controversial identities

7.2.1 Key features of identity

Before defining and examining the distinction between controversial and failed identities, it is necessary to return to the notion of identity explicated in detail in Chapter 4, and to summarize some key features (see section 4.2). Identity is the totality of my self-conceptions. It is not a list of social categories (e.g., researcher, teacher, man, Buddhist, Māori) but the way in which these categories figure in my understanding of myself. Though you might learn something about a person from knowing that she is a teacher, you can learn a lot more from understanding how she takes being a teacher: is it a vocation or just a job that pays the bills? Is it important for research or for producing learned individuals? People find themselves embedded in certain collective categories, and their understanding of who they are arises from the way in which they are situated, and situate themselves, in relation to these categories. People also reject certain categories and seek to understand themselves in terms of new ones. Or they may endorse a

---

[1] Falling outside the scope of recognition and misrecognition owing to impaired capacities for identity formation may coincide with diminished moral and/or legal responsibility. However, even though they may coincide, they do not necessarily do so: not all individuals who require support to author a self-understanding cease to be responsible from a moral and/or legal perspective. These two determinations raise different issues and the question of moral responsibility in the sense in which it is connected to legal repercussions and clinical capacity is not my concern. There is a voluminous literature that tackles these issues; recent examples include Sullivan-Bissett et al. (2017); see also Radden (1996).

collective category yet endeavor to change its social meaning and value.[2] This reflexivity with regard to identity underpins its contemporary problematization: identities are not fixed and can change, which is also the reason that they are contested in a way that might not have been possible in other historical periods.

Another key point about the notion of identity developed in Part II is that our self-conceptions are not inert with respect to action; they play a key orientating function in our life as agents. As argued in section 4.2.1, an essential feature of human agency is the capacity to form strong evaluations, which are reflective endorsements or sanctions of our desires that do not depend on the possibility of satisfying them but on the standards we have set ourselves. For example, strong evaluations are involved every time we refrain from or engage in an action not for instrumental reasons but on the basis of a judgment that the action is "bad," "base," "ignoble," or "meaningful," "commendable," "good." They stand outside our desires and inclinations and form the standards that enable us to evaluate them. For example, if I understand myself as a secular scientist, it is expected that the values embedded within this self-conception will have a significant impact on the choices I make in my life: it delimits my field of action and gives it meaning and purpose.

From this we can draw two key features of identity: (1) Identity, within certain limits, is achieved not given—we have a say in how we understand ourselves and how this understanding develops over time. (2) Our self-conceptions inform action through a process of deliberation or are retrospectively invoked to justify it (by giving reasons for our actions).

7.2.2 When things go wrong: On gaps in social validation

The two features of identity noted in the previous section correspond to two ways in which things can go wrong: (1) Even though we have a say in how we understand ourselves, we do not have absolute say and can be wrong about who we think we are: I might think I am of Māori descent when the truth is that I am not; I might think I am a good pianist when the truth is that I am a mediocre one. (2) Our self-conceptions can fail to inform action appropriately (e.g., in some cases of ambivalence), or can inform it in a way that reduces our well-being (e.g., owing to my (false) belief that I am a good pianist, I apply to every job opening in the London Symphony Orchestra and receive a string of rejections; my self-esteem suffers). In the remainder of this chapter I only consider the first problem, leaving aside the second problem concerning the connection between self-conceptions and action. The reasoning behind this decision is twofold: first, my concern is with the judgment that a person is wrong about who they think they are, and the nature of the mistake they are involved in. Second, even though the connection between self-conceptions and action raises important issues pertaining to moral and legal responsibility, decision-making, and pragmatic rationality, these issues are not unique to allegedly (or actually) mistaken self-conceptions or,

---

[2] Once a person is invested in a collective identity by making it central to her understanding of herself, it becomes important to her how this particular collective identity is publicly valued and understood (see section 4.2.4).

in general, to allegedly (or actually) mistaken beliefs.[3] Recent work on delusions and irrationality, for example, argues that there is no more a necessary connection between delusions (and epistemic irrationality more generally) and reduced pragmatic rationality, than there is between epistemic rationality and improved pragmatic rationality (e.g., Craigie and Bortolotti 2015; Sullivan-Bisset et al. 2017). For these two reasons, the focus henceforth is on the first problem: the achievement of identity and the ways in which this can go wrong.

The first problem underpins the gaps in social validation that feature in the many demands for recognition that we see today. This is the gap between my understanding of myself and other people's understanding of me. Among the recent examples are the ongoing disagreements surrounding transgender identities, where some radical feminists are refusing to accept that male-to-female transgender individuals are women, with trans-women perceiving this as a form of misrecognition. Such gaps in social validation are described by Robert Pippin (2008b, p. 71) as follows:

> In any . . . commitment to a claim or course of action there is a possible gap between my own self-certainty, my subjective take on what is happening and what is called for, and the "truth," often manifest when it is apparent that others attribute to me commitments and implications of commitments other than those I attribute to myself. The experience of such a gap, itself a kind of social pathology, is what Hegel appeals to as the engine for conceptual and social change, a struggle or striving for reconciliation and mutuality in such a context.

Pippin's succinct description goes to the heart of the issue we are dealing with here (see Chapter 3, sections 3.4.2 and 3.5.2). In every interpersonal interaction it is always a possibility that the identity I claim for myself would be seen by others as invalid in some way; in their eyes, I am wrong about who I think I am. As a person striving for recognition, I insist on my claim and demand that others recognize me for who I am (or how I wish to understand myself): a struggle for reconciliation is born. But we cannot regard all such gaps in social validation as occasions to work toward reconciliation. Sometimes this gap is simply an outcome of one side committing a mistake that needs to be called out as a mistake. Accordingly, not all demands for recognition are within the scope of recognition. For example, even though my belief that I am a good pianist, according to certain standards, is false, it is the kind of claim that can be considered

---

[3] Pragmatic rationality refers to "decision-making that promotes the agent's well-being or success in pursuing their goals" (Craigie and Bortolotti 2015, p. 393). To be pragmatically rational is to be effective in realizing my intentions in the world (whatever these happen to be) and/or to act in ways that promote my well-being. Success and well-being need not coincide, for the former only requires that I achieve the ends I had set myself, without those ends necessarily contributing to my well-being as judged from a particular standpoint (Craigie and Bortolotti 2015, p. 388, note 1). "Well-being" is a philosophical (ethical) concept and can be conceived in various ways including hedonism, desire-fulfilment, and objective list theory (see Crisp 2006; Rice 2013). Whatever the conception in place, a key point in judgements of well-being is that they are not restricted to what the agent reports (unless one adopts a purely subjective view); as Crisp (2013, p. 411) notes, well-being refers to "what makes people's lives go well *for them* (where 'for them' is not to be understood as 'from their point of view' or 'in their opinion')."

within the scope of recognition—I could make the case that the standards are discriminatory, or that I am a good pianist within the cohort of self-trained pianists. On the other hand, my belief that I am of Māori descent (I am not) cannot be considered within the scope of recognition, for that would imply that failing to recognize me as Māori can be an instance of misrecognition, and hence a social harm and a possible injustice, when it is obvious that it cannot be that.

These examples show that getting it wrong about who one is does not necessarily remove that person from the scope of recognition: some mistakes call, at least in principle, for revising the category in question (the good pianist), while some mistakes cannot call for that (the Māori descendant). Maintaining this distinction is crucial, for without it *all* demands for recognition would be rejected as they would all be judged to be based on a mistake of which the collective category is innocent. We can, therefore, conceive two kinds of cases: cases where subjects are wrong about who they think they are but where this can potentially call for revision of the collective category with which they identify (I refer to these as *controversial identities*); and cases where subjects are wrong about who they think they are but where this cannot call for revision of the collective category with which they identify (I refer to these as *failed* identities) (in such cases there may be a further suggestion of impairment in the person's ability to form an identity). And the question therefore becomes: *Can we sort out those mistakes that can be considered within the scope of recognition (controversial identities) from those mistakes that cannot (failed identities)?*

7.2.3 **Method**

Before outlining the method for addressing our question, several clarifications are due pertaining to what is meant by the scope of recognition, and the requirement that must be met in order for a claim to be within that scope.

The scope of recognition: For a claim to enter the scope of recognition is for it to merit attention as to whether it is accorded the appropriate status concerning its validity. This is no guarantee that the claim will be acknowledged as valid, only that it is the kind of claim that merits a social or a political response whatever these turn out to be. When a claim enters the scope of recognition, attention shifts from the capacities of the person making the claim to the category with which the person is identifying—its range, meaning, and boundaries.

The requirement that must be met in order for a claim to be within the scope of recognition: The self-conception that is the subject of the demand for recognition, and which already appears from a certain social vantage point as an inaccurate view of oneself, must involve a mistake (the supposed basis of its inaccuracy) that can, in principle, be addressed through social and political action by questioning and modifying the collective category with which the person identifies: it must be a *controversial* and not a *failed* identity.

Method: Returning to the question of sorting out controversial from failed identities, my approach to answering it is to work my way through some identity claims and assess the mistake in which these claims are implicated (section 7.3). I chose to work with claims that can be described as delusional. There are three reasons for this decision: (1) These are the kind of claims I am interested in given the ultimate concern of Chapters 7 to 9, which is to examine the argument that madness can be grounds for identity. (2) Delusional identities are vociferous demands for recognition: a common feature of delusions is the subject's insistence that others validate their belief. (3) Delusions demonstrate major epistemic faults and hence one could be tempted to think that were they to enter into a person's self-conception we could only have a failed identity. If we can demonstrate otherwise in the hard case of delusions, then we might be able to achieve some progress.

Two provisos: The first proviso pertains to the aspect in which an identity is mistaken: one can be wrong about who one is in a factual and/or evaluative manner. For example, I may believe that I am a Knight when I am not, and I may believe that I am a brave Knight when I am a cowardly one. We might regard the former mistake to be a more serious one than the latter. And it could be argued that it is much easier for evaluative mistakes to be accommodated within the scope of recognition, after all the meaning of bravery is fairly subjective and can change. Perhaps, then, we could try to map the failed/controversial distinction onto the factual/evaluative distinction. Promising as this may sound, this is not an approach I will pursue, partly due to the contested nature of the fact/value distinction, a distinction routinely attacked either by demonstrating the value-ladenness of facts or the factual nature of values (see Appiah 2005, p. 181). What I intend to do is to consider the hard case—claims that would normally be considered "factual"—and examine the controversial/failed identity distinction in this light. The reasoning is that for those who endorse the fact/value distinction, showing that some factual mistakes can be accommodated within the scope of recognition is likely to be sufficient as a demonstration that evaluative mistakes also can. And for those who do not accept the distinction, nothing is lost.

The second proviso is a further distinction between, on the one hand, the identification as such (and whether it is controversial or failed) and, on the other, the coherence of the collective category with which the person is (allegedly) wrongly identifying. It is one thing for a person to wrongly identify as an alien abductee (and for this to constitute a failed identity), and another to question the validity of the category "alien abductee." In what follows, I am only concerned with the former problem; the latter will concern us in Chapter 10, section 10.3.2.

7.3 **Delusional identities**

7.3.1 **Clinical definitions and the criterion of sharedness**

Without doubt, the most extreme example of getting it wrong about who one is, is a delusional identity, the sort where one believes oneself to be the Queen of England, or considers oneself to be the latest in the line of Abrahamic prophets. It might be tempting to regard delusional identities as paradigmatic examples of failed identities, but does this necessarily apply to all delusional identities, or can some of them be regarded as controversial identities?[4] In answering this question I presuppose an understanding of delusions that incorporates the following features: a delusion is held with strong

---

[4] Delusions can be classified across a range of dimensions according to: (1) *Origin*: primary versus secondary delusions. (2) *Content*: for example, grandiose, persecutory, religious,

conviction; it is resistant to change and to counterevidence; it is a belief with which the subject is excessively preoccupied; it is poorly grounded in being supported by insufficient or irrelevant reasons (it is an irrational belief); it may or may not be associated with harm to the person or others; it may or may not be false and/or bizarre.[5]

Clinical definitions of delusion add another feature: lack of sharedness; a belief must not be diagnosed as a delusion if it is shared among a person's culture or subculture.[6] Sharedness, however, is better thought of as an exclusionary criterion rather than a feature of a delusion. As an exclusionary criterion it serves two useful and connected purposes: first, it focuses clinical interest on those who are likely to be harmed by their beliefs, and deviation from a shared reality is an indication of probable harm; second, it indicates that clinical psychiatry is not after the pathologization of cultural beliefs no matter how irrational or bizarre they are. For some authors, this exclusionary criterion is arbitrary: if we were consistent we would regard any belief as a delusion if it satisfies the relevant criteria irrespective of how many people hold this belief. In *Delusions and the Madness of the Masses*, Reznek (2010) makes this argument, taking issue with what he referred to as the "community axiom" (and what I have been referring to as the criterion of sharedness). Reznek abandons this axiom and proceeds to describe as delusional the beliefs of large swathes of the world's population: belief in the paranormal, Christian Creationism, end-of-the-world ideology and other cults, 9/11 conspiracy theories, Jewish belief in the Promised Land, Muslim fundamentalist ideology, and others:

....

nihilistic, and delusions of misidentification. (3) *Scope*: monothematic versus polythematic. (4) *Relation to other beliefs*: circumscribed versus systematized. In the text I am not concerned with the particular classification of a delusional identity but with analyzing its status (i.e., whether it is a failed or a controversial identity).

[5] It has proven difficult to provide a set of necessary and sufficient conditions that would satisfy every instance of delusion. Delusions appear to be a heterogenous phenomenon—a syndrome rather than a symptom (Gilleen and David 2005). For example, delusions of persecution can be poorly grounded, but what about delusions that concern a person's inner states such as delusions of thought control? Such delusions cannot be subjected to the same epistemic questioning as a persecutory delusion that concerns events in the world. Another problem with attempts to provide an encompassing definition of delusion is the continuity between delusions and irrational beliefs in general: "ordinary" and "everyday" beliefs frequently demonstrate poor consistency and integration, are justified on the basis of limited or irrelevant evidence, and are resistant to counterevidence (see Craigie and Bortolotti 2015; Sullivan-Bisset et al. 2017). There appears to be continuity between beliefs that tend to be picked out as delusional and those that are not considered so. Demonstrating such continuity, however, does not necessarily end the quest for a definition; we could continue the search for what sets delusions apart from ordinary irrational beliefs.

[6] The *Diagnostic and Statistical Manual of Mental Disorders* warns that religious beliefs are not delusions if "ordinarily accepted by other members of the person's culture or subculture (i.e., it is not an article of religious faith)" (APA 1994, p. xxiv). We can replace "religious beliefs" with any other kind of beliefs—the key issue for the DSM stipulation is not to mistake cultural beliefs—of any kind—for psychopathology (see Rashed 2013a).

The whole world is mad, with irrationality pervasive throughout the normal population. The failure of reason seems to characterize normality, and no person seems free of delusional ideas . . . We all seem to have succumbed to the sleep of reason, spawning delusional ideas and making monsters of us all. (Reznek 2010, p. 188)

Reznek's position is problematic in three ways: (1) It stretches the language of psychopathology to the point where it becomes meaningless. Terms like "delusion" and "sickness" when applied to groups in expressions such as "the delusional masses" or "sick societies" are metaphorical extensions of their meaning in the individual case: they cannot be taken literally. To describe a society as "sick" is to indicate our disapproval of its state of affairs, so much so that it resembles a sick person. In many cases, applying these terms to groups amounts to no more than an insult. Of course, the various concepts of mental disorder are meant to pick up something about an individual's inability to function, including the inability to fulfill social roles and to be part of a shared reality; this point alone reveals the absurdity of applying these concepts to whole communities. (2) It promotes scientific methodology as the only method by which communities must form and revise beliefs: any beliefs that do not conform to "contact with reality" in light of the scientific method are delusional. The leap from *failure to follow the scientific method* to judging as delusional those who do not shows that Reznek regards the scientific method not only as a particularly successful way of constructing observations and theories about the world (which it is), but as an ideology that everyone must follow. Such a leap ignores the complicated ways in which beliefs are actually formed and the many roles aside from scientific rigor that belief plays in people's lives (see Rashed 2013c, pp. 139–44).[7] (3) It conflates the origin of a delusional belief with the mechanisms of its transmission to others. There is a difference between a person who on seeing a blue car pass in front of his house becomes convinced that the world will end in ten years (a delusional perception), and the one thousand followers he subsequently attains. His belief is poorly grounded in the sense that he has no good reasons for it, and strictly speaking it is a delusion. His followers, on the other hand, though they can be justifiably accused of being gullible, evince a recognized mode of social learning: believing and following a charismatic individual (and placing aside our critical faculties) is not always admirable, but it is not thereby delusional.[8]

For these reasons, Reznek's attempt to extend the concept of delusion to entire communities does not work. However, I do share with Reznek the starting point, which is that the concept of delusion and the criterion of sharedness must be kept apart (unlike in clinical psychiatry). But while he utilizes this to argue that whole communities can be deluded, I take it in a different direction. Delusion must be disentangled from sharedness in order to create a conceptual and normative space whereby we can conceive of and respond to demands for recognition. Every demand for recognition is a perception of a mistake by both sides. If I claim to be the latest in a line of Abrahamic prophets

---

[7] For further details, see my review of Reznek's book in *Metapsychology*, online: http://metapsychology.mentalhelp.net/poc/view_doc.php?type=book&id=6180

[8] See Radden (2011, chapter 5) for an excellent overview of the various ways in which delusions can be shared.

my interlocutor is likely to consider me delusional, and I am likely to consider her wrong in her disbelief. My identity claim is unshared, and what I want to achieve is to have others validate it (i.e., for my claim to be shared). I may or may not succeed in this: sharedness (or its absence) is an outcome of an interaction and not a diagnostic criterion. If we take lack of sharedness as a diagnostic criterion then we are no longer in a position to evaluate those interactions, given that the issue is precisely whether that belief should be shared. Therefore, the question we must ask is this: When does a delusional identity merit consideration within the scope of recognition—when can it be considered a candidate for what should be shared (i.e., a controversial and not a failed identity)?

7.3.2 The President's son

Kamal is a twenty-two-year-old man who lived with his parents in the Dakhla oasis of Egypt (Rashed 2012).[9] He believed that his real parents were Hosni Mubarak (then President of Egypt) and Suzanne Mubarak, the First Lady. Meanwhile, his actual parents with whom he lived were farmers of modest means. This is how his belief had started:

> I was watching television and I saw Suzanne [the First Lady, referred to by the state media as "Mama Suzanne"]. She was on channel 1 or 2 I can't remember. It was like a conference, and there were several young girls and boys, but they weren't her children. She was saying "thank God, now I am not worried about any of you, and he, he has grown up into a man. He is unwell now but will get better soon." She was supporting me; she was saying "my child lives in a place with sand and mountains in a deserted house and his father [Mubarak] passes over him in a plane. He plants cactuses and flowers and spends time in a square next to a big mosque [El-Midan]. He is older now and insha'allah I will get him married. I know where he is, and I know of him." At one point I wanted to leave the room and as I walked towards the door the channel changed on its own, and this movie was playing, "Shams El-Zanatee" [Shams means sun], why this movie? And I understood, they mean this town, the sun shines here a lot. I wanted to go outside and look up at the sky, I thought they must have been videoing me through the satellites, they could see me, that's what I thought at the time, that's how she knows everything about me. She could see me while giving her speech. Since that day and my head, my head, I knew it must be me, she means me.

This experience prepared the ground for a virtual encounter with Mubarak a few days later. On that occasion the President was giving a speech broadcast live on television.

> My father was there in a big hall and one thousand people were clapping. He was speaking of the "simple peasant," the "peasant" [reference to Mubarak's rhetoric that the government's policies are tailored to the needs of the peasants and the underprivileged]. He means someone specific but he doesn't want to show it. He was referring to me. [And what about Abbas, your father?] I knew he wasn't my father. [And Nafisa, your mother?] I was raised in Gomhoreyya [Republic] Street, Mubarak's street.

----

[9] The research on which this case study is based was conducted under ethical approval from University College London (UCL Ethics Project ID Number: 1521/001). Identifying data has been changed, and informed consent has been obtained from participants.

Kamal's convictions lead him, on two occasions, to intercept ministerial motorcades moving across town and demand that he be taken to his "father" at the presidential home in Cairo. When Mubarak visited the nearby town of Uweinat in 2007, Kamal walked to Dakhla military airport after learning that the President would be landing there. Kamal did not keep his convictions to himself and would frequently argue with people in town about his real parents. Unfortunately, though not altogether surprisingly, this led to ridicule by others and to gradual social isolation.

In time, Kamal learnt to avoid arguing with people about his real parents, despite still believing that his father and mother were the President and the First Lady. On our last meeting, he made his sentiments and doubts clear:

> I am strongly attached to him. I feel a link between us. I never met him but my heart is strongly attached to him, and I love my mother, Suzanne. If all the people do not love him, I still will. [Is Mubarak aware of you?] He knows what I think, he knows I want to be united with him, and he wants to come back to me, but something distances us from each other, I don't know what it is. He is kind, I know him, he has a kind heart. It's the people who have the wrong idea of him. Why would he visit hospitals then? Why would he talk to patients, or mention the peasants in his speeches? I don't care about the money, the position, I just want my parents. For a long time and I haven't had their love, haven't been in their bosom.

As we were parting I asked Kamal why Mubarak had not attempted to contact him. After several pauses and hesitant attempts, he explained that Mubarak had in fact contacted him and sent him money, but it was stolen before it got here, an explanation that ended with a request:

> If you meet my father or any of the people with him in Cairo could you tell them about me, lead them to me?

We can see in Kamal's claim that he is the President's son, and in his insistence that others agree with him, a demand for recognition: he wants his claim validated. Is his claim a failed identity that must be rejected outright, or is it a controversial identity in the sense that we might want to consider modifying the category with which he is identifying so that it includes him? It is obvious, in this case, that his claim is a failed identity; he cannot receive the validation he desires. On what basis have we made this assessment? Assuming we are using the word "son," as Kamal does, to refer to the biological offspring of specific individuals, then Kamal can only be recognized as the President's son in the case that he actually is (i.e., only if his claim is true). Truth and falsity are appropriate terms to use here as his claim is one that can have a truth value: he either is the President's son or he is not; there is a fact of the matter that is open, in principle, to public verification; there are methods to prove or disprove paternity, methods over which there are significant consensus (such as conducting DNA tests and consulting official documents). Kamal's claim that he is the President's son is therefore a failed identity, and it fails *on its own terms*.

As it happens in this case, and in many other cases, we do not get around to confirming the truth or falsity of an identity claim yet continue to regard it as likely to be false. In Kamal's case, his claim is highly implausible: a poor, young farmer from an oasis in the heart of the western desert is the son of the most powerful man in Egypt? And even if the claim is plausible, the way in which it is argued for—the reasons by which it is justified and defended—cast huge doubt on the likelihood of its truth. In the philosophical literature on delusions, it would be said that the belief is epistemically irrational.[10]

A belief is epistemically rational to the extent it is formed on the basis of sufficient evidence and is responsive to counterevidence (see Bortolotti 2009). On this definition Kamal's claim, and delusional beliefs in general, are quintessential examples of failures of rationality: they are held with conviction despite poor evidence, and when the subject is confronted by counterevidence he or she props up the delusion with ad hoc hypotheses lacking in good evidential support. As can be seen in the aforementioned quotes, Kamal arrived at his belief through a series of delusional perceptions, ideas of reference, and persecutory delusions (as they would be referred to in descriptive psychopathology). The evidence cited by Kamal in support of his claim that Mubarak and Suzanne were his parents falls extremely short of what would generally be regarded as good evidence for parenthood, if not being irrelevant. For example, he believed that the First Lady's speeches included coded messages for him, her son, messages of comfort and patience. He grew up in *Gumhuriyya* Street (the Arabic word for Republic), and his middle name is the same as the President's, two facts he marshaled in further support of his claim. Not only did Kamal consider these experiences and facts as evidence for his parentage, he also rejected all possible alternative explanations for them. When pressed to explain obvious inconsistencies in his story he would come up with random hypotheses: when asked why his "father" had left him in a small town more than a thousand kilometers from Cairo, he would say that Mubarak was keen to avoid rivalry between him and his brothers (the President's two sons); when shown a birth certificate confirming his real parentage, he would dismiss it as a fake; when asked why the man who claimed to be his father would do such a thing, Kamal would argue that this man had been paid by the President's office to keep it a secret.

Kamal's story demonstrates a range of epistemic shortcomings and reasoning errors: forming a belief on the basis of limited and irrelevant evidence; holding onto his belief with conviction despite counterevidence; when challenged, defending his belief through the addition of hypotheses for which there is no convincing evidence; and jumping to conclusions when interpreting information to support his hypothesis. A key point to note is that epistemic rationality and irrationality concern the grounding of the belief and not its truth or falsity. "Epistemic rationality provides norms that

---

[10] The connection between mental disorder and rationality has long been recognized (see Edwards 1981; Radden 1985; Foucault 2001; cf. Bortolotti 2015). In the case of delusions, for example, irrationality is part of the definition of these phenomena (see Bortolotti 2013). The meaning of rationality with which the recent literature operates involves several distinctions, in particular between procedural, epistemic, and pragmatic rationality (see Bortolotti 2009, 2013, 2015; Bortolotti et al. 2012; Craigie and Bortolotti 2015). Procedural rationality refers to consistency and integration among an agent's intentional states; epistemic rationality refers to the process of belief acquisition and revision; and pragmatic rationality refers to decision-making that serves the agent in achieving its goals and/or enhances its well-being.

govern the formation, the maintenance, and the revision of beliefs" (Bortolotti 2009, p. 115); one may arrive at a false belief despite following those norms (though if one is epistemically rational this would prompt revision of the belief), and one may coincidentally arrive at a true belief despite violating them. Thus, Kamal's belief is epistemically irrational *even if* he really is Mubarak's son.

Focusing on epistemic rationality/irrationality rather than truth/falsity is a wise approach to adopt in the diagnosis, investigation, and explanation of delusions. One reason behind this is that it would be highly impracticable to examine the truth or falsity of certain delusions—think of an elaborate persecutory delusional system that is not sufficiently bizarre to be dismissed outright, yet is too complex to be actually investigated. Another reason is that some delusions cannot have a truth value, there being no possible investigations relevant to determining their truth or falsity (see section 7.3.4). However, given the distinction that we are trying to make between failed and controversial identities, what matters in the case of claims that can have a truth value is not the quality of their grounding but whether or not they are true or false. Establishing this requires, first, that we agree with the claimant on the meaning of the category (in the case of Kamal this was the meaning of "son") and, second, determine in accordance with that meaning whether the claim is true or false. If it is false, then the claimant is wrong on their own terms. In such cases the mistake in which the person is implicated is not one that can be corrected by modifying the category with which the person is identifying. In fact, when a person is wrong on their own terms, such modification is not, strictly speaking, demanded by that person. In the foregoing procedure, epistemic irrationality can only ever be a pointer to the likelihood of a claim being false; its mere presence is not sufficient to dismiss outright a particular identity claim as a failed claim.

7.3.3 On being black when one is white

On June 10, 2015, Rachel Dolezal was being interviewed by a reporter for a local news channel in Spokane, Washington State. At the time, Dolezal was head of the local chapter of the National Association for the Advancement of Colored People (NAACP), chair of the Office of the Police Ombudsman Commission, a part-time instructor in African studies at Eastern Washington University, and an activist and campaigner for Black Lives Matter. After a few minutes inquiring over a range of harassment claims Dolezal had made, the reporter asked her: "Are you African-American?" Stunned, she replied a few moments later by saying "I don't understand the question." The reporter asked again: "Are your parents white?" At that point Dolezal walked off the interview. What happened next was a rapid dismantling of her life. After it transpired that Dolezal was born in 1977 to white American, fundamentalist Christian parents of Czech and German ancestry, yet has been identifying and living as a Black person since 2006, she resigned from her position as Chair of the Spokane NAACP, lost her University teaching post, and many of her friends stopped speaking to her. She was subjected to threats, hate, and ridicule on social media, newspapers, blogs, and television shows. Many described her as an unstable delusional woman; some African-Americans accused her of exploiting their suffering for her own gain; others described her self-styling by braiding her hair and tanning her skin as cultural-appropriation and an example of blackface; and a minority of commentators quietly suggested that it might be the right time to have a debate about race. There is much to be said about why Dolezal, a white European-American woman, would choose to identify as Black. In her autobiography (Dolezal 2017) and in a detailed interview (Sunderland 2015), she describes an early, gradual, and lifelong involvement with African-American individuals and Black culture.

In the early 1990s, Dolezal's parents adopted four black children in a short space of time.[11] While still a teenager, she played a significant role caring for them. She endeavored to surround the children with books and images in which they could see themselves, especially that the town where they lived was almost exclusively white. She took to braiding her adopted sister's hair and began educating herself about "Black culture." At high school she came across a book on racial reconciliation and, impressed by the ideas within, got in touch with one of the authors: an African-American man called Spencer who lived with his biracial family in Jackson, Mississippi. Spencer agreed to be her mentor and she moved to Jackson to attend Belhaven Christian College. Dolezal became close to Spencer's family and attended their church regularly to the point where people assumed she was his daughter; she subsequently called him her dad. At the time, she recalls, she only spent time with black students and became involved in black student's associations. She played a role in starting the first African-American Studies course at the college. Students assumed she was a "light-skinned black girl." Remarking at this period in her life, Dolezal says: "I wasn't white! It's so hard to explain this to people: I don't feel white. I didn't hang out with anybody white in Mississippi." A parishioner at the church which she attended, and with whom she lived for some time, would later recall: "she knew in her heart that she was supposed to be born black. She felt that she had a stronger connection to the black race. Her struggle was tear-jerking real." In 2000 Dolezal married an African-American man and had one son with him. She enrolled and was given a place at historically black Howard University where she continued her interest in Black culture and history. Her husband did not understand or appreciate this interest and Dolezal's autobiography paints him as a controlling man. Their relationship broke down and in 2005 she filed for divorce. By 2006 Dolezal, now a single woman, started tanning her skin and doing her hair in braids. She also stopped correcting people when they assumed she was mixed-race or black, after all this cohered with how she felt about herself. It was the first time, she says, that she began living an authentic life, a life interrupted on June 10, 2015.

Does this retrospective narrative provide sufficient reasons for Dolezal's identification as Black? Many people, like Dolezal, live their lives in deep and sustained interaction with people from different races, but this does not lead them to identify as members of the opposite race. There seems to be a missing ingredient in Dolezal's story, an ingredient that would explain why she would make, as her critics would see it, such a preposterous claim. In the aftermath of her "exposure," many commentators populated the missing ingredient by arguing that she was a "delusional" or "mentally ill" person. In a CNN opinion piece, the author argued that Dolezal had created around herself a delusional world, and whatever her reasons for doing so happen to

---

[11] Direct quotes in this paragraph are from Sunderland (2015).

be, she should not be celebrated for her beliefs.[12] For one blogger, Dolezal's commitment to her "delusion" was horrifying.[13] Another article considered Dolezal's belief an extreme case of self-deception, manifesting in the subject "creat(ing) a new reality." The same article entertained the possibility that she might have body dysmorphic disorder.[14] A *Washington Times* opinion piece began by noting that wishful thinking is something we do engage in, but in Dolezal's case it had deteriorated into delusion.[15] Add to this numerous posts on social media to the effect that her belief is a delusion and that engaging with her merely reinforces it.

Whether or not Dolezal's belief *really* is a delusion (in the sense that it would be diagnosed as such by a trained clinician) is something that cannot be established without directly interviewing her: armchair diagnosis is notoriously inaccurate and possibly unethical. However, in the "court of public opinion," as we have seen, one of the more prominent responses to her had been that she is delusional or mentally ill. To frame her belief in this way is to say that there is nothing in her claim to be Black that merits consideration (i.e., it is a failed identity, a clear mistake arising, in part, from a psychological defect). It is not a mistake that can be rectified by questioning our conception of the collective category with which she is identifying. To what extent is this a valid judgment?

We can see in Dolezal's claim that she is black, and in her continued adherence to and defense of this claim even after almost universal condemnation, a demand for recognition. Yet she has not—and seems unlikely to—receive the validation she desires. The response to her has been so final and forceful that one is left with the idea that she had committed a fundamental mistake, and one that cannot call for further consideration. In terms of the distinction we have been working with, Dolezal's claim would be a failed identity and it is so because it is false: she is not black. Aside from a position that rejects the very notion of race, all disagreements around the boundaries of a racial category presuppose that questions pertaining to racial classification are ones that are capable of an answer: in other words, they can have a truth value. If I claim to be of Uyghur descent, there are certain publicly available investigations to prove or disprove my assertion. Let us assume *for the sake of argument*, and along with many of Dolezal's critics, that to claim Black identity one has to be African-American (which is to have ancestors who were born in sub-Saharan Africa and were brought to America during slavery). If that is the criterion of membership of Black identity, and if Dolezal claims to be black in the sense of being African-American, then her claim is a failed identity,

[12] Why the fascination with Rachel Dolezal? CNN, June 18, 2015. Online: http://edition.cnn.com/2015/06/18/opinions/opinion-roundup-rachel-dolezal/index.html

[13] Online: http://jezebel.com/the-strangers-rachel-dolezal-profile-is-so-good-we-neve-1794463350

[14] How scientists explain Rachel Dolezal. Think Progress, June 12, 2015. Online: https://thinkprogress.org/how-scientists-explain-rachel-dolezal-4a2ed99165ef/

[15] Identifying with delusion. *The Washington Times*, June 17, 2015. Online: http://www.washingtontimes.com/news/2015/jun/17/editorial-rachel-dolezal-identifying-with-delusion/

and it fails on its own terms. But Dolezal has been very clear that she does not identify as African-American, she identifies as Black (Dolezal 2017, Prologue).[16] She disentangles being black from being African-American and in this sense is presenting a contentious conception of what it is to be black in modern America, a conception that would include within its boundaries a woman with European ancestry. What, according to her, are the elements of this conception?

In the prologue to her autobiography *In Full Color*, Dolezal (2017) asks these questions about the bases of racial classification:

> How do you decide whether certain people are white or Black? What's the determining factor? Is it their DNA? Is it their skin color? Is it how other people perceive them, or is it how they perceive themselves? Is it their heritage? Is it how they were raised, or is it how they currently live? Does how they feel about themselves play a role, and if so, how much? . . . does the idea of separate human races have any sort of biological justification, or is it merely a creation of racism itself?

On these questions—judging from a range of interviews and writings—Dolezal adopts an antiessentialist, experiential, and cultural conception of race. Her antiessentialism is expressed clearly in these passages:

> Other people are operating on an autopilot that race is coded in your DNA, that there are different races of human beings and those races are called black, white, etc. As opposed to race is a fiction that was invented . . . What I believe about race is that race is not real. It's not a biological reality. It's a hierarchical system that was created to leverage power and privilege between different groups of people.[17]

For Dolezal, how you feel, the experiences you have lived through, and your ability to choose are more fundamental to your racial identity than the strictures of your birth:

> How I feel is more powerful than how I was born. I mean that not in the sense of having an easy way out. This has been a lifelong journey . . . Nothing about whiteness describes who I am.[18]

> Yes, my parents weren't Black, but that's hardly the only way to define Blackness. The culture you gravitate toward and the worldview you adopt play equally large roles. As soon as I was able to make my exodus from the white world in which I was raised, I made a headlong dash toward the Black one, and in the process I gained enough personal agency to feel confident in defining myself that way. (Dolezal 2017, Prologue)

---

[16] In an interview she explained: "African-American is a very short timeline if we're talking about people who have ancestors who were here during child slavery, biologically connected to those ancestors. Which I know that I don't have." From: Rachel Dolezal: "I wasn't identifying as black to upset people. I was being me." *The Guardian*, December 13, 2015. Online: https://www.theguardian.com/us-news/2015/dec/13/rachel-dolezal- i-wasnt-identifying-as-black-to-upset-people-i-was-being-me

[17] Rachel Dolezal: "I wasn't identifying as black to upset people. I was being me." *The Guardian*, December 13, 2015. Online: https://www.theguardian.com/us-news/2015/dec/13/rachel-dolezal-i-wasnt-identifying-as-black-to-upset-people-i-was-being-me

[18] See footnote 17.

A key aspect of being Black is identification with an ongoing struggle:

> For me, Blackness is more than a set of racialized physical features. It involves acknowledging our common human ancestry with roots in Africa. It means fighting for freedom, equality, and justice for people of African heritage around the world. (Dolezal 2017, Epilogue)

Dolezal draws an analogy with individuals struggling with their gender identity and seeking to be recognized for who they feel they are. She invokes the term transracial as equivalent to transgender and hopes for a time when fluidity in racial identity will be accepted in the same way that fluidity in gender identity is beginning to be accepted in some communities:

> If the narrative of fluid, non-binary gender identity is now widely accepted, Dolezal believes the same should apply to race. "It's very similar, in so far as: this is a category I'm born into, but this is really how I feel." Is racial identity as fluid as gender? "It's more so. Because it wasn't even biological to begin with. It was always a social construct."[19]

With this conception in mind, we can reask the question: Is Dolezal's claim a failed or a controversial identity? First, note that the reason we are asking this question is that Dolezal appears to have committed a mistake. Every demand for recognition implies that a mistake has been committed by both sides implicated in this demand: the recognizer and the recognizee. Dolezal demands recognition as black; others deny her that recognition. How is this situation to be rectified? This depends on the nature of the mistake: the kind of mistake implicated in a failed identity is when the person is wrong on her own terms. Kamal (section 7.3.2) was wrong on his own terms, and so would have been Dolezal if she had claimed Black identity on the basis of being African-American. But as we have seen, she hadn't. She claimed Black identity on the basis of a radical conception of this social category, a conception that would include her. This amounts to saying that Dolezal's claim is a controversial and not a failed identity. That does not mean, however, that it is a claim that must be accepted; it only means that it should be considered as a challenge to prevailing conceptions, as a set of ideas we may want to listen to and debate. These ideas can certainly be rejected but this would be due to problems with the ideas themselves, with no necessary implication that the person's ability to form an identity is impaired.

Would we have arrived at the same conclusion if a similar claim was made by a "white" woman, Grace, who lived in England in the late nineteenth century? Would her claim to be black on the basis of the claim that race is something you can partly choose be seen as anything but insanity? It is unlikely that Grace's claim would have been viewed as anything else. Perhaps the reason we are able to arrive at the view that Dolezal's claim is controversial (and not failed) is because categories of race (and gender) have become, in Brubaker's (2016) terms, unsettled, in flux and, in Tuvel's (2017) term, malleable. For some people (most of whom would be academics and

---

[19] Rachel Dolezal: "I'm not going to stoop and apologise and grovel." *The Guardian*, February 25, 2017. Online: https://www.theguardian.com/us-news/2017/feb/25/rachel-dolezal-not-going-stoop-apologise-grovel

intellectuals) the idea that race is a social construct is familiar. For Grace, however, there is no such precedent. In Victorian England, race was not a social construct, and a person espousing such views would not be judged kindly. There is also a question concerning how Grace arrived at such views. Dolezal, an African studies lecturer, was aware of arguments on the status of race, and her ideas were shaped by this. But where did Grace get her ideas from? Was it an epiphany, perhaps akin to a delusional perception? Was it an outcome of deep thought about the issue?

The point I want to highlight through this comparison is that the plausibility of a particular conception of a social category depends on the extent to which the innovation in question develops already existing ideas into something new. Arguably, this is what Dolezal had done, though for her critics—many of whom reject the view that race is a social construct—her claim is a delusion and her views on race attempts to justify her belief. On the other hand, given the cultural milieu in which Grace existed, the plausibility of her claims would have amounted to zero. But plausibility is one thing and innovation another: Grace's claim is an innovation irrespective of its plausibility in a particular context. That it is so is given in the fact that she is presenting a controversial conception of a particular social category, which is also what Dolezal sought to do. If we collapse plausibility and innovation—if we stipulate that only those claims that are already plausible are to be considered innovations—then we would be unnecessarily restricting innovation to that which is already (partially) accepted. On the other hand, if we accept the proposal offered here, then all innovations amount to controversial identities and hence can be considered within the scope of recognition (whatever the ultimate outcomes of such consideration). In this respect there is no difference between the claims of Grace and Rachel Dolezal: both are presenting controversial identities.

7.3.4 Communion with God

Abeo is a twenty-nine-year-old woman who was born in a West African country.[20] She lived with her father in the United Kingdom for the past 15 years. Prior to her engagement with mental health services, she was reportedly in good health and had no past medical or psychiatric history. Her circumstances were no different to many people of her age and social background: after completing high school she did a number of jobs until she finally settled in the sales section of a department store. She had several close friends and recently had been in a relationship. According to both Abeo and her father she had always been religious. She attended weekly sermons at a Pentecostal church in London, her father's church, and was inclined to adjust her life to Christian teaching.

Two months prior to admission to a mental health unit she began missing the weekly sermons and instead would spend long hours reading the Bible. She got disillusioned with her church, describing their sermons as "empty" and "uninspiring." Around that time she got in touch with another church in her native country, one that emphasized a personal understanding of God through experience. She began isolating

---

[20] Consent was obtained from the person whom this case study concerns. Identifying information has been removed or altered.

herself, engrossed in reading and listening to recorded sermons. She got rid of many of her possessions justifying that by saying that she wanted to purify herself of material needs. She stopped going to work and made a habit of daily extended walks. She avoided going to her father's church claiming that there was no point or value in going there anymore. Four weeks prior to admission she began to have intense experiences where she would hear God talking to her, consoling, advising, and at times ordering her to get rid of her possessions. She began having a direct experience of the "Spirit" in her body to the point, at times, of feeling "taken over." She surrendered to these experiences and did not doubt their authenticity at any moment. Her father was hugely concerned by these experiences and by what he described as an unexplainable and sudden change in her behavior. He tried to dissuade her from pursuing these new-found practices and appealed for support from the London-based church. The church pastor considered Abeo's behavior to be harmful and excessive, and made it known that it was not endorsed by his church. A few days prior to admission she began a prolonged fasting episode to "further cleanse her soul." She was physically challenged by the fasting and was found confused and disoriented in a public place, upon which an ambulance was called and a mental health act assessment arranged.

When she was assessed by a psychiatrist and social worker she said that for the past four weeks she had been in direct communion with God, that God had spoken to her telling her to get rid of her belongings, give up her job, fast, and change her life as a way of getting closer to Him. When the clinicians challenged the authenticity of the voice, she responded that she had no doubts it was from God. She also mentioned that she sometimes experienced her actions as directly controlled by God, and that she would feel the "Spirit" moving her body. She said that she had finally understood what God was and had felt on to something significant in her life. She was considered to present with second-person auditory hallucinations, command hallucinations, volitional passivity, and significant risk to self in the context of recent social/occupational deterioration, and in the absence of validation by her father and the church that this was a genuine religious experience. She was consequently placed under a section of the mental health act.

After admission she continued to resist all forms of treatment. She was unable to grasp the reason for her incarceration and considered the whole process to be a test from God. One week into the admission, and after mental state assessments and nursing observations confirmed persistence of the previously mentioned symptoms, the clinicians were convinced that a diagnosis of "acute psychotic episode" was justified, upon which medication was forced on her. Several days later she no longer resisted medication, and two weeks after that she acknowledged, for the first time, that she might have been ill. In terms of her symptoms, she no longer heard the voice of God, no longer felt the expectancy of a major change in her life, and was transformed into an unmotivated and indifferent young woman.

This is an important case-study to analyze for a number of reasons. In my essay *Religious Experience and Psychiatry* (Rashed 2010), I examine Abeo's story at length in the context of a critique of the two central justifications for a psychiatric diagnosis: social dysfunction and absence of cultural congruence. Here my concern has to do with Abeo's understanding of what she was going through, and whether her self-conception amounts to a controversial or a failed identity. To begin we can note that Abeo understands herself to be in communion with God, yet receives no validation for this self-conception, not from her father, or from the London-based church, and certainly not from mental health services. The consensus is that she is not having a religious experience: she is mentally ill. They consider Abeo to be wrong about who she thinks she is; she presents a failed identity. In Kamal's case (section 7.3.2) we were able to arrive at a similar conclusion because his claim is one that can have a truth value and hence it is possible, in principle, to determine whether it is true or false. But can Abeo's claim *I am in communion with God* have a truth value?

Abeo's claim, and religious and spiritual beliefs in general, can only have a truth value if one is already committed to the basic concepts in which such claims are presented, including the possibility of causally efficacious supernatural agents. Such a position requires that we accept that there is a valid category referred to as "communion with God," and that there is a correct and an incorrect way of inhabiting that category. To entertain the truth or falsity of the claim that one is in communion with God is to accept that the concept of God has an actual referent, and that it is possible to verify whether a particular claim of communing with that referent is true or false. For those who hold such prior beliefs, the claim will appear for them as capable of being true or false, but probably only answerable by those who possess the relevant kind of knowledge, such as religious figures and authorities; only they can answer the question for us, for only they would know if someone really is in communion with God, or is in fact bedeviled by the devil, or is faking it (as we have seen in Abeo's case, her London-based church was able to proclaim that her experiences were not genuine religious experiences). On the other hand, if one rejects the basic concepts in which the claim is presented, then it cannot be assigned a truth value: we understand what the claim means, but we cannot comment on its truth or falsity. Is it really the case that religious claims cannot have a truth value?

The epistemological status and the meaning of religious claims is a huge scholarly topic. As is well-known, metaphysical (including religious) claims have been rejected in the past by the logical-positivists who regarded all such claims as meaningless. In the classic text *Language, Truth and Logic*, A. J. Ayer (1946) employed Hume's famous distinction from *An Inquiry Concerning Human Understanding* to argue that two kinds of propositions constitute the entire class of meaningful propositions. The first are analytic propositions that concern, in Hume's terminology, "relations of ideas;" they are necessarily true as they "record our determination to use symbols in a certain fashion" and do not make a claim about the empirical world (Ayer 1946, p. 31). The second are empirical propositions that concern "matters of fact" and which are hypotheses that can, in principle, be refuted or rendered probable through experience. For a statement to express a genuine empirical hypothesis there must be some possible observations relevant to determining its truth or falsity: the principle of verification.[21] On this basis, Ayer sought to reject much of what was regarded as central to

---

[21] Ayer (1946, p. 35) defined the principle of verification as follows: "a sentence is factually

philosophical enquiry, most notably metaphysics.[22] Metaphysical assertions, claimed Ayer, are literally meaningless as they are neither analytic statements nor empirical hypotheses; the latter since there can be no observations that are, in principle, relevant to proving or refuting a metaphysical assertion such as the assertion that there exists a transcendent, supraempirical reality.

Logical-positivism received many criticisms. One key criticism concerned the validity of the principle of verification (e.g., Quinton 1991, p. 48). The principle restricted meaningfulness to propositions that can, in principle, be empirically verified and to analytic propositions that are true by virtue of definition. But the principle, clearly, is not an empirical hypothesis. The other possibility then is that the principle is analytic; that is, it offers a definition of the term "meaning." However we can understand the words that make up the definition, and understand that its truth logically follows from the meaning of these words, without accepting it as a valid definition of the term "meaning." Hence, the principle itself stands in need of proof and defense.[23] Other philosophers argued that Ayer's stringent criterion of meaning and his empiricist outlook were "needlessly austere," and that while curbing the "conceptual extravagances of speculative metaphysics" is to be lauded, the constraints Ayer placed on what should count as intelligible human thought were too severe (Foster 1985, p. 297). Another critic communicated a similar view when he wrote that Ayer's principle of verification (and the restriction of meaning that resulted from its application) "exceeded its useful purgative role in such a way as to clearly constrict our understanding and to thereby 'diminish thought'" (Sutherland 1991, p. 87).

It is important to distinguish two claims embedded in the principle of verification: the first is a delimitation of those propositions that can have a truth value, and the second is the claim that only propositions that can have a truth value are meaningful. It is the second of those claims that is problematic and which the criticisms cited here seem to have a problem with. The first claim, on the other hand, only concerns whether it is possible to establish, in principle, the truth or falsity of a proposition. We can accept that only analytic propositions and empirical hypotheses can be tested as to their truth or falsity (the former as a matter of definition and the latter through empirical verification). But why limit *meaning* to those kinds of propositions? Clearly that is a stipulation by the logical-positivists that one can reject. We could argue, for example, that the meaning of a proposition arises from the way in which it is connected to other

---

significant to any given person, if, and only if, he knows how to verify the proposition which it purports to express—that is, if he knows what observations would lead him, under certain conditions, to accept the proposition as being true, or reject it as being false."

[22] As understood by Ayer and the logical positivists, metaphysics is a mode of philosophical inquiry that seeks knowledge inaccessible to the empirical sciences. Metaphysicians seek an understanding of the ultimate nature of reality, the nature of Being; in general, of truths that transcend the world of science and commonsense. The logical empiricists rejected this notion of metaphysical knowledge.

[23] Another criticism concerned Ayer's sense-data theory of perception and its reliance on the "the myth of the given," in Wilfrid Sellars' memorable expression.

propositions, is embedded in certain practices, and in how it allows explanation and prediction of behavior. Construed thus, religious language is clearly meaningful both personally and culturally. It may not be capable of having a truth value (within a certain definition) but it is not thereby meaningless.[24] Accepting this carries important implications for our assessment as to whether Abeo's claim to be in communion with God amounts to a failed or a controversial identity.

A claim that cannot have a truth value cannot be a failed identity since there is nothing against which we can determine the nature of the mistake in which the subject is implicated. Despite this—or perhaps because of it—religious beliefs, including Abeo's claim, come in all shapes and inspire huge disagreement with limited chance for resolution. Look at Abeo's case: the London-based church and her father rejected her claim, while mental health services redescribed her experiences in medical language thus violating them completely—"she is in communion with God" became "she is psychotic." On the other hand, the church in her native country validated her claim and actively encouraged her to pursue this communion. Who is right? Well, as we have seen, this is not the right kind of question. What is happening in a situation like this is that we have several authorities, religious and otherwise, each of which deploys its own theological or scientific criteria and descriptions under social pressures (perceptions of risk to self and/or others) and political pressures (complex dynamics between the domain of the church and the domain of medicine) (see Rashed 2010, pp. 193–6). Who prevails, ultimately, has to do with who has sufficient resources and power—or persuasive ability—to enforce their vision.[25] What we have then is a paradigm example of a problem that should be considered within the scope of recognition, for the disagreement here concerns whose description is to prevail. If that is what's at stake, then Abeo's claim needs to be considered and not rejected outright: it amounts to a controversial and not a failed identity.[26]

7.3.5 On being dead when one is alive

The Cotard delusion is a nihilistic delusion that, in extreme, involves the belief that one is dead. In some cases, the belief refers to being emotionally dead, signaling a radical loss of vitality and connectedness to the world; at other times "dead" is intended

------

[24] Radden (2011, p. 97) makes a similar point when she writes: "If we accept that beliefs about supernatural matters can be neither true nor false, we must still consider their force and applicability as metaphorical language."

[25] In fact it is a possibility that, had the context been different, she might have been regarded as a religious innovator and a spiritual figure (see Littlewood and Lipsedge (2004) and Littlewood (1997, 1993) for case studies and analyses of factors that may transform "psychopathology" [in the medical sense] to religious innovation).

[26] The same analysis would apply if Abeo's identity was based on a delusional perception. For example, if one morning she saw a traffic light switch from green to amber and in that moment became convinced that she was sent by God to warn of some impending disaster, her belief would still be within the category of beliefs that cannot have a truth value. According to the analysis in the text, it would therefore be a controversial identity, though perhaps one that is unlikely to find more than a few converts.

literally and coterminous with this literality some persons refuse to eat (since dead people do not need food) or demand last rites and burial (as dead people would normally receive). In some case reports, when persons with the Cotard delusion are challenged—when it is pointed out to them, for example, that dead people cannot move and speak—they acknowledge the strangeness of their situation yet continue to believe that they are dead.[27] The Cotard delusion subverts its truth in its very utterance, since only people who are alive can speak, and what they say cannot logically include that they are literally dead. It is an example of a logically impossible identity claim; it violates the law of noncontradiction whereby an entity cannot simultaneously be x and not-x.

It could be pointed out that the definition of death is generally contested, with competing criteria for establishing when death should be considered to have occurred. There are definitions of death that require total failure of brain function, including the brainstem; others require that the heart and lungs stop functioning; others yet require irreversible loss of consciousness irrespective of brain stem and/or cardiopulmonary function. Each approach raises distinctive practical, moral, and legal issues. But whatever the criteria, these competing definitions are trying to get clearer on when death should be considered to have occurred in people who have lost the majority of their physiological functions (first and foremost consciousness), and frequently the ability to maintain vital functions without external support: in other words, whatever else death may be, it does not include a person who can speak. The person with the Cotard delusion is not dead, hence whatever debates there are surrounding the definition of death will not include that person.[28] As an identity claim, the Cotard delusion commits a fundamental mistake; it is a failed identity since the very expression of it undermines it.

7.4 **A methodology for distinguishing failed from controversial identities**

In section 7.2.2 I noted that every demand for recognition—all gaps in social validation—involves the perception by each side that the other is committing a mistake: I think I am x whereas you think I am y; I demand that you see me as x; you consider my demand. Given this, I formulated the question we had to address as follows: can we sort out those mistakes that can be addressed within the scope of recognition (controversial identities) from those that cannot (failed identities)? The implication here is that a failed identity involves a mistake that cannot be corrected by

---

[27] The following are a selection of case reports and analyses of the Cotard delusion: Young and Leafhead (1996); McKay and Cipolotti (2007); Graham (2010, ch. 9).

[28] Worth noting is the cultural phenomenon of zombification that can be found in Haiti (see Littlewood and Douyon 1997). A similar notion can be found in modern fiction and movies where it is usually referred to as the "living dead." The Cotard delusion is not an instance of the cultural phenomenon of zombification: the latter is the belief that a person who had died had been revived in order to be enslaved as a zombie; the Cotard delusion refers to a person who is alive but claims to be dead.

revising the category with which you identify, while a controversial identity involves a mistake that can, in principle, be corrected in that way: Can we reconceive the category *x* to include you, or are there uncontroversial reasons by which you must be excluded from that category? To explore these questions, I set out to examine them in the case of identities that can be described as delusional. A delusional identity would seem to be the paradigm case of a failed identity, an identity that is mistaken and cannot call for revision of the relevant category. But does this apply to all delusional identities, or can some instances be conceived of as controversial identities? By describing and analyzing four case studies we arrived at a tentative methodology for answering the question whether a particular delusional identity is controversial or failed. This methodology is derived from a limited number of case studies and is therefore decidedly tentative, but it is a start (see Figure 7.1). What are the elements of this methodology?

When confronted with an identity claim accompanied by a demand for recognition, we first need to ask if the claim is logically possible. If it is not, then it is a failed identity; the case discussed in section 7.3.5 is of this kind. If the claim is logically possible, then we ask if it can have a truth value: If we were to inquire whether that claim is true or

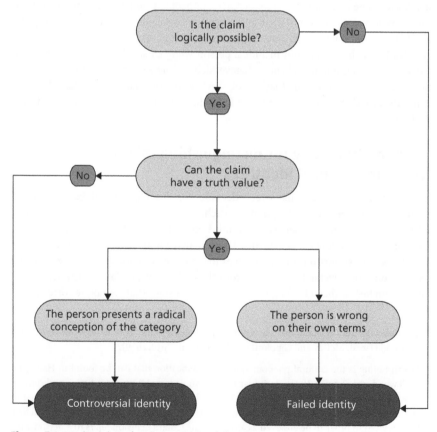

Figure 7.1 Methodology for distinguishing failed from controversial identities.

false, is there a fact of the matter that would enable us to arrive at an answer? The cases discussed in sections 7.3.2 and 7.3.3 fulfill this requirement. If the claim can have a truth value, what we need to do next is to get clear on the nature of the alleged mistake:

(i) The person is wrong on his own terms. M claims to be x because he has y; he accepts along with others that having y justifies belonging to x; but he does not have y where determining y-ness is a matter over which there is consensus (this would be a failed identity).

(ii) The person is wrong in that she is presenting a radical conception of the category in question. M claims to be x because she has z; others do not accept that having z justifies belonging to x; M is presenting a radical (innovative) conception of x that would accommodate her in virtue of having z; that conception is rejected by others (this would be a controversial identity).

Note that cases of the first type will not always be easily ascertainable; that is, even if it is clear that a person is claiming to be x because he has y (and is not presenting a radical, new conception), it might not always be feasible to establish the truth or falsity of his y-ness, but it must be possible in principle. On the other hand, claims that cannot have a truth value are simpler to determine: as I have argued in section 7.3.4, such claims cannot be failed identities. They amount to a presentation of a point of view that stands alongside other points of view; it can be debated, shared, or rejected, and in this sense it can be considered within the scope of recognition. Putting all this together, we can see that a delusional identity is not necessarily a failed identity: each claim must be analyzed on its own terms, and the methodology offered here is an approach to doing so.

It could be objected that the qualification *"over which there is consensus"* (stated in the description of the first kind of mistake an agent can make) sneaks in the status quo and limits people's chances in having their claims heard. Their claims are cut-off from the start by the judgment of consensus, the very consensus they are trying to change. In response to this objection, we can say three things: (1) It is unavoidable that we employ standards for assessing claims. It is so because if we forego all standards we also forego the concept of recognition. The structure of recognition juxtaposes an individual self-conception with a collective category to which this self-conception appeals. If all such appeals were automatically validated, then the collective category would have no criteria for membership: it becomes absolutely permissive and hence empty. Not only would this undercut demands for recognition, it would also be extremely counterintuitive; it would mean that anyone can make any sort of identity claim and for this to be immediately valid. (2) The term "consensus" as I use it here applies to relatively unobjectionable claims. For example, there is consensus over the following: to be someone's biological son you must share 50 percent of their DNA; to be African-American you must have a connection to ancestors who were born in sub-Saharan Africa. Furthermore, both claims can be verified in principle, though this might be difficult in practice. If I claim to be someone's son or to be black on the basis of fulfilling these definitions when I actually don't, then I am wrong on my own terms. If I claim either category on the basis of offering a new conception of "son" and "black," then I am not wrong on my own terms but

I might be considered wrong in how I am using these categories; my claim amounts to a controversial and not a failed identity. (3) On the basis of this final point, we can see that by distinguishing *being wrong on one's own terms* from *being wrong in terms of one's conception of the category* we allow for demands that fall in the latter camp to be considered within the scope of recognition. As such, demands that appear to be committing a fundamental mistake can actually be a radical critique to existing categories and hence a possible challenge to the status quo.

7.5 **Conclusion**

The primary question considered in this chapter (and in Chapter 8) is whether madness can be grounds for identity. In section 7.1 I identified three requirements for identity formation while pointing out that, in accordance with widely acknowledged views, madness cannot meet those requirements and hence cannot be grounds for identity. To what extent is this claim true?

This chapter focused on the first requirement: the identity claim that is the basis of the demand for recognition must involve a mistake that can, in principle, be resolved through social and political action by modifying the collective category with which the person is identifying; it must be a controversial identity. Delusional identities, so the argument would go, commit a fundamental kind of mistake and constitute failed identities. The case studies examined in this chapter indicate that this is not necessarily the case. Some delusional identities can, in fact, be conceived of as controversial identities and hence are within the scope of recognition. Accordingly, even though the person is presenting an unorthodox identification with a specific category—an identification that can be described as delusional—such presentation can initiate debate surrounding the inclusiveness, exclusiveness, and overall meaning of the category in question. However, each claim has to be examined on its own merits as to whether it is a failed or a controversial claim. This chapter offered a tentative methodology for doing so, a methodology that can be tested in relation to other identity claims. The key elements of this methodology are to ask: (1) Can the claim have a truth value, and if the answer is yes, (2) is the person wrong on their own terms or are they offering a radical conception of the category with which they are identifying? If the latter—if they are pushing new ground—then even though we might ultimately reject these views, we are presented with a controversial and not a failed identity. In conclusion, delusions (as a key phenomenon of madness) can, in some cases, be grounds for identity.

Chapter 8

Mad identity II: Unity and continuity of self

8.1 **Introduction**

In Chapter 7 I identified three requirements for identity formation that must be met in order for an identity claim to be the kind of claim that can be considered within the scope of recognition: it must be a controversial and not a failed claim; it must be an expression of a unified mental life; and it must persist over a sufficient period of time. The first requirement was examined in Chapter 7 in relation to delusions. The task for this chapter is to examine the second and the third requirements in relation to, respectively, passivity phenomena and the discontinuities of self often experienced by individuals diagnosed with schizophrenia and bipolar disorder. The main issue concerns the impact of certain phenomena on the unity and the continuity of self.

In *Divided Minds and Successive Selves* Jennifer Radden (1996, p. 11) draws a distinction between two ways in which we can speak of the unity of self:

> Normally, a oneness and harmony to the heterogeneity of the experiences of a person *at a given time* allows us to say that they are all the person's experiences. Distinguishable from this is the normal connectedness between a person's experiences *as they are scattered over time*—the linked and enduring nature of sets of traits and experiences through time that allows us to say they are all attributable to the same person.

The former refers to the *unity* of self at a time inviting questions such as "are these (present) experiences all mine (hers)?", and the latter refers to the *continuity* of self over time inviting questions such as "am I (is she) the same person now as I (she) was at some earlier time?" (1996, p. 12).[1] The account of identity summarized in section 7.2.1 and described in detail in section 4.2 requires both kinds of unity of self. Implicit in this account is the requirement that my mental life is unified at any given point in time; that my mental states are experienced as mine, that a particular desire or thought—no matter how unsavory I judge it to be—is still *my* desire and thought. A self that cannot, at the very least, identify with its own mental states cannot develop an encompassing

---

[1] Unity and continuity are also referred to, respectively, as diachronic and synchronic unity of self (see Radden 1998, p. 659).

understanding, precisely because elements for this self-understanding are not being acknowledged, let alone evaluated.[2] Identity also requires continuity of self over time, as our self-conceptions are not momentary happenings and are expected to persist over time: they are defining of a person. Certain instances of mental disorder, as noted in section 7.1, undermine unity and continuity of self and hence undermine two key requirements for identity formation. This chapter explores the nature and extent of these problems, and whether or not they are fatal to the claim that madness can be grounds for identity, a claim upon which rests the coherence of Mad identity as a route recognition.

8.2 **(Dis)unity of self**

8.2.1 **Unity of self**

Unity of self is ordinarily transparent, and it is evident that we only become aware of it when we can no longer take it for granted. What kind of everyday experiences can bring this about? Radden (1996, p. 16) cites several examples, key among which is ambivalence. Ambivalence is a familiar psychological state involving conflict among a person's desires.[3] It manifests in huge difficulties deciding what to do, and these difficulties can be intractable, lasting years and never achieving proper resolution. There are many reasons why we may find ourselves in a situation like this. Perhaps we are ambivalent due to the pull of equally important, yet incompatible, commitments. We may feel that to decide one way or another is to foreclose an emotionally resonant, valuable option. An example of this would be the attempt to honor two life-scripts with which one identifies, scripts which circumstance had brought into conflict with one another. A person can be confronted, for instance, by the impossibility of reconciling her vocational ambitions with her wish to be a dutiful daughter who now has to care for her ailing mother. In other cases, ambivalence is not so much an artifact of mutually incompatible paths, but an indication of a deeper psychological conflict. A person in an abusive relationship may find herself ambivalent about ending it. On the one hand, she can see that her spouse is regularly trying to control, coerce, and undermine her, all sufficient reasons, in her view, to leave him and seek a fulfilling life elsewhere. On the other hand, she resists the idea of ending it for fear that this would hurt their two young children. She is conflicted over which impulse to follow: that which arises from her desire to be fulfilled and happy, or that which arises from her sense of duty toward her family. With continued psychological and emotional assaults on her confidence, ambivalence can become implicated with self-deception. She may say to herself that her spouse is only doing this because he cares for her, and that, after all, he is not a bad person; she may justify remaining in the relationship by saying that she is not worthy of a better person. These examples show that conflict among one's

---

[2] What it is to identify with a mental state is a complex determination (see section 8.2.3). For the purpose of this initial discussion, to identify with, say, a particular desire is to acknowledge that it is one's own and to place it alongside one's other desires and beliefs.

[3] The conflict of relevance here is among a person's second order desires, which are evaluations whose object is a first-order desire (see section 4.2.1).

desires or over courses of action, as Radden (1996) points out, is a "commonplace and natural experience." It comes in degrees of course, and ambivalence in the context of an abusive relationship is certainly among the more distressing and tragic experiences of ambivalence.

Do these examples indicate breakdown in the unity of self? In Radden's (1996, p. 11) description of unity, cited earlier, she refers to it in two ways: as involving *oneness* and as involving *harmony* among a person's experiences. Harmony (and disharmony) apply to elements that have been brought together under a prior unity, for how else would we perceive their copresence as harmonious (or not) had they not been already conceived of, or experienced as, belonging to this unity? It is this prior unity that we can refer to as the *oneness* of the heterogeneous elements. An orchestra, for example, is unified in the sense that all its elements add up to one thing: the orchestra as such. Within this unity, the orchestra can be disharmonious if the various elements, the musicians, are unable to work together in such a way that produces harmonious music. The oneness of an orchestra, on the other hand, can break down if an alien instrument is brought into its midst, an instrument that none of the musicians are able to accept as part of their ensemble. Breakdown in oneness, then, refers to the refusal (or inability) to accept (or identify) a particular element as part of a particular entity's heterogeneity. It is that, and not disharmony, that the expression disunity must be reserved for.

Returning to ambivalence, I propose that cases of the sort described earlier evince disharmony and not breakdown in the oneness of self: so long as there is an experienced conflict among my desires, unity of self in the sense of oneness of self is implied; how else would I experience a conflict had it not been that I identify with my desires? If we follow this line of thought, it would be more accurate to characterize ambivalence as a disharmonious unity.

If disharmony is not the marker of disunity we are left, as argued previously, with persons' identification with their mental states, with lack of identification being evidence for disunity. Some relatively commonplace experiences get us close to this: for example, when someone is intensely in love it is possible to be moved by emotions powerful enough to evoke the experience *as if* one is driven against one's will. Infatuation does not take us right to disunity, however, because the persons involved continue to identify with their mental states: even though the desire is too powerful and seems to have caught me off guard, it is still my desire, and I am already justifying it with reasons (such as the uniqueness of my lover, or our suitability for each other). At the point where I no longer identify with the desire, the *as if* element is gone and it ceases to be experienced as mine. That is the point where we can talk about disunity of self. Examples of disunity of self, in the sense of lack of identification with one's mental states, are evident with certain religious experiences and abound in the mental health literature where they are grouped under the umbrella term "passivity phenomena."

8.2.2 Passivity phenomena

Passivity phenomena are paradigmatic examples of disunity. With these phenomena the subject does not experience the familiarity that people ordinarily have in relation to their thoughts, volitions, impulses, or feelings. In descriptive psychopathology, passivity experiences are among the first-rank symptoms of schizophrenia and include thought insertion and volitional passivity (see Sims 2003, pp. 164–71). Thought insertion is commonly expressed as the belief that the thoughts a person is experiencing are not her own, with further elaboration as to the source of agency to which these thoughts belong. With volitional passivity the subject does not experience her actions as emanating from her own will, attributing them to some outside agent who is controlling her. Some examples:

> I have never read nor heard them; they come unasked; I don't dare to think I am the source but I am happy to know of them without thinking them. They come at any moment like a gift and I do not dare to impart them as if they were my own. (Jaspers 1963, p. 123)

> When I reach for the comb it is my hand and arm which move . . . , but I don't control them. I sit watching them move and they are quite independent, what they do is nothing to do with me . . . I am just a puppet manipulated by cosmic string. (Graham and Stephens 1994, p. 99)

> I wasn't confused and I wasn't disillusioned by anything. I feel I was receiving something. I could feel it. You sense things when you know something. I do believe it is possible to communicate telepathically. At one stage I was with people and they would give us a sign to say I was. I was definitely receiving thoughts. It wasn't my own thoughts made up in my own mind. You can tell the difference. I know my own mind, I know my own self. It's hard to express. Just that you can communicate to people with your mind, without using your mouth. I was recepting [sic] people's thought patterns. It's not as if it's my own thoughts being made up in my own mind.[4]

If passivity phenomena undermine unity of self, then they also undermine one of the requirements for identity formation. The argument can proceed as follows: (1) passivity phenomena undermine unity of self (they constitute a failure of the subject to identify with its mental states); (2) unity of self is a requirement for identity formation (to arrive at an encompassing self-understanding, the subject must be able to identify with its mental states—volitions, impulses, and thoughts—and not attribute them to someone else; failing this, the quality and depth of that self-understanding would be seriously diminished); (3) given this, passivity phenomena undermine a key requirement for identity formation, which suggests that the subject may not yet be within the scope of recognition. In what follows I examine the first premise, for the argument hinges upon it. What is immediately clear from a first pass is that passivity phenomena undermine unity of self only under the assumption that the mental states with which the subject is failing to identify are ones with which the subject should identify; their failure or inability to do so is what constitutes disunity of self. I want to argue that this assumption is more complex than it might seem at first, and that in some cases "passivity" phenomena rather than constituting disunity of self can actually be the basis for a complex and potentially enriching self-understanding. Before making this argument

---

[4] This report is cited in the *Oxford Handbook of Philosophy and Psychiatry* online clinical-case resource. Online: http://fdslive.oup.com/www.oup.com/booksites/uk/booksites/content/9780199579563/clinical/fulford_cases_section1.pdf

and tracing its implications (sections 8.2.4 and 8.2.5), I introduce a key distinction from the philosophical literature on passivity phenomena.

8.2.3 **Ownership and authorship**

Philosophical analyses of passivity phenomena draw a distinction between ownership and authorship of mental states. With reference to thought insertion, ownership refers to "the capacity for acknowledging a thought as one's own," and authorship refers to "endorsement of the content of that thought via reason giving" (Bortolotti and Broome 2009). Phenomenologically, thought insertion displays a failure in both dimensions and hence a failure in self-knowledge (Bortolotti and Broome 2009; Gunn 2016). In typical reports of thought insertion, such as those cited in section 8.2.2, subjects report that the thoughts they are experiencing are neither authored by them nor their own. Analytically, however, the main issue is not ownership, but authorship.

In her analysis of thought insertion and "ego-alien states," Radden (1996, pp. 255–66; 1998) describes such states as examples of "disownership" and identifies two ways in which we can understand this notion: logical (grammatical) and psychological. Logically, argues Radden, our experiences are necessarily owned by us. This is guaranteed by the grammar of "experience" which precludes the possibility of having experiences that are not our own (Radden 1998, p. 666). Phenomenologically, thought insertion is a heterogenous phenomenon. Some people report that their experienced thoughts are not their own; others report only loss of authorship. Notwithstanding the diverse phenomenologies of thought insertion, the key point is that ownership is guaranteed by the fact of the subject having first-person access to the reported experiences. If ownership is "logically guaranteed," as Radden (1998, p. 670) puts it, then the key issue with passivity phenomena lies in the dimension of authorship (see also Graham and Stephens 1994). If ownership concerns the agent in whom the experience occurred, then authorship concerns the agent who produced the experience—two determinations that ordinarily would refer to the same agent.[5] With thought insertion (and passivity more generally), ownership and authorship come apart, for while it is me who is necessarily undergoing that experience (a logical matter), I do not experience being the one who produced it (a psychological matter). Concluding her analysis, Radden (1998, pp. 670–1) writes:

> So these patients' inviolable ownership of their experiences is compatible with their believing those experiences—falsely, but not incoherently—to be other selves' experience. It is also compatible with their believing them to be, and or experiencing them as alien, and or believing them to emanate from an alien source.

....

[5] With reference to thought insertion, Bayne (2013) describes ownership and agency (authorship) as, respectively, the no-subjectivity and the no-agency accounts. In the former, subjects deny that thoughts of which they are aware are actually theirs. In the latter, subjects deny only that they are the agents of the thoughts of which they are aware. Bayne is non-committal on which account is correct. However, I agree with Radden that ownership is logically guaranteed, which would make the no-subjectivity account incoherent: to be introspectively aware of a thought is the same as being the one who is thinking it. Who the author of that thought is, is a separate question.

I agree with Radden's account and with the crucial distinction between ownership and authorship. It allows us to identify the basis of the assumption underpinning the claim that passivity phenomena undermine unity of self. This can now be stated as follows: *under normal conditions a person should be the author of all of her mental states*; lack of authorship undermines unity of self. Putting it this way shows that we are talking about an ideal, a measure of normal experience: any cleaving of ownership from authorship is a violation of this ideal and evidence of disunity of self. How has this ideal come to be so intuitive to the extent that it is presupposed by theoretical discussions on passivity phenomena?

8.2.4 Passivity phenomena and cultural psychology

The ideal of unity of self requires that ownership and authorship must not come apart: if they do we have disunity of self and hover close to the realm of psychopathology.[6] As an ideal, it concerns the *right* way persons should relate to their mental states; it is underpinned by a normative psychological theory that does not permit external authorship of mental states. It is a theory that puts a premium on maintaining clear boundaries between self and other, where other agents cannot, as it were, encroach upon and influence my mental life (except indirectly, say through conversation). It is also a *cultural* psychological theory in the sense that its presuppositions are relative to a specific context.[7] Remarking upon this psychological perspective, Fabrega (1989, p. 53) writes:

> [The ideal self is] autonomous, separate, sharply bounded and wilful. It originates or is the source of its own activity, and outside influences cannot control it. Properties of the self include thoughts (as well as actions and feelings), which are like language statements that are a part of the mind, and the self owns and controls them. They are secret and private things no one except the self can know about.

Though we may disagree with some of the details of this description, the general picture is readily identifiable. Such normative assumptions about the ideal self provide the measure by which passivity experiences, and other symptoms of "schizophrenia," are considered to be abnormal. In light of such a psychological theory, any cleaving of ownership from authorship is bound to be seen as a disunity of self, followed by inquires as to why this had occurred.[8]

....

[6] Note that in so far as auditory verbal hallucinations (AVH) involve misinterpretation of inner speech as external voices, a similar analysis can be offered for AVH as offered here for passivity phenomena.

[7] In *Psychiatric Judgements Across Cultural Contexts* (Rashed 2013c, pp. 139–44) I examine, through a historical/genealogical account, such a cultural psychology in its relation to the epistemological stance that accompanied the rise of modern science. Psychiatric norms and the folk psychology underpinning them are based on distinctive brands of normality and relationships to reality, or what we can call modes of engagement with the world.

[8] All such inquiries begin with the premise that subjects are misidentifying their mental states (e.g., their "inner speech" or thoughts). Given this premise, the inquiry then becomes an investigation into an absence and not into a positive phenomenon: the question becomes "Why is this person misidentifying her own mental states?". And the various approaches give their own distinctive answer (e.g., psychodynamic, cognitive, or neuropsychological).

If we adopt a different cultural psychology, one where under certain conditions external agents can directly influence one's thoughts and actions, then ownership and authorship can come apart without this necessarily implying a threat to unity of self, but an *addition* to the self. Consider the following story of Mahdi, a thirty-two-year-old man I met while conducting fieldwork in the Dakhla oasis of Egypt (Rashed 2012). This is Mahdi's account of his involvement with a female *jinni* (a "spirit"):

I have a woman cohabiting with me for several years, ten years. When she first appeared I was not able to stay at home; I would run away and walk the town all night. I am *mekhawy* [attached/in a relationship with a *jinni*].

In the beginning when she used to appear I would be terrified, but she beautified herself along the years. In the beginning I wanted to go to a Sheikh to get rid of her, but she began to help me, she cares about me. For example she would tell me the personality of the person in front of me, and if a person would hurt me I would just leave and find some excuse. I show people nothing but a surface, but I know a lot and I understand people.

She only appears at night when everyone is asleep. I go to my bedroom and she spends the night with me. We copulated several times. To the extent that her love for me makes her complicate the engagements I enter. To the extent that I would be at the coffee-house and she would tell me "go check on this woman you love, see her true nature." Or, she would put thoughts in my mind that my fiancé is not to be trusted. I would go and find that it was true, that she was standing with a man talking. And this happened several times, and she was always right. She can read my thoughts and know what is worrying me. Once I was visiting my fiancée in her house, and her father left us to talk in private. We were just about to hold hands when I suddenly slapped her, but it was not me who did that, she [the *jinni*] gets very jealous.

[How often does she talk to you?] Most of the time, but it increases when there is a problem. She tells me the personality of the person in front of me, and advises me. Could you know who to trust and who not to trust? You can't know yourself, but she tells me. I could ask for anything, thousands of pounds, cars, but I don't want to let her control me. But I am so used to her now. When she goes away for a few days, I miss her.

In descriptive psychopathology, Mahdi's account recalls several key psychiatric symptoms including: auditory hallucinations (second-person and command hallucinations), thought insertion, volitional passivity, and passivity of impulse.[9] Within the psychological perspective outlined earlier, all of these symptoms indicate marked disunity of self, evident in that Mahdi does not experience himself as the author of some of his mental states. If we stay with Mahdi's account, however, a different picture emerges. As he had told me, he is *mekhawi*, an Arabic term derived from the root for

---

[9] Mahdi told me that the *jinni* accompanies him "morning and night, any time." When I explored this with him the nature of the jinni's presence became apparent. He "knows" that she is always with him and he, sometimes, experiences her "presence" by his side in the absence of any auditory or visual signs of her presence. This recalls the feeling, occasionally reported both with psychotic and non-psychotic states, of "being beside oneself, alongside oneself or having another self" (Sims 2003, p. 217).

"brother"; it refers to a state of closeness, even intimate involvement between two individuals. In the cultural context of Dakhla, it is acknowledged that this state can occur between a human being and a *jinni*, usually of the opposite sex. It may be suspected, for example, if a young man or woman refuses eligible suitors for no good reason. It is thought that the infatuated *jinni* affects the person's moods and perceptions in the presence of a suitor to facilitate a refusal, thus keeping the person for her- or himself. Sometimes the *jinni* would make its presence explicit, talking to the person and appearing to them in bed at night. The persons affected may resist this presence, this relationship, if it hampers marriage or their ability to carry out duties in general, or otherwise they may accept it if it brings some benefits.

So there is a cultural script, underpinned by a distinctive cultural psychology, that allows for these kinds of unusual but nonpathological influences on the self. This script structured Mahdi's experiences, giving them both personal and social meaning. Neither Mahdi, nor members of the community who endorsed this script, considered these states as indicators of disunity of self; rather there was influence and interaction with an agent that was not of the self. If we look at Mahdi's account from this perspective, what emerges is a complicated relationship with the spirit, a relationship that has the ingredients of dramatic human interactions: care, control, fear, jealousy, love, insecurity, loss; a much richer picture than would be possible through the vocabulary of disownership and disunity. Given this distinctive cultural psychology, Mahdi's experiences appear as an enrichment and not as a breakdown of self.[10] What implications does this carry for judgments of disunity of self?

8.2.5 Judgment of disunity: The role of context and activism

In the foregoing analysis, the judgment that there is disunity of self depends, in part, on the cultural psychological assumptions in place concerning the possibility of external authorship of mental states. It also depends on the perspective from where this judgment is issuing; as Radden (1996, p. 12) notes, "the self's disunity and discontinuity may be understood introspectively and from the more detached perspective of the public stance." A public perspective where external authorship of mental states is not possible will regard passivity experiences as evidence of disunity of self—this perspective is exemplified by scientific theories of schizophrenia and psychosis. Conversely, a public perspective where external authorship is possible will not see in passivity experiences evidence of disunity but of an addition to the self—this perspective can be found, among other contexts, in the community of the Dakhla oasis I referred to earlier.

---

[10] Pointing out the cultural psychological basis of judgements of disunity does not commit us to endorsing a rival cultural psychology; that is, we do not have to believe in spirits and other ethereal beings in order to accept that Mahdi's experiences, in the context of a particular cultural psychology, represent an enrichment and not a breakdown of self. The confrontation of rival cultural psychologies (and hence of worldviews) is a separate matter. It is a confrontation where one worldview can seek to demonstrate its superiority vis-a-vis the other in relation to a defined set of concerns (see Rashed 2013c).

The subjective perspective is more complex, as subjects' prior beliefs concerning the possibility of external authorship will impact on how they relate to their experiences. Recall that a defining feature of passivity experiences is the loss of the usual sense of authorship we have in relation to our mental states, a loss that is frequently made sense of by invoking other external agents, or authors, of our mental states. Given this, if the subject does not ordinarily believe that external authorship of mental states is possible, then passivity phenomena can generate a state of dissonance between the subject's prior beliefs and current experiences. Conversely, if the subject has a prior belief that external authorship is possible—like Mahdi in the aforementioned example—then a state of dissonance need not arise. The duality of perspectives (public versus subjective), and the complexity of subjects' relationship to their experiences, create a range of possibilities for disagreement. Pulling these possibilities together, I want to consider four scenarios that shed light on judgments of disunity of self and the role of context and activism in this. The scenarios have been simplified in order to focus the discussion on key elements (see Table 8.1).[11]

In each scenario there are two opportunities for dissonance: there is the possibility of *internal* dissonance issuing from discrepancy between the subject's current experiences and prior beliefs concerning external authorship; and there is the possibility of *external* dissonance (or lack of congruence) between the subjective and the public judgments on whether there is disunity of self. In the first scenario there is no dissonance of either type. In the second scenario there is no internal dissonance, but there is external dissonance. Diagnostic procedures in psychiatry have allowance for the second scenario, evident in the advice that experiences and beliefs shared with members of a person's cultural community must not be regarded as psychopathology, even if they resemble psychiatric phenomenology.[12] External dissonance in the second scenario may therefore be an artifact of employing the wrong context to assess other persons' beliefs and experiences.[13] There is no immediate reason why Mahdi, simply by virtue of moving from Dakhla to London, should bear the brunt of a mismatch in psychological and other assumptions between the context in which he grew up (and whose assumptions he internalized), and the one in which he now finds himself. The second scenario thus calls for suspension of judgment subject to further ethnographic and individual understanding of the situation (see Rashed 2013a, 2013c, pp. 134–6).

The third scenario is the situation of most mental health consultations where clinician and patient share the cultural psychological assumption that external authorship of mental states is not possible. Consider, for example, Sarah, an English person who

---

[11] Note that there are other issues at play aside from belief in the possibility of external authorship of mental states. For example, even though this belief exists in Dakhla, there are criteria for fulfilling the relevant kind of experience. It is possible for a person's report that her thoughts are influenced by a "spirit" to be rejected by the community or the relevant experts: "spirits" communicate in specific ways and not every claim to be in communion with "them" is valid.

[12] See Chapter 7, footnote 6.

[13] Elsewhere I explore what a right context of judgement might be, how to determine this, and why congruence with a relevant cultural context matters at all (see Rashed 2013a).

Table 8.1 Scenarios of unity and disunity of self with passivity phenomena

	1: Cultural congruence	2: Cultural incongruence	3: Mental health	4a: Medical response	4b: Social response
Is external authorship possible from public perspective?	Yes	No	No	No	No
Is external authorship possible from subjective perspective?	Yes	Yes	No	No	Yes
Does the subject experience internal dissonance?	No	No	Yes	Yes	No
Is there a subjective judgment of disunity?	No	No	Depends on outcome: 4a or 4b	Yes	No
Is there a public judgment of disunity?	No	Yes	Yes	Yes	Yes
Is there external dissonance (lack of congruence)?	No	Yes	Depends on outcome: 4a or 4b	No	Yes
Example	Mahdi among his community in the Dakhla oasis	Mahdi in conversation with mental health professional	Sarah in conversation with mental health professionals	Sarah after adopting a medical view of her experiences	Sarah in engagement with activism
Outcome	Overlap in subjective and public judgments	Disagreement in judgments with the need to seek the right context	Either medical response (4a) or social response (4b)	"Insight" is gained with agreement in judgments. Internal dissonance is entrenched	Disagreement in judgments occasioning a demand for recognition

grew up in Cambridge and moved to London as an adult. Consistent with the context in which she grew up, Sarah does not ordinarily believe that external authorship of mental states is possible. Her experience of thought insertion is putting a strain on this, resulting in internal dissonance. The public judgment is likely to be that there is disunity of self, a judgment with which Sarah may or may not concur, for she is not yet certain as to whether what she is experiencing indicates disunity of self. In other words, she is not yet sure whether her experiences invalidate her prior assumptions or whether those assumptions invalidate her experiences. Accordingly, the third scenario can proceed in two ways (scenarios 4a and 4b in Table 8.1).

The approach that tends to be pursued in the majority of psychiatric consultations is to encourage Sarah to regard the psychological theory by which external authorship is not possible as the measure of her experiences (scenario 4a). This is for Sarah to accept that she deviates from normative psychological standards and that these standards invalidate her experiences (practically, this involves describing Sarah's experiences in the language of psychopathology and offering her a diagnosis; if this approach is successful it would be said that she has gained "insight"). This might produce agreement on the question of disunity of self (and therefore resolve the external dissonance), but it might not resolve the internal dissonance. If anything, it could entrench it further by prioritizing psychological standards that continue to contradict her experiences (assuming Sarah does not opt for treatment that might stop these experiences).[14]

The second way in which the third scenario can proceed is represented in Table 8.1 by scenario 4b. In that instance, a question is raised whether the psychological standards deployed are the right measure of judgment. Recall that in the second scenario we did the same, but whereas the goal there was to seek the most appropriate context of judgment (ethnographically speaking), in this scenario that context may not yet exist and needs to be *created*: this is where activism has a role to play. The various counternarratives of psychological diversity advanced by activists can be regarded as attempts to create contexts of judgment that are more appropriate to people undergoing experiences such as passivity phenomena and auditory hallucinations ("voices"). For example, Sarah may get together with other people who have similar experiences and construct alternative understandings of passivity phenomena that allow for external authorship of mental states. Sarah cannot do this on her own, for part of the force and potential legitimacy of a counternarrative is that it is shared among a group. In creating such a context, the first achievement would be to resolve the internal dissonance, for there would no longer be a mismatch between her beliefs and her experiences. Scenario 4b, therefore, is similar to the second scenario in that there is no internal dissonance while there is external dissonance (lack of congruence). But whereas in the second scenario an attempt is made to seek the right context of judgment, in scenario

---

[14] The following report, cited in Gunn (2016, p. 562), shows a similar transformation to the one described in the text, from entertaining the possibility that one's experiences indicate "telepathy" to regarding them as part of "psychosis": "Often, in a quiet place, and all the time at night when I am alone, I experience thoughts that do not 'feel' like my own. It's like they come out of a part of my brain that is not the part that controls my 'normal' thoughts and into my awareness from there. It is hard to describe. These 'false thoughts' are usually about random subject matter and usually make little sense, but are extremely distracting. Back when I first experienced them, I thought I was psychic and that I was picking up other people's thoughts (telepathy?). However, now I know that they are a part of psychosis because I experience them around the times I hallucinate."

4b activists construct alternative contexts and demand recognition of various counter-narratives as valid alternatives to medical and psychological understandings of passivity phenomena. If this final objective is realized, then scenario 4b becomes identical to the first: there would be neither internal nor external dissonance, and no grounds for claiming disunity of self.

8.2.6 Conclusion

By analyzing the claim that passivity phenomena undermine unity of self and hence a person's encompassing self-understanding, we have seen the complexity of such judgments and the role of context and activism in this. Clearly, the claim that persons should be the authors of all their mental states, though intuitive, oversimplifies the issues and takes for granted a set of cultural psychological assumptions. Once we account for the perspectives in place and the assumptions underpinning them, we are able to get a clearer picture: there are situations in which a person can experience passivity phenomena without this constituting disunity of self (scenarios 1 and 2 in Table 8.1). There are also situations that bring us closer to the discourse of psychopathology where we can talk about passivity phenomena being a threat to identity formation (scenarios 3 and 4a). But even in those cases, the possibility of creating new contexts of judgment through activism can transform such situations to ones in which there is no disunity (scenario 4b). Given this, and returning to the problem that led us here, we cannot make a general statement that passivity phenomena always undermine unity of self and with it a key requirement for identity formation. If that is the case, then passivity phenomena do not necessarily remove the subject from the scope of recognition, in fact the very same phenomena can play a key role in a person's self-understanding. And in cases where they appear to remove the subject from the scope of recognition, activist counternarratives can have a therapeutic role in bringing persons within this scope, an idea developed in Chapter 9 (sections 9.4.2 and 9.5).

8.3 (Dis)continuity of self

8.3.1 Continuity of self

In addition to requiring *unity* of self at a time, identity claims that can be considered within the scope of recognition require *continuity* of self over time. To clarify the notion of continuity, Iris Murdoch's (1999, pp. 80–1) description of how we encounter others is a good place to start:

> When we apprehend and assess other people we do not consider only their solutions to specifiable practical problems, we consider something more elusive which may be called their total vision of life, as shown in their mode of speech or silence, their choice of words, their assessment of others, their conception of their own lives, what they think attractive or praiseworthy, what they think funny . . . what, making two points in the two metaphors, one may call the texture of a man's being or the nature of his personal vision.

Murdoch's expectations of other people are ambitious—How many among us have a clearly articulated "total vision of life"?—but the key point remains: when we talk about identity we are talking about self-conceptions that are overarching and have a temporal dimension; we expect them to be enduring: tomorrow I anticipate that I will continue to hold the values, beliefs, and plans that I endorse today. If we eliminate the temporal dimension, we would lose this notion of identity and would be left with a succession of barely connected snapshots. One is reminded of the original View-Master stereoscopes that were popular in the 1960s, 1970s, and 1980s, where the user would repeatedly flick a button to move and view a reel of small color photographs usually of beautiful vistas and tourist attractions. Each photo on the reel was a self-contained, vivid 3-D image and shared with the others a flimsy connection such as being photos of "Paris" or of "The Sahara." Nevertheless, each photo could be viewed on its own without this rendering it any less vivid, beautiful, or self-contained.

Evidently, though, this is not a satisfactory view of identity: a snapshot of a person at a given moment in time can only make full sense in terms of how it derives from *that* person's past, and how it connects to *his* or *her* future. It can only make sense, that is, if there is continuity of self over time. It is because most people assume such continuity, that even though a person may revise her values, beliefs, and plans (and change drastically in the process), she *remains the same person even as she changes*. This final assumption appears necessary in order for us to be able to understand ourselves—and for others to understand us—in a certain way, but is it a legitimate assumption to make? The issue pertains to the persistence of numerical identity over time, a vexed and long-debated issue formulated by Derek Parfit (1984, p. 202) as follows: "what makes a person at two different times one and the same person?". Typically, answers to this question proceed by providing a set of necessary and sufficient conditions for numerical identity, an endeavor that gets very complicated very quickly.[15] Notwithstanding these attempts, continuity of self over time is a necessary view to maintain from a pragmatic point of view. This means that we need to construct such continuity in order for goods that are coterminous with it to be available to us, and fundamental among these goods is the very notion of agency.

In an important essay Christine Korsgaard sidesteps the metaphysical problems associated with the question of the persistence of numerical identity in favor of a pragmatic view. She argues that even if it can be established that "there is no deep sense in which I am identical to the subject of experiences who will occupy my body in the future . . . I nevertheless have reasons for regarding myself as the same rational agent as the one who will occupy my body in the future" (Korsgaard 1989, p. 109). These reasons are practical and not metaphysical in nature. Korsgaard begins her argument by noting that much of what we do can only be accomplished over a period of time. All action takes us into the future, and many of our valued projects and plans occupy months, years, and sometimes a lifetime; for example, being a friend, spouse, or parent,

---

[15] Standard views divide into those that explain persistence in terms of physical continuity (a spatiotemporally continuous body), and those that explain it in terms of psychological continuity (inheritance of memories, beliefs, connections between current intention and future action, and so on)—see Olson (2003) for an overview. Physical continuity explanations are subject to fatal counterexamples, and psychological continuity has been famously attacked by Parfit (1984), who argued that this sort of identity relation is not what matters for our survival over time.

developing a career, writing a book, finishing a degree, or training for a marathon. In committing ourselves to such projects "we both presuppose and construct a continuity of identity and of agency" (1989, p. 113). The argument is this: a deliberative choice made in the present is made on the basis of reasons; our choices and our most-valued projects extend beyond the present moment into the future, and so do our reasons for choosing them; my present self therefore identifies with my future self in order to be able to make a choice now (since choosing now commits it to those reasons in the future), and for something like a project or life-plan to be practically possible (since long-term projects place demands on our future conduct that we will need to buy into when that moment arrives); in this way continuity of self over time is maintained, and the necessity for doing so arises from the demands of practical reason.[16]

Korsgaard's approach is notable in that it argues for continuity of self over time by demonstrating the necessity of such a conception for our concept of agency. In a commentary on Korsgaard's argument, Radden (1996, p. 201) puts it like this: "a merely present self cannot encompass or match the instigator of life plans and actions, whose perspective spans more than the present moment." If my present self is unable to identify with my future self—if, for whatever reason, I am unable to conceive of myself as unified over time—then the goods that would otherwise be potentially available to me would be foreclosed. I would not be able to instigate and pursue projects on the grounds that I would not be able to assume that my future self will buy into the reasons, values, and goals of my present self. "Only the notion of a unitary self," Radden (1996, p. 196) notes, "will permit us to preserve the concepts and distinctions surrounding our sense of ourselves as voluntary agents, planners, and goal-directed actors." But the notion of a unitary self permits of degrees, and the consideration of some mental health conditions in the following sections will show that the assumption of continuity of self over extended periods of time is one that cannot always be made (e.g., in cases of dissociative identity disorder and bipolar disorder). Given this, we can ask with Radden, how much continuity is sufficient for preservation of our valued concepts? In this case, how much "continuity [is] sufficient for agency"? (Radden 1996, p. 229). If we understand agency, as we do here, as the capacity to instigate and pursue projects, then continuity of self is sufficient in so far as it allows the pursuance of projects. The question therefore becomes one of time frames: How long is a project, a few months, years, or an entire lifetime?

Radden (1996, p. 229) objects to the idea that the concept of agency can only be sustained under the assumption of continuity of self over an entire lifetime; she writes:

> The features of human agency linking earlier and later moments of a life, thought and action, plan and execution, expectation and outcome, need not span a human lifetime to be meaningful. We make and execute plans for an hour away or a day or five years, and to do so seems to require the same concept of agency, and all it implies, as the one we employ when we plan for a lifetime.

---

[16] Bratman (2007, p. 21) makes a similar point, arguing that we do not just act from moment to moment, "we form prior plans and policies that organize our activity over time. And we see ourselves as agents who persist over time and who begin, develop, and then complete temporally extended activities and projects."

The idea is this: many of our projects occupy variable periods of time, and because projects—irrespective of their lengths—exhibit the same features of agency, the continuity of self sufficient to sustain the concept of agency does not require the span of a lifetime. I agree with Radden on this point: conceptually, agency does not require the perspective of a lifetime. Socially and evaluatively, however, it requires more than the perspective of a few minutes at a time, or is it a few hours, or a few days? The point is that there is no clear-cut answer possible here, and the question of how long a project should be falls back on what societies and individuals value. A brief glance at communities around the world and across time would show that friendship, companionship, vocational accomplishment, and parenthood—to name a few long-term projects—are valued almost universally, though people vary in what they consider to be of primary importance. And where certain projects are not valued at all—where, say, notions such as "career" and "marriage" are ridiculed—that would be in favor of other long-term perspectives on life. "Living in the moment," elevated to a dictum, is the project to end all projects, and hence becomes itself a form of long-term accomplishment. While the concept of agency does not require the perspective of a lifetime, socially and evaluatively most forms of human accomplishment are time-intensive, and will require continuity of self coterminous with them.

It follows that if a person, for whatever reason, is unable to construct continuity of self, he or she would lose out on the ability to instigate and pursue projects and to maintain an identity over time. Certain instances of mental disorder can manifest in discontinuity of self, interrupting a person's identity. This can be noted, for example, when an individual's personality changes to such an extent that it becomes difficult to sustain the idea that she remains the same self she was before. In a lay sense, discontinuity of self is picked up against something apparently stable, which is continuity of the person's body, the issue being that the self that inhabits this body now appears radically different from the self that inhabited this body at an earlier point in time. Examples of such discontinuity abound in the clinical literature and in the beliefs and practices of many communities around the world. In what follows I consider discontinuity as it manifests in schizophrenia and bipolar disorder, but in order to get a better sense of what it involves I begin with a brief discussion of cases where it is dramatically demonstrated: spirit possession and, its naturalized cousin, dissociative identity disorder (DID, also known as multiple personality disorder).

8.3.2 Spirit possession and dissociative identity disorder

Spirit possession refers to a broad set of beliefs, experiences, and practices that are ubiquitous in most regions of the world (see Rashed 2018b). The defining feature of spirit possession is the involvement of a noncorporeal agent with a human host in a variety of ways. Those agents are usually referred to as spirits and include a host of assumed ethereal beings such as ghosts of departed ancestors, demons, and divine entities. Spirit possession can be helpfully mapped into two forms: pathogenic and executive (Cohen 2008). Pathogenic possession refers to the belief that a spirit has intruded into a person's body causing various kinds of physical and psychological changes; it does not involve identity alteration, and spirit intrusion is invoked as a causal explanation of certain desired/undesired states. On the other hand, executive possession refers to a state in which the host's identity and agency are displaced by that of the spirit. This form of possession can involve either a partial or a full displacement of the host's identity. With partial displacement, only certain aspects of the host's behavior are attributed to the spirit. With full displacement, the person's body becomes a medium through which the spirit or spirits speak and act. During such episodes the person is likely to be in a trance state; he or she would not have full conscious awareness of the episode and, subsequently, limited memory of it. Executive possession, in the form of full displacement, clearly demonstrates discontinuity of self; the person is eclipsed by the spirit, which is conceived of as a being in its own right with a name, a religion, a vocation, and a personality.[17]

Executive possession recalls another condition: dissociative identity disorder (DID). In DID the person has several personality states (or "alters"), any one of which assumes control at a given moment, and each has its own "relatively enduring pattern of perceiving, relating to, and thinking about the environment and self."[18] Spirit possession and DID share many points of similarity: radical identity alteration, discontinuity of self, total or partial loss of control over behavior, and limited memory of such states (Bourguignon 1989, 2005). Spirits differ from alters in key ways: a spirit is a public phenomenon and ideas about it are constructed socially—it is not conceived of as internal but external to the person's psyche. On the other hand, an alter is commonly seen as a personal, psychological entity that reflects aspects of the person's psyche. Further, while both possession by a spirit and switching from one alter to another can occur spontaneously, the emergence of the former is typically associated with ritual contexts. Nevertheless, both phenomena appear to fulfill Radden's (1996, p. 41) helpful typology of criteria for multiplicity of selves:

> 1. *Separate-agency*: Separate selves will have separate agendas. 2. *Separate-personality*: Separate selves will exhibit distinct, nonagential personality traits singly or jointly. . . . 3. *Continuity condition*: Separate selves will persist through time. 4. *Disordered-awareness condition*: Disordered awareness on the part of at least one self will result in disordered memory in the subject in excess of that found in normal people.

How do these criteria fare in the case of schizophrenia and bipolar disorder?

8.3.3 Schizophrenia

Schizophrenia is widely considered to manifest in radical changes in self-awareness and personality, hence the question of continuity of self over time is raised. In *General Psychopathology*, Karl Jaspers (1963, p. 126) cites the following narrative given by a man after the onset of psychosis:

---

[17] For further accounts of spirit possession, see Cohen (2007, 2008) and Rashed (2012, 2018b). For DID, see Littlewood (2004) and Clark (2013).

[18] *Diagnostic and Statistical Manual of Mental Disorders IV-TR*, American Psychiatric Association (2000).

When telling my story I am aware that only part of my present self experienced all this. Up to 23rd December 1901, I cannot call myself my present self; the past self seems now like a little dwarf inside me. It is an unpleasant feeling; it upsets my feeling of existence if I describe my previous experiences in the first person. I can do it if I use an image and recall that the dwarf reigned up to that date, but since then his part has ended.

More recently, Wells (2003, p. 299) writes about a young woman's experiences of what he describes as the "early stages of schizophrenia." She told Wells that she was "in the process of becoming someone else, that her self had left her, somehow, that she was fundamentally different than she had once been and discontinuous with that person" (2003). She expressed this impending loss in those words: "I know I'm still myself, but it doesn't feel that way. Where I was is filled with noise and voices, and there's—it's a small area, the brain, but there's a huge emptiness there that I used to fill" (2003).

In contrast to the sense of uncertainty presiding over these narratives, for some individuals the new person they are becoming is identified and named. Identity-delusions, where a person comes to believe that he is a prophet, a monarch, or some powerful and/or famous person, are of this kind. The new identity emerges as a revelation, and aspects of the past are reinterpreted to support the new self-understanding.[19]

Returning to the criteria for multiplicity of selves described by Radden, we can see that the first three criteria apply to these cases. Both describe the emergence of a new self that is discontinuous with the previous self. We can assume that, in time, the new self will have distinct agency and personality (in the case of identity-delusions it already does). What seems to be lacking is criterion 4: the "disordered memory" criterion. In contrast to DID where one self may not have awareness of the other selves (or alters), in these cases the present self is aware of the loss of the original self, thereby indicating that it is remembered. What we have here then is not *multiplicity* of self, but *discontinuity* of self and the emergence (gradual or sudden) of a new one.

It is important to be clear about what is being said here. Discontinuity of self can manifest in two directions: as the inability to identify with one's past self or with one's future self. The former is evident in the cases mentioned earlier: the narrative is from the perspective of the present self looking at what it once was, at a past self that has been, or is being, consigned to a side role: "the dwarf reigned up to that date, but since then his part has ended." This rift suggests that the present self would struggle to identify with the past self, and hence may not identify with past values and projects. This can result in suspension of relationships, commitments, and other long-term

---

[19] In the following excerpt, Craig Hamilton (2005, p. 2), a news reporter who was just about to start covering the Sydney Olympics, describes how it dawned upon him that he was Jesus Christ (he speaks from the vantage point of someone who had gained insight): "Now, if this tale is not weird enough already, then try this: in my mind I had become Jesus Christ reincarnate. This is delusion on the grandest scale. The Jesus notion hadn't struck me like a lightning bolt but, rather, taken shape as a result of the escalating mania throwing off grandiose delusions . . . All the events of my life to that point had been readying me for this occasion, or so I thought. In the two days before arriving at the railway station my Olympics planning had changed. I had a new assignment. It was perfectly clear: I was going to change the world. My gospel for the global audience was disarm, feed the hungry and love one another."

projects a person was engaged in. Discontinuity of self can also consist in the inability to identify with one's future self; to what extent is this a problem here? Let us return to DID, a condition where this problem is particularly notable, and then reconsider schizophrenia.

Wells (2003, pp. 300–3) describes the case of Mary, a woman in her thirties with severe DID. Mary experiences multiple personality states with spontaneous switching from one to the other. She also experiences memory gaps across the different states and significant loss of continuity in her life. For example, she finds it difficult to maintain a relationship with her daughter:

> I've been cheated . . . Almost eighteen years have gone by since my daughter was born, and I haven't even had the opportunity to live most of it. Somebody else got my fucking time, and I don't care which part of me it was. (Wells 2003, p. 301)

Loss of continuity placed huge challenges on their relationship; her daughter had told her once "how hard it was to go to school when she did not know who would be at home [which alter] when she returned" (Wells 2003, p. 300). We have seen that in order to continue discharging our obligations with regard to our different roles, we need to construct a continuity of self (and therefore of agency) over time. As discussed in section 8.3.1, identifying with one's future self is necessary for preserving a rich concept of agency. If I know that tomorrow I may be taken over by a different personality state, one with its own pattern of perceiving and relating to the world, then my ability to commit to projects that take me into the future will be compromised. In a commentary on Mary's situation, Kennett and Matthews (2003, p. 309) interpret these difficulties in similar terms:

> Ordinarily we can rely on our later selves buying into the projects of our earlier counterparts because the rational dispositions driving activities in their support are preserved over time, and simply because the later self conceives of itself as bearing the same relation to the project as before. It conceives of itself this way because it conceives of itself as being the same owner of the project. But once again, the path ahead for a switching DID sufferer cannot supply such a continuity of conception, and so quite explicit commitments now to complete plans then will not always be sufficient to complete one's projects.

With schizophrenia, prompted by the examples outlined earlier, there is no suggestion that the person is unable to identify with his or her future self in the same way that we find in DID.[20] On the other hand, as already noted, there may be difficulties autobiographically uniting present and past selves.

8.3.4 **Bipolar disorder**

With bipolar disorder, a different kind of discontinuity of self is apparent. Bipolar disorder is characterized by alternating states of manic and depressed mood, each associated with distinctive levels of psychic and motor activity (see Sims 2003, pp. 313–22).

---

[20] What could be problematic is loss of trust that one will persevere into the future without radically changing again, and without confidence in this it is possible that the person loses the motivation to instigate and carry through long-term projects (see Kennett 2009).

With mania, the person's mood is elevated for a variable period of time and is associated with rapid activity of thinking (flight of ideas), and fast, uninterruptible speech (pressure of speech) to express the multitude of one's thoughts (2003). During a manic episode, the person is restless and distractible with uncharacteristically high energy levels. They can become increasingly optimistic about life and may start grandiose or unrealistic projects—which they rarely finish—while abandoning prior commitments such as their job. Typically, during manic episodes persons engage in behaviors that are risky and out of character (at least as judged by others). They may, for example, partake in a series of sexual encounters or spend the family money to buy, on a whim, an expensive object. All these changes suggest that with bipolar disorder the differences between the person's self during a manic episode and his or her depressed (or normal) self are sufficiently notable so as to warrant talk about discontinuity of self.

Radden (2004, p. 138) argues that bipolar disorders "challenge the customary continuity we associate with normal multiplex persons" in such a way that invites "a description of the manic and depressed selves as more than mere aspects of a single identity."[21] Elsewhere (Radden 1996, pp. 62–6), she discusses the case of Mr. M, a thirty-three-year-old postal worker who is married and a father of two. One day he announced that he was "bursting with energy" and that he was "wasting his talent" in his job as a postman. He stayed up all night working an elaborate plan for a business venture. Next day he quit his job and, using the family savings, bought a large amount of tropical-fish equipment convinced that he had figured out a way to make millions by modifying this equipment. Mr. M, writes Radden (1996, p. 63), has become "provocative, optimistic, reckless, ambitious, and energetic," a contrast with his traits both before and after the episode.

There appears to be a clear disconnect between Mr. M's traits and behavior before, during, and after the manic episode. Does this disconnect amount to discontinuity of self? Immediately we have to qualify the question: Who is asking? In the vignettes cited earlier to demonstrate discontinuity of self in persons diagnosed with schizophrenia, it was the persons themselves who noted a rift with their earlier self. But if we were to ask Mr. M during his manic episode, he might not report discontinuity. In fact, he had already given reasons for the sudden change in behavior: he is wasting his talents at his current job, and he has figured out a way to make more money.[22] Things will look different when he returns to his usual mood and self, or if he experiences a depressive episode. At that point, the manic episode and the associated behavior can appear to him entirely out of character; as Radden (1996, p. 65) puts it, the whole episode becomes something that happened to him, rather than something that he did. By contrast, the family and colleagues of a person experiencing a manic episode are likely to judge, from the start, that he had changed to the point of being discontinuous with his earlier self. The partner of a man discussed by Wells (2003, p. 298)—a man

---

[21] "Normal multiplex persons" are those majority of people who go through complex, heterogenous personality and mood states, yet demonstrate unity in this diversity.

[22] Radden (1996, p. 65) makes a similar point: "from Mr. M's point of view at the time, it is clear that he took this personal alteration to be normal. His new knowledge and ideas naturally led to his changes."

experiencing manic episodes—was very clear about this: "he's not my husband . . . I like him fine, but he's a different person." When relatives, colleagues, and the person him- or herself report discontinuity between the manic and earlier (or later) selves, they are not normally saying that the person has been replaced by an identical looking impostor who happens to have a different personality; what they are saying is that the "normal" self has been temporarily eclipsed by an episode of "illness." Discontinuity in the case of bipolar disorder is therefore a judgment that can be made by family and friends, as well as by the person himself once he is no longer in a manic phase and is able to regard that phase as an external imposition on him, perhaps due to "illness."

8.3.5 **Overcoming discontinuity of self**

How can discontinuity of self with schizophrenia and bipolar disorder be overcome? The first thing to note is the pattern in place: with schizophrenia, discontinuity is longitudinal, evident in difficulties autobiographically uniting past and present selves. With bipolar disorder, discontinuity is cyclical, evident in difficulties autobiographically uniting the manic, depressed, and baseline selves. Accordingly, overcoming discontinuity in each case calls for different solutions. One way to proceed here is to consider phenomena that exhibit a similar *pattern* of discontinuity of self, yet are not regarded as psychologically abnormal: two candidates are ideological conversion and falling in love, which correspond (in terms of the pattern in place) to schizophrenia and bipolar disorder, respectively. Upon identifying the features by which these phenomena remain outside the realm of psychopathology, we can examine whether these features can be employed to overcome discontinuity of self with schizophrenia and bipolar disorder. To anticipate a discussion that will occupy us in Chapter 9, section 9.4.1, two such features are evident: phenomena such as ideological conversions are not ordinarily considered in the realm of psychopathology in the case that (1) they are accompanied by a narrative that unites past and present selves and hence bridges the discontinuity, and (2) this narrative retains some social intelligibility. The counter-narratives of psychological diversity advanced by activists can potentially fulfill those features and hence can play a therapeutic role in overcoming discontinuity of self and bringing back persons within the scope of recognition.

8.4 **Conclusion**

Unity and continuity of self are two requirements for forming and maintaining an identity. It is widely noted that certain mental health phenomena undermine both requirements and hence undermine identity formation. If that is the case, then these phenomena cannot be grounds for identity, a conclusion that would render incoherent the notion of Mad identity. This chapter examined this argument and we can now state some conclusions. (1) With regard to passivity phenomena and unity of self, the judgment that the former necessarily undermine the latter is underpinned by a specific set of cultural psychological assumptions. Once we allow for different assumptions, it becomes apparent that judgments of disunity are complex, with a range of possible scenarios. In some of those scenarios, passivity phenomena are conducive to an enriched, and not to a diminished, self-understanding; in others they lead to a dis-unified self; and in others the issue of whether passivity phenomena are a break-down or an enrichment of self has to be worked out through activism and therapy. (2) Discontinuity of self with schizophrenia and bipolar disorder can be a hindrance to the temporal unity of the self. While this certainly is a problem with regard to madness and identity formation, it is a problem for which there can be solutions evident in the possibilities for overcoming discontinuity outlined in section 8.3.5.

Can madness be grounds for identity? Given the arguments of this chapter, the answer to this question is that it can be as a matter of possibility. There is no doubt that in many cases madness lies beyond the limits of recognition. If madness is to constitute the grounds for identity—if the possibility described here is to become an actuality—then work needs to be done to bring it within this limit. This is the kind of work represented by scenario 4b in the case of disunity of self (Table 8.1), and by attempts to overcome discontinuity of self. Chapter 9 investigates what this work would look like, and whether it is possible for madness to be sufficiently ordered such that it can be brought within the scope of recognition *without becoming something else* (i.e., without ceasing to be madness).

Chapter 9

Madness and the limits of recognition

9.1 **Introduction**

Over the course of Chapters 7 and 8 we have been exploring whether madness can be grounds for identity. We identified three requirements that must be met by any identity claim: it must be a controversial and not a failed claim; it must be an expression of a unified mental life; it must persist over a sufficient period of time (section 7.1). Madness can only be grounds for identity in so far as it satisfies those requirements. Chapter 7 examined the first of these requirements in light of delusional identities, concluding that such identities, in some cases, can be understood as controversial (and not failed) identities; that is, the identity claim involves a mistake that can be addressed by revising the collective category with which the person is identifying; it is a claim that can be considered within the scope of recognition. Chapter 8 examined the second and third requirements. We found that madness (in the form of passivity phenomena) can undermine unity of self, and the conditions of schizophrenia and bipolar disorder can undermine continuity of self. But we have also seen that (1) judgments of disunity are complex and it is possible for passivity phenomena to result in enrichment, rather than impoverishment, of self; and (2) there are ways of overcoming discontinuity of self. Hence, even though madness, by virtue of impairing the requirements for identity formation, lies at the limits of recognition, it is possible to bring it back within those limits. This chapter investigates how this can be done.

9.2 **The limits of recognition**

The claim that madness lies at the limits of recognition arises from the following argument: every demand for recognition presents an identity and demonstrates that it is not accorded the appropriate status (it is not socially conceived of or valued in the right way); identity formation presupposes certain capacities; in cases where those capacities are impaired (such as with certain phenomena of madness) identity formation cannot proceed adequately; in such cases the question of recognition is not yet the right one to raise, not until the person is in better possession of the required capacities. All of this means, the argument can continue, that the demand for recognition of Mad identity is, at best, misguided and, at worst, irrelevant. It is misguided because it overestimates the capacities of those to whom the demand could apply. Yet, if it excludes those individuals and includes only those who are in possession of their capacities, it would be stipulating itself into irrelevance or, more precisely, would be relevant to a very small group of activists. These would be the individuals who are making a demand for recognition and who play a key role in constructing counternarratives of psychological diversity. They are likely to have lived experience of mental health phenomena and to have experienced difficulties with mental health institutions. These activists are sufficiently empowered and are instrumental in changing social perceptions of madness. If the kind of Mad activism investigated in this book is to have further reach than this group, then it must be shown how it can be relevant to those who do not already fall within the limits of recognition (and who would need support to overcome various impairments to identity formation).

That recognition has a limit was inevitable. The clue to its inevitability can be found in key words in the previous paragraph: to talk about impaired (or disrupted or adequate) capacities is to invoke normative standards concerning the range within which those capacities are supposed to function relative to the fulfillment of valued goals: typical goals include the formation of a rich and coherent identity, and being an effective and autonomous agent. The general point here is that normative moral and political theories—including the theory of recognition—put forth a range of goods (or aims) underpinned by a range of capacities, both to ground the theory and to provide a measure of its success or failure. For example, in Kant's moral theory, a good will is motivated by respect for the moral law; it acts out of duty and not on the basis of contingent inclinations or externally imposed principles: it is an autonomous will. Achieving an autonomous will is the good—the aim—of Kant's moral theory. In order to be autonomous, the will must legislate for the laws that bind it, and it can only do so a priori, that is, through exercising its capacity for reason (see section 3.2). Kant's moral theory requires an individual who is capable of reason. Of course, such a theory can accommodate the challenges individuals may face in exercising their capacity for reason and the temptation to act on their desires and inclinations, but it does so with the understanding that the addressee of the theory is a being who is capable, in principle, of rational autonomy. Individuals perceived to lack such capacities are outside the scope of the theory: they constitute its limit and not the range of its possible enactment.

For a very long time, this has been the fate of madness, variously equated with "unreason," "disintegration," and "irrationality." Understood thus, madness cannot be brought within the ambit of a normative moral theory that presupposes a certain kind of person. If the "mad" are not considered capable of rational autonomy, they would not be considered moral subjects but recipients of treatment, a point which doubly justifies doing things to the "mad person" as well as excusing the "mad person" from the constraints of our moral theories and ethical frameworks. And within the theory of recognition, as suggested earlier, the "mad" may not appear as candidates for recognition but as recipients of care and treatment, a suggestion borne out of the observation that madness disrupts capacities considered key to identity formation.

The exclusion of madness is something that Michel Foucault (2001) had made much of in his sweeping account of insanity in the age of reason. "In the serene world of mental illness," he wrote,

modern man no longer communicates with the madman: on one hand, the man of reason delegates the physician to madness, thereby authorising a relation only through the
abstract universality of disease; on the other, the man of madness communicates with
society only by the intermediary of an equally abstract reason which is order, physical and
moral constraint, the anonymous pressure of the group, the requirements of conformity.
As for a common language, there is no such thing. (Foucault 2001, p. xii)

Mad activism seeks to end this exclusion. In this respect, finding a voice for madness
and constructing counternarratives of psychological diversity are key endeavors. But
these emerging voices are facing the obstacles described here: How can the voice of
madness be reconciled with normative theories that appear to exclude it? Is it possible
to bring madness within the limits of the theory of recognition (and in this way to
further support the case for society to take seriously and to address the demand for
recognition of Mad identity)? There are two possible solutions here: (1) Extend the
limits of recognition by relaxing the normative requirements of the theory (section
9.2.1). (2) Order madness by overcoming impairments to identity formation, these
impairments being the obstacles to madness lying within the limits of recognition
(section 9.2.2).

9.2.1 **Extending the limits of recognition**

To extend the limits of recognition is to relax the requirements for identity formation.
I examine this in relation to one such requirement: continuity of self. As discussed
in Chapter 8, continuity of self is a necessary requirement for agency; in order to be
able to instigate and pursue projects over time, my present self needs to be able to
identify with my future self. Continuity of self is not all or nothing, however, and in
section 8.3.1 the answer to the question of how much continuity was sufficient fell back
on how much value we placed on the projects and commitments that we engage in
as agents. From a social perspective, most valued human accomplishments take long
periods of time, and mental health conditions that undermine continuity of self also
undermine one of the necessary conditions for partaking in such accomplishments.
It follows that one way of extending the limits of recognition is to give up on the idea
that time-intensive projects set the bar for successful agency, and to hold with equal
value a life proceeding in shorter episodes. The theory could then allow for more discontinuity of self than otherwise possible, and hence can accommodate a wider range
of individuals. How far can we go with this idea?

   In his ethnography of a shelter for homeless "mentally ill" individuals in downtown
Boston, Robert Desjarlais (1996, p. 71) writes that the residents "struggle along" in a
"routine existence marked by stress, fear, and distractions."[1] For many of the residents,
life is a "constant focus on daily concerns," "a succession of engagements, which can
include a constant but purely episodic unfolding of events" (1996, pp. 86–7). The temporal dimension is key here, and Desjarlais contrasts the state of "struggling along"
with the concept of "experience" as ordinarily understood. The former is defined by

---

[1] Individuals in Desjarlais' study had mental health diagnoses including schizophrenia and
bipolar disorder.

actions that take "temporally finite forms in which future, present, and past need not have much to do with one another," while the concept of experience "entails an aesthetics of integration, coherence, renewal, and transcendent meaning—of tying things together through time" (1996, p. 87). Struggling along, for Desjarlais, arises from the nature of homelessness and street life, and also from the consequences of "mental illness." The upshot is that individuals live from one moment to the next, with the possibility of future planning significantly hindered. Kennett (2009, p. 96) notes a similar issue when she asks:

> What if we find we can no longer rely . . . on our future selves being appropriately affected by our present plans and decisions? What if our projects, large and small, were at constant risk of derailment? What if even those traits and dispositions which we might think of as fundamental to our characters . . . were in danger of being masked or reversed?

The answer that Kennett (2009, p. 97) offers is that lack of confidence in an individual's "power to see through valued plans and projects" may be demoralizing, "and the person lives an impoverished life dominated by short-term considerations." For persons in such situations, the issue is not that they have chosen to "live in the moment" but that they are confined to the moment. While we can certainly extend the limits of recognition (in the dimension of continuity of self) by relaxing the conditions for successful agency, we can only go so far as it begins to appear that agency is being curtailed not exercised. In order to go further with our concern of bringing madness within the limits of recognition, we must now consider the second option noted earlier: ordering madness by overcoming impairments to identity formation.

9.2.2 **Ordering madness**

In Chapter 8, impairments to identity formation were cashed out in terms of disunity of self and discontinuity of self. Individuals who experience such impairments owing to mental health phenomena can enter the scope of recognition if these impairments are resolved and identity formation can proceed adequately. There are various ways in which we can understand "resolution." Resolution can mean treatment in the medical or psychological sense where, roughly, the goals are either elimination of the phenomena through psychopharmacological treatment, or their reinterpretation in accordance with a psychological framework such that the person is considered to have gained insight. Given the problem we are dealing with, this meaning of resolution will not do, since it requires elimination or radical transformation of the thing for which recognition is sought into something else. Resolution must be understood in more complex terms as a dialectical process governed by two requirements:

(1) Preserve something of madness.

(2) Resolve the impairments to identity formation.

Only if these two requirements are satisfied can madness be brought within the scope of recognition not as something else, such as a psychiatric condition or a psychological construct, but as itself. This may sound like an attempt to square the circle—How can you order madness without it ceasing to be madness?—but it only sounds so if we view the process of resolution in the usual one-sided manner: resolution here is dialectical and will change both the subjective narratives *and* the social narratives of madness. To talk of *narratives* is appropriate: the demand for recognition of Mad identity is essentially a demand to demedicalize madness, and to replace dominant medical and psychological narratives with a range of counternarratives of psychological, emotional, and experiential diversity (henceforth referred to as Mad narratives). We need to investigate what kind of narrative can satisfy the two requirements of the dialectical process noted here earlier. Where a narrative fails to satisfy the first requirement—where it fails to preserve something of the phenomenology of madness—there is no need to investigate how it fares in relation to the second requirement, since satisfaction of this first requirement is a necessary condition: these narratives can be rejected as a solution to our problem. Accordingly, a successful narrative must satisfy both requirements. In what follows, the narratives are outlined schematically with brief indications of their content, the purpose being, primarily, to express the nature of their approach to madness.

9.3 Narratives of madness

9.3.1 Subjective narratives

By subjective narratives of madness, I mean persons' accounts of their experiences and elaboration of their beliefs, the very same accounts that clinical psychiatry and psychology would then redescribe and organize into symptoms or processes. Subjective narratives preserve the madness—they *are* the madness; an expression of the person's world that might not be well articulated and might not afford a deep understanding of what is going on, but it remains their personal attempt to render their world to themselves and others. While subjective narratives can satisfy the first requirement, they cannot satisfy the second. They cannot do so because reports of passivity experiences and of radical and unexplained breaks in one's self-conception over time—that is, the contents of the subjective narrative—are themselves taken as evidence of impaired capacities for identity formation. Subjective narratives of madness cannot satisfy the second requirement unless they change and *become ordered* in some way, for example, by being placed in a broader interpretive context. However, as argued earlier, the change in question cannot be at the expense of losing madness entirely by making it into something else. Professional narratives sacrifice precisely that requirement.

9.3.2 Professional narratives

By professional narratives I mean any systematic approach to madness, whether this is medical, psychological, or psychoanalytic, to name a few key approaches.[2] By systematic I mean that the narrative in question provides (or seeks to provide, or presupposes that one day it will arrive at) a total view of the phenomena, from an understanding of their genesis to a framework for their treatment.

---

[2] See Geekie and Read (2009, chapter 5) and Read and Dillon (eds.) (2013, parts I and II) for an overview of various professional accounts of madness.

In terms of their fundamental logic, professional narratives of madness are either divisive or integrative. Divisive narratives enact a "hypostatic abstraction," a process by which a predicate is transformed into a relation: instead of honey *is* sweet, we say honey *possesses* sweetness.[3] Clinical diagnosis is divisive in this sense: it transforms a human suffering into a human (plus) suffering. Instead of saying Ahmad is depressed, we say Ahmad has depression; instead of saying Maria is schizophrenic, we say Maria has schizophrenia. Given this move, expressed mental content plays a specific function: by providing access to the person's subjectivity it allows for diagnosis, prognosis, follow-up, and identification of risk. Mental content remains ontologically separate from the person, a separation that allows efforts to be directed at treating or curing the affliction without the distraction of personal moral judgments. Diagnosis as hypostatic abstraction diverts moral judgment from the person and onto the presumed disorder: instead of the person being "disagreeable," we have a "terrible" illness. This allows the medical setup, as well as some psychological approaches, to operate on disorders, persons being current—and sometimes permanent—unfortunate carriers of disorder.

By contrast, integrative narratives regard phenomena of madness as alienated mental content (a point that can apply to thought insertion and auditory verbal hallucinations), or as arising from psychological processes of which subjects need to be aware (a point that can apply to manic states and grandiose beliefs). In terms of theoretical frameworks, there are many: for example, alienation can be understood psychodynamically as the defensive objectification, and exclusion, of mental states that threaten integrity of self and self-esteem; it can also be understood phenomenologically as the appearance into consciousness of phenomena that are normally tacit in the background of awareness. The task, clinically, is not to further objectify those mental states by placing them, as it were, alongside the person—something that may be encouraged by a psychiatric diagnosis—but to find ways of integrating this content with a self that continues to experience it as other-than-self.

Neither the divisive nor the integrative narratives can satisfy the first requirement identified here (preserving something of madness). Both kinds of narrative subvert the person's speech of its actual semantic referents in favor of the framework embraced by that person's interlocutor. For example, if I express that "*Mostafa is putting thoughts into my head*," my interlocutor would translate this to "*he has a psychotic disorder*" if the strategy was divisive or "*he is failing to recognize that he is the author of his own thoughts*" if the strategy was integrative. The upshot of either move is that the subjective narrative is redescribed in such a way that it loses its basic meaning: it is transformed into something else entirely. Therefore, professional narratives would not do as a way of ordering madness.

9.3.3 **Mad narratives**

By Mad narratives I am referring to accounts that have been developed by activists and people with lived experience in order to make sense of madness; we have already

---

[3] See Charles Peirce (1958, paragraph 235 of volume 4). The term "hypostatic abstraction" was employed by Peirce in his mathematical logic (see also 1958, paragraph 534 of volume 5).

encountered aspects of these narratives in Chapter 1. Mad narratives are unique in that they are constructed to make sense of madness as it is experienced by individuals and not of madness after it has been redescribed in medical or psychological language. They are, thus, more faithful to madness and, in this sense, are more likely to satisfy the first requirement: preserving something of the phenomenology of madness. They are also in a position to satisfy the second requirement by playing a role in resolving impairments to identity formation. Mad narratives are constructed to correct for professional narratives (and their inadequacy vis-a-vis the experience of madness) and for subjective narratives (and their idiosyncratic character). They are worked out in a group and hence are more likely to achieve a degree of social intelligibility (see section 2.2.5). Even though they are unlikely to perfectly coincide with a subjective narrative, they offer a blueprint for a person to make sense of her experiences and to be able to adopt a broader and unifying perspective on what is happening to her. Mad narratives, therefore, can offer a means of ordering madness and bringing it within the scope of recognition. Before I examine how this can come about (in section 9.4), I offer some details on three Mad narratives. In approaching these narratives, my aim is not to defend or critique their basic claims, but to outline their elements. How society ought to respond to them is a further issue to be considered in Chapter 10.

Spiritual transformation

Narratives of spiritual transformation have long been associated with madness, most famously, perhaps, in the writings of R. D. Laing. For Laing (1967) schizophrenia involves a fragmentation of the ego that can lead to a breakthrough and an existential rebirth. The idea that "breakdown can be the entrance to breakthrough" has been expressed more recently by Sascha DuBrul (2014, p. 267), one of the founders of the Icarus Project. Similarly, Seth Farber (2012, p. 9) in *The Spiritual Gift of Madness* notes that in the experiences of some people "madness . . . has value, it has the potential to shed light on the human situation, to promote spiritual growth." Spiritual approaches to madness are not surprising given the commonality of spiritual concerns in the accounts of service users, activists, and others with lived experience. For example, Sally Clay (1999, p. 27) writes that "becoming 'mentally ill' was always a spiritual crisis, and finding a spiritual model of recovery was a question of life or death." In their study *Making Sense of Madness*, Geekie and Read (2009, p. 57) report that "one of the most pervasive features of how participants spoke about their experience . . . was their interest in spiritual aspects." Spirituality, for the participants, covered broad ground, and the authors define it as

> an inclination to view the experience of psychosis . . . in terms of a broad framework of meaning, pertaining to how the individual views his or her relationship with the universe. That is, a tendency to place the psychotic experience in a metaphysical context where it is considered to reflect something of existential or moral significance for the individual. (Geekie and Read 2009, p. 85)

Narratives of spiritual transformation also recognize that contemporary beliefs about and approaches to mental health (whether psychological or medical) deny the spiritual dimensions of madness and can even regard these dimensions as evidence for mental illness. First-person accounts abound with examples where mental health profession-als suppressed people's attempts to make sense of their experiences in spiritual terms, either through forced treatment or the categorical refusal to engage with their views. Such suppression was experienced as a significant harm; a tragic loss of something valuable, and an interruption of an important transformation, leaving people confused and lost.[4] Following from this, narratives of spiritual transformation lament the state of contemporary, "advanced-capitalist" societies where the notion of "experiences on a journey" has been lost. This is contrasted with other communities and historical peri-ods where there is/was a social space for spiritual approaches, and an understanding of the transformative potential of madness:

> For centuries . . . people have experienced extreme mental states. In most societies, altered states of mind have held a place of respect, and have served to give spiritual meaning to the culture. In indigenous cultures, for example, the shamanistic tradition involves an indi-vidual's journey through his or her own mind. This journey is typically painful and even turbulent, but, because the people who experience it are guided through it by spiritual elders and the community itself, they emerge from their ordeal with new-found wisdom and the power to heal. (Clay 1999, pp. 31–2).[5]

Narratives of spiritual transformation seek to address these shortcomings by repopu-lating our cultural repertoire with spiritual ideas about madness. These ideas range from Eastern mystical and spiritual traditions (e.g., Peddie 2014) to radical ecological perspectives (e.g., Fletcher 2017). The latter, for example, reject the fundamental sepa-ration between humans and the natural world, and see humanity as fundamentally connected to nature. They understand extreme mental states as expressions of, and continuous with, the state of the ecosystem and the well-being of all life on Earth. Irrespective of their specific content, spiritual narratives share the structure of a radi-cal transformative process: breakdown of the habitual experience of body/self/world; disintegration of the self/spiritual death; guided attempts at reorganizing experience through the content of a particular spiritual narrative; in successful cases this leads to transformation and spiritual rebirth. This final outcome recalls the concept of *meta-noia*, a concept employed by Carl Jung to refer to "a fundamental change of attitude" (1970a, p. 379), "transformation of mind" (1970b, p. 192), and "a rebirth of the spirit" (1970a, p. 276).

"Dangerous gifts"

The view of madness as a "dangerous gift" has been popularized by the Icarus Project (see section 1.4.2). The narrative embraces the Janus-faced nature of madness: on the one hand associated with distress and difficulties in social functioning, on the other associated with the potential for creativity and unique vision. I present the narrative through the words of one of the founders of the Icarus Project, the artist and activist

---

[4] See, for example, *From the Ashes of Experience: Reflections on Madness, Survival, and Growth* (Barker, Campbell, and Davidson 1999). See also Chapter 7, section 7.3.4, and Rashed (2010).

[5] See also Chapter 1, section 1.4.2.

Jacks McNamara who was diagnosed with bipolar disorder as a young woman.[6] The narrative rejects the illness model and the accompanying notion that people must be cured (rather than guided through their experience).

> I don't feel like there's this foreign, evil thing operating in me and my goal is to eliminate it and tame it into submission. . . . One of the most distressing things about the disease model of mental illness in our culture, to have any periods of darkness or suffering is wrong. It means you're off the track. It means you need to be fixed.

The idea that there is something valuable to acquire from the unique thought process associated with certain kinds of madness is central to the narrative, and so is the understanding that when this is not controlled in the right way, the individual could suffer.

> We have been given a sensitivity, a temperament, a disposition which can grant us access to a lot of beautiful things, and can also be extremely painful and destructive. It's our responsibility as individuals to try to learn how to take care of our dangerous gift. . . . We need to stop putting all the focus on treatment on how can we make you stop being the person you are. How can we stop telling you that you are wrong if you experience these things. And how can we instead help you to learn how to handle your sensitivities. That you might make the transition from having these sensitivities overwhelming you, to having these sensitivities be giving you information you can use.

Being able to see connections among events and experiences that otherwise would seem disparate is part of the potential value of certain forms of madness, a value expressed in the notion of a dangerous *gift*:

> something that happens for a lot of us who get labelled as bipolar is we have these kaleidoscopic tendencies in our brains, where we can't filter out as much of the world as a lot of people do, and it's like we have 500 antennas out in every direction all at once, and we're bringing in tons and tons of information on all these different channels: the dead flower over there, and the shadow over here, and this person over there, and the love letter over there, and the map over here, and the apocalypse over there, and Walmart down there, and the ocean and the children, and . . . in my mind, they're all connected, and they're not separable.

The "dangerous gift" narrative, unlike an illness narrative, does not redescribe or invalidate the experience of madness, but places it in an interpretive context that gives it meaning and value while recognizing the difficulties people can face.

"Healing voices"

The Hearing Voices Movement (HVM) has been successful at advancing a perspective on voices that challenges the psychiatric view. Instead of regarding voice-hearing as a psychopathological phenomenon that ought to be treated, the HVM portrays it as a normal and meaningful human experience connected to a person's life story. Voices are regarded as '"messengers' that represent important information about life problems, and which can therefore be utilized as a means of solving social and emotional

---

[6] Quotes are from the documentary *Crooked Beauty* (2010), the first movie in the *Mad Dance Mental Health Film Trilogy*, directed by Ken Paul Rosenthal.

conflict" (Longden, Corstens, and Dillon 2013, p. 164). Underpinning this is the idea that the problem is not the voices as such, but the relationship the person develops toward them. Voice hearers are encouraged to communicate with their voices in order to understand their origin and meaning, and to be able to cope with and learn from them. The notion of "healing voices" encapsulates this potential for growth.[7] In her TED Talk, *The Voices in My Head,* Eleanor Longden describes how she interacted with her voices: [8]

> I would set boundaries for the voices, and try to interact with them in a way that was assertive yet respectful, establishing a slow process of communication and collaboration in which we could learn to work together and support one another . . . each voice was closely related to aspects of myself, and . . . each of them carried overwhelming emotions that I'd never had an opportunity to process or resolve, memories of sexual trauma and abuse, of anger, shame, guilt, low self-worth. The voices took the place of this pain and gave words to it.

The narrative of "healing voices" does not commit to a particular view on the source of voices; voice hearers are encouraged to develop their own understandings. Some may understand voices as spirits from a different world that have come to communicate with them; others may understand them as belonging to departed relatives and friends; others may view them as divided parts of their own self. Whatever the presumed source, the key points are that voices provide information the voice-hearer can use, and that developing a relationship with the voices is key to being able to cope with them and to utilize them for personal growth.

9.4 Overcoming impairments to identity formation

As argued in the previous section, only Mad narratives can, in principle, fulfill the two requirements for ordering madness: (1) preserve something of the phenomenology of madness; (2) resolve impairments to identity formation. Professional narratives stumble at the first requirement and subjective narratives stumble at the second. It remains to be seen how Mad narratives can play a role in ordering the subjective narrative in such a way that resolves the impairments in question (and hence satisfy the second requirement). In what follows I demonstrate this in relation to the two problems discussed in Chapter 8: discontinuity of self and disunity of self.

9.4.1 Overcoming discontinuity of self

In section 8.3.5 I proposed that overcoming discontinuity of self with schizophrenia and bipolar disorder requires, in principle, a narrative that can unite aspects of the self and bridge the discontinuity. This, in turn, depends on the pattern of the discontinuity: with schizophrenia discontinuity is longitudinal and the difficulty lies in auto-biographically uniting past and present selves; with bipolar disorder discontinuity is

---

[7] From the documentary *Healing Voices.* Directed by P. J. Moynihan (2016).

[8] From Eleanor Longden's TED Talk: *The Voices in My Head* (2013). Online: https://www.ted.com/talks/eleanor_longden_the_voices_in_my_head/up-next

cyclical and the difficulty lies in autobiographically uniting the manic, depressed, and baseline selves. These patterns of discontinuity are evident in other experiences that are not ordinarily considered within the scope of psychopathology. Radical change in personality and values can take the form of a longitudinal discontinuity, and one way in which this can be overcome and made sense of is through the notion of "ideological conversion." Repeated and intense emotional attachment is a form of cyclical discontinuity that can be overcome and made sense of through the notion of "falling in love." Part of the reason that these experiences are not typically considered psychopathological is because they are socially intelligible (Radden 1996, pp. 19–20). Accordingly, the kind of narrative that can, in principle, overcome discontinuity with schizophrenia and bipolar disorder must unite the various aspects of self while retaining some social intelligibility. My contention is that certain Mad narratives can achieve this goal, even if the question of ultimate intelligibility has to be worked out socially within the framework of recognition (see Chapter 10). In what follows I develop further the view that the *patterns* of discontinuity subsumed under the notions of ideological conversion and falling in love are similar to those reported and observed with, respectively, schizophrenia and bipolar disorder.[9] In each case, I propose a candidate Mad narrative that can, in principle, resolve this discontinuity.

With the kind of discontinuity reported in schizophrenia, what is required is a narrative that can unite past and present selves despite their radical differences (see section 8.3.3 for examples of such discontinuity). A model for this is ideological (or religious) conversion. A person may radically transform, and quite rapidly and deeply, from being pious and religiously observant, to being hedonistic and secular. Or, conversely, from being open-minded and liberal, to being an intolerant religious zealot. Conversions of this sort, as Radden (1996, pp. 19–20) notes, "point to one way in which personality change may be both radical and rapidly occurring in those who are psychologically normal." The key is for the transformation to remain intelligible. A person may fall under the grip of a powerful ideology at a time of confusion and vulnerability, or may undergo an intense experience that reorders his identity. From the perspective of the person himself, he may be able to identify a key moment or revelation when the change began, and for this moment to constitute a link between his old self and his new self. Most people can understand—though many may not approve of some of the resultant behaviors—a person who, upon witnessing violent maltreatment of animals for the first time, transforms from being a carnivore to a militant animal-rights activist. Ideological conversion, if it is to be construed as psychologically "normal," has to be accompanied by some intelligible narrative that can explain the transition.

A Mad narrative that can play this role in the case of the longitudinal discontinuities often seen with schizophrenia is that of spiritual transformation (see section 9.3.3). Narratives of spiritual transformation—irrespective of their specific content—bring a sense of unity over time. They can provide the narrative thread that connects past and

---

[9] I am only referring to the *pattern* of discontinuity of self, and not to the nature, severity, or implications of the subjective experiences. The latter, obviously, are very different in the conditions known as schizophrenia/bipolar disorder than they are with ideological conversion/falling in love.

present selves despite their radical differences, and hence they can make that transition intelligible. This thread is provided by the notions of disintegration/death followed by reorganization/rebirth of one's self/soul in accordance with the content of the spiritual narrative in question. In the absence of a unifying narrative thread, as we have seen in section 8.3, individuals can experience radical discontinuity with no possibility of connecting past and present selves.

With the kind of discontinuity evident in bipolar disorder, what is required is to bring the different phases—manic, depressed, baseline—under an overarching narrative (see section 8.3.4 for examples of such discontinuity). A model for this is "falling in love."[10] The experience of sudden, intense, and often inexplicable emotional attachment and physical attraction to another person is something that many people undergo several times in their lives. When a person is "in love" he or she is taken over by powerful emotions and their outlook and behavior can change drastically—they may become extremely optimistic about life and may engage in behaviors that are risky in light of their own standards as they stood *before* they fell in love. Observers such as close friends and family tend to note this change in personality, sometimes with concern; it is no coincidence that in some communities falling in love is likened to being possessed—taken over—by another person. When the attraction ends, as it inevitably does, and the person "falls out of love," they now can see nothing but the faults of the same person who had been previously idealized. A reversal in outlook ensues, optimism about the future is gone, motivation is dampened, and decisions taken while in love seem rash. These two contrasting states—"in" and "out" of love—are balanced by a third baseline state where it is possible to take a more objective stance toward one's experiences, until the person falls in love again and the saga repeats itself. The notion of "falling in love" subsumes these three states: it allows for all the different states to be aspects of the same person: it allows for continuity of self and for repeatability of the experiences.

A Mad narrative that can play a unifying role similar to the "falling in love" narrative is that of the "dangerous gift" (section 9.3.3). It allows for the person to go on emotional and cognitive "flights" where a multitude of connections are made among events and objects in the world; it allows for this to go too far with the person crashing in confusion, despair, and depression; and it allows for a baseline state where one can reflect on, and try to make sense of, the other two states. This baseline state can be the standpoint from where the narrative of the "dangerous gift" is initially adopted. The dangerous gift narrative, unlike the illness narrative, can allow for the different phases of "bipolar disorder" to be seen as part of a continuous self and, hence, as reconcilable to each other.

9.4.2 Resolving disunity of self

In section 8.2 I argued that disunity of self in relation to passivity phenomena is not an objective feature of the phenomena, but a judgment that assumes a particular

---

[10] I refer here to the state otherwise known as infatuation. I do not refer to nonromantic love or to the kind of loving relationships that develop over a lifetime.

cultural-psychological theory. It is only relative to particular assumptions about self, the boundaries of self, and the possibility of external authorship of mental states that one can judge whether or not passivity phenomena constitute disunity of self. Resolving disunity, therefore, amounts to transforming the assumptions underpinning the judgments themselves. Consider the situation of a typical mental health consultation, one where both the clinician and the patient share the cultural-psychological assumption that external authorship of mental states is not possible (this is represented in Table 8.1 by scenario 3). The clinician considers the patient's report of thought insertion to constitute disunity of self. The patient ordinarily does not believe that external authorship of mental states is possible, yet at the same time his experiences of thought insertion are putting a strain on this assumption. This can go in two ways: either he prioritizes the assumption that external authorship is not possible (and agrees with the clinician that thought insertion amounts to disunity of self) (Table 8.1, scenario 4a), or he rejects this assumption and endorses a narrative whereby external authorship of mental states *is* possible (and disagrees with the clinician on the question of disunity) (Table 8.1, scenario 4b). Resolving disunity of self, therefore, begins by adopting the position in scenario 4b, and endorsing or constructing with others a narrative that can allow for a more appropriate context of judgment for passivity phenomena (see section 8.2.5 for details). Are there Mad narratives that can, in principle, bring about such resolution?

The narrative that can bring about such resolution will have to allow for external authorship of mental states. In many cultural communities around the world, and in the case of Mahdi that I discussed in section 8.2.4, such a narrative exists in the form of spirit possession beliefs and practices. Spirit possession is an example of a cultural narrative by which passivity phenomena can be judged to constitute an enrichment and not a disunity of self. But beliefs about spirits and possession are not a fundamental part of the cultural repertoire of many of the people engaged in Mad activism in North Europe and North America. If so, what other sense to "external authorship of mental states" can there be? Consider the "healing voices" Mad narrative, which I outlined earlier. The narrative advocates that people communicate with their voices and learn from the information they bring. In this advice we find implicit acknowledgment that the voices are *external* to the person, not necessarily in the sense that they belong to other beings (such as spirits), but in the sense that they are external to the person's locus of awareness. It is precisely in virtue of this externality that the person can regard the voices as independent and hence as capable of bringing to him or her original information and insights. I contend that a Mad narrative informed by this notion of externality can allow for passivity phenomena to constitute an enrichment rather than a disunity of self, in the same way that the "healing voices" narrative allows this for voices.

9.5 **Making the difference between subjective narratives and Mad narratives**

So far in this chapter I have been exploring ways of bringing madness within the scope of recognition. Much of the argument centered on what I have been referring to as *ordering madness*; an endeavor whose fulfillment requires two conditions: preserving something of the phenomenology of madness, and resolving impairments to identity formation. I identified Mad narratives as capable, *in principle*, of fulfilling these two conditions and addressing the shortcomings of subjective and professional narratives. But *in principle* is one thing and *in practice* another; Mad narratives have the potential to order madness, but for this to be evident in practice it needs to inform people's actual attempts to make sense of their experiences. In other words, we need to make the difference between subjective narratives and Mad narratives.

Individuals experiencing phenomena of madness are actively engaged in attempts to make sense of their experiences (e.g., Barker et al. 1999; Larsen 2004; Roe and Davidson 2005; Geekie and Read 2009; Rashed 2012). This process is affected by many factors such as the nature and intensity of the experiences, the available narratives, individual creativity, and the input of others including that of family members and the designated experts (see Rashed 2012). For individuals diagnosed with schizophrenia or bipolar disorder, attempts to make meaning might produce idiosyncratic subjective narratives. These narratives tend to be taken by others as evidence of impairment in the various capacities for identity formation (section 9.3.1). In the case of individuals diagnosed with schizophrenia, for example, Phillips (2003, pp. 327–31) notes two types of subjective narrative: the delusional and the fragmented. With delusional narratives, the subject organizes his or her lived experience in a self-narrative that revolves around an increasingly systematized core of persecution or exaggerated self-importance. A fragmented narrative, on the other hand, is a failed narrative, a consequence of the subject's inability to transcend intense emotional experiences and cognitive challenges. In such cases, individuals require support to construct a narrative that can order their experiences. If we are concerned with ordering madness in the terms defined in this chapter, then what needs to happen, in practice, is for individuals to begin to reinterpret their experiences and to rethink their self-understanding in light of a Mad narrative.

Assisting individuals with constructing an identity is a recognized aim in the literature. In *Towards Humanism in Psychiatry*, Jonathan Glover (2003, p. 532) writes that one aim of a humanist psychiatry "is to improve people's damaged or impaired capacity for living a good human life." Among the many factors that enter into a good life, Glover considers "self-creation" to be of fundamental importance. "Self-creation" recalls the account of identity described in section 4.2: people find value in defining themselves, in deciding what kind of person they wish to become, and in having some say in how they relate to the collective categories in which they find or place themselves. In the case of mental health conditions that impair identity formation, a humanist psychiatry can help individuals restore "self-creation" (Glover 2003). Reflecting a similar concern, Jennifer Radden (2003, p. 359) argues that "some of the task of attributing and constructing self-identity may be one that can be undertaken by others when the patient's own identity-constructing capabilities are compromised." This task can be adopted among the goals of therapy (Radden 1996, Chapter 13). In his essay *How Do I Learn to Be Me Again?* Grant Gillet (2012, p. 249) writes that when people are ill, they need a "guide, an informant" who engages them in a "reasoned, respectful discussion . . . that enables [them] to assume and enact identities and to live out life stories each with its unique value."

In what kind of fora can individuals diagnosed with schizophrenia and bipolar disorder be assisted with "self-creation," with constructing and maintaining an identity informed by a Mad narrative? Glover and Radden suggest therapeutic endeavors of the kind one would see in clinical practice. These are, of course, of crucial importance, and it would be welcome to see more of these endeavors informed by diverse narratives. Gillet's suggestion of the need for a "guide, an informant" casts a wider net and highlights the important role of the many mental health groups and networks. The Hearing Voices Movement (Longden et al. 2013), Open Dialogue, and Soteria (Thomas 2013), the Icarus Project (DuBrul 2014), and Psychology in the Real World groups (Holmes 2013)—to name just a few examples—are all avenues where people can get together and develop a *shared understanding* of their experiences; in such cases people act as guides and informants to each other. A Mad narrative just is a shared understanding; in this chapter I outlined three but there are many more that exist today and many, no doubt, that will be formulated in the future. "Self-creation" then requires that one is supported in developing a personal understanding of their experiences that retains a basis in a broader, shared narrative. Each person, however, will have different needs and will require different levels of support. Persons who experience unusual phenomena (such as passivity phenomena and voices) but are able to interact socially, join groups, and develop with others a new, shared understanding of their experiences require less support than those who experience social withdrawal, persecutory fears, and struggle to interact with others.[11] Determining the level of support that is required and the interventions that can be helpful is to be accomplished on the ground and on a case-by-case basis. But if the overall aim of the process is to reconcile a person's subjective narrative with a Mad narrative, then it might ultimately succeed in ordering madness and bringing individuals within the scope of recognition.

9.6 **Conclusion**

We can now consider a final answer to the question initially raised in section 7.1: Can madness be grounds for identity? In Chapter 8 we answered this question in the affirmative but only as a matter of possibility. It remained to be seen just what is required for madness to be grounds for identity in practice. Given that certain phenomena of madness can impair the ability to form and maintain an identity, madness can be brought within the scope of recognition once it is ordered in some way and these impairments are overcome. Ordering madness requires the satisfaction of two conditions: (1) Preserve something of the phenomenology of madness, and (2) resolve impairments to identity formation. As argued in this chapter, Mad narratives can, in principle,

---

[11] Clinicians who work in acute settings or with individuals with chronic conditions might not recognize in this chapter a place for their clients or patients. They may, for example, see individuals who have severe thought disorder and are unable to communicate, and others whose sense of self is fragmented to the point where the very question of identity cannot be raised. For those individuals, the kind of support they need is not so much to author an identity but to regain basic cognitive and psychological functions. This is an important point, and anyone who has worked on a mental health unit would agree with it. Nevertheless, Mad narratives have benefits that go far beyond the cohort of individuals who are already well enough to be able to participate in therapeutic endeavors and in group activities (see section 10.5).

fulfill these two requirements. In practice, making the difference between subjective narratives and Mad narratives requires that individuals are supported in their attempts at constructing an identity that can make sense of their experiences. Where this is successful, madness can be said to be ordered. In conclusion, madness can be grounds for identity, and hence within the scope of recognition, once it is ordered in line with a Mad narrative. The notion of Mad identity is not incoherent. We can now consider the final question: Does the demand for recognition of Mad identity possess normative force and, if it does, how should society respond to it?

Part IV

Approaches to Mad activism

Chapter 10

Responding to the demand for recognition of Mad identity

10.1 **Introduction**

Part III considered the first question identified in the Introduction to this book: Can madness be grounds for identity? With a range of qualifications in place, our answer was that it can: the notion of Mad identity is not incoherent. We can now consider the second question identified in the Introduction: Does the demand for recognition of Mad identity possess normative force and, if it does, how should society respond to it? I begin by restating what the demand is about. We have examined this in Chapter 1 (section 1.4) through the writings of activists: the demand is for society to acknowledge that madness can be grounds for identity, and to recognize the validity and value of a range of counternarratives of psychological diversity, or Mad narratives as I have been referring to them (section 9.3.3). These include narratives such as "dangerous gifts," "spiritual transformation," and "healing voices." Mad narratives come up against prevalent professional and lay narratives, many of which in one form or another indicate deficit, disorder, irrationality, disease, or illness, to name some notions associated with madness. From the perspective of Mad activism, professional and lay narratives are instances of misrecognition; misrepresentations of the meaning of madness that prevent people from finding themselves at home in the social world.

Conceiving the issue in terms of the confrontation of narratives is correct, but this must not tempt us to think that the solution is to move words around. As if replacing the word "disorder" with the word "order" is sufficient; as if we have not seen over the past many decades how the adoption of neutral or even positive terms does not prevent people from using them as terms of abuse. The latest example of this is in the United Kingdom, where in an effort to fight stigma, the term "mental health" has replaced the term "mental illness" in some public discourse, only for "mental health" to now be heard in use as a slur: "do not listen to him, he has mental health." Accordingly, in order for the demands of Mad activism to be addressed, significant transformations need to occur in the beliefs and values that inform popular and professional thinking about, and attitudes toward, madness. As Jennifer Radden (2012) has argued, ideas about "mental illness" are not floating on the surface of our conceptions of rationality, responsibility, personhood, and agency but rather are constituted by them (see section 1.5); for example, in order to explain why a group of people disvalue the experience of hearing voices (which they might describe as auditory hallucinations), our explanation has to invoke deeply held norms that touch on what it is to be a self and in control of one's mental life. In this sense we can understand Thomas and Bracken's (2008, p. 48) perceptive remark that Mad Pride discourse is "reshaping our views of what it is to be normal, to be human." The change required for addressing Mad activism's demand for recognition is profound and not to be taken lightly. All of which adds to the stakes of asking whether the demand for recognition of Mad identity possesses normative force; whether society ought to take it seriously and attempt to address it.

Essentially, then, the two questions before us are: (1) Should anything be done in response to Mad activism's demand for recognition? (section 10.3); and (2) what is it that should be done? (section 10.4). Following this, I articulate the outcome of successful recognition in terms of a broadening of our cultural repertoire as it pertains to madness. Mad narratives can become a cultural form of societal adjustment—a "cultural adjustment"—that can benefit many people in society (section 10.5). Before these issues can be addressed, I begin with a summary of the theory of recognition detailed in Part II, with a focus on the normative force of demands for recognition in general.

10.2 **Normative force of demands for recognition (a *précis* of Part II)**

In Part II I presented a philosophical and political account of recognition that could enable us to understand, justify, and address demands for recognition. A key idea is that recognition is not an empirical or a metaphysical concept, but a philosophical articulation of what it is to be a free agent; being a free agent requires that my self-conceptions, beliefs, and reasons for action are recognized as valid, and for this recognition to issue from those whom I recognize in turn as free agents (section 3.4.2). "Free agent," on this account, is a normative status "dependent on social recognition" (Pippin 2008b, p. 68); it is socially achieved and ascribed, and it can be denied others just as much as it can be bestowed upon them. If we accept this view, as I suggest we do in section 3.5, then we have a philosophical concept that we ought to employ in thinking about freedom and social relations. Once we begin to do so we need to say more about why misrecognition is a wrong that may require social or political redress. Chapter 5 presented an answer to this question by inquiring over the consequences of misrecognition; the consequences of being consistently related to as an agent whose self-conceptions, reasons for action, and beliefs are invalid. As parsed out in section 5.2, misrecognition can result in two social harms (collectively generated and maintained harms): social disqualification and identity impairment. Social disqualification begins with the denial that you are an authority on yourself or the world. You can become epistemically marginalized and your ability to be an effective agent is compromised (in the sense of an agent who is able to realize its point of view in the world). Identity impairment refers to the psychological consequences of misrecognition and which I have outlined in section 4.4 through the work of Axel Honneth. Recognition, according to Honneth, is one key (empirical) condition in the development of positive self-relations in the dimensions of self-confidence, self-respect, and self-esteem. The denial of recognition can impair the development of identity in these dimensions.

If social disqualification and identity impairment are social harms, and if repairing social relations in the direction of mutual recognition can play a role in alleviating these harms, what is the right kind of response here? Chapter 5 explored two responses: political reform and reconciliation. The case for a political response to mis-recognition can begin by specifying the social harms in question as impediments to human flourishing, and it can continue by arguing that it is unjust to deny people the conditions to flourish. Whether or not it really is an injustice to deny people adequate recognition (where such denial cannot otherwise be justified) is a question that requires further examination (as I indicate in section 5.3.3). Notwithstanding, given the requirement that recognition is freely and genuinely offered, political institutional responses based on incentive and/or coercion are not adequate as a response to mis-recognition, though political action can play a role in creating the right conditions for people to meet. Which brings us to the second response to misrecognition: the achievement of interpersonal reconciliation. Reconciliation involves an acceptance of the other, an accommodation between individuals realized in the social contexts in which they interact and the narratives that inform these interactions. Reconciliation is both an outcome and an attitude. As I argue in section 5.5, the outcome of reconciliation cannot be forced or guaranteed. On the other hand, the recommendation here is to approach others with an attitude of reconciliation, which is to acknowledge that their ability to find satisfaction in the social world matters as much as my own (which is the ability to enact their identity and projects and to receive confirmation of their validity and worth).[1]

Repairing social relations as a way of responding to demands for recognition requires, as a first step, that we adopt an attitude of reconciliation toward others, and this can be aided by certain kinds of political activity (see section 5.5). Reconciliation can be encouraged through political interventions such as educational campaigns that introduce positive narratives of the social identities in question, or by the extension of legal rights to groups previously denied them. In general, political interventions that aim to humanize certain groups in society may prime social relations in the direction of reconciliation. The more one is able to adopt an attitude of reconciliation toward those demanding recognition, the more their claims can be heard and the validity and value of their self-understandings considered.

10.3 Does the demand for recognition of Mad identity possess normative force?

Should anything be done in response to Mad activism's demand for recognition? In general, demands for recognition possess normative force if it can be demonstrated that, owing to social relations that fail to recognize them as successful agents, individuals are experiencing the social harms of disqualification and identity impairment. If we consider the particular case of the demand for recognition of Mad identity, the presence of social harms owing to misrecognition is amply evident. After all, public representations of madness as deficit, disease, and disorder are directly socially disqualifying. When activists talk about "being silenced" and about the struggle to "find a voice," a key obstacle are precisely those representations. Similarly, on the question

---

[1] See section 5.4.2 for some ways of thinking about why we should approach others with an attitude of reconciliation.

of the development of identity, for some people, being consistently subject to the discourses of disorder and illness—in general to the idea that there is something wrong with the mind—can eventually undermine self-confidence and self-esteem.[2] However, the presence of social harms satisfies only the first step in our determination of the normative force of a demand for recognition. The second step is to see if there are no *other reasons* by which the denial of recognition is justified; a further process of adjudication is therefore required. In what follows I consider three reasons that may deflate a demand for recognition of normative force: the identity for which recognition is demanded is trivial, morally objectionable, or irrational.

10.3.1 Trivial and morally objectionable identities

In some cases, the identity for which recognition is demanded is trivial. It is trivial in the sense that even though it may go deep in a person's self-understanding, it does not play a fundamental or irreplaceable orientating function in their life as agents. So-called life-style enclaves (Bell 2005, p. 230) such as golf-club memberships and (arguably) fan clubs can fall under this category. For example, if all Bryan Ferry fans were to organize and demand recognition of the validity of their musical tastes, others might be justified in judging such claims trivial, putting aside that Bryan's fans would struggle to get recognition for that particular musical choice. This is not to underplay the huge commitment people can develop toward a musical band—suicides have been known to happen—but to point out that such commitment is voluntary and wavers as the years go by: yesterday I might have died for *The Beatles*, tomorrow I might die for *Wavves* (this is purely hypothetical). Further, these commitments are localized in a way that misrecognition of the identity in question would not disqualify the person in a global manner, but only in the more limited area of, say, musical taste: it would not constitute a social harm. Contrast this with identifications based on race or gender and the sense in which identities based on "life-style enclaves" are trivial can become apparent. Is Mad identity trivial? The intensity of certain mental health phenomena, the importance that these phenomena can assume for people, their impact on people's lives, the obvious sense in which they are not voluntary, the fact that they challenge key concepts such as agency, self, and responsibility, and the far-reaching consequences of misrecognition in terms of social harms—all of this shows that Mad identity is not trivial.

In other cases, the identity for which recognition is demanded is morally objectionable. Within the framework of recognition, a morally objectionable identity is one whose demand for recognition is undercut by the fact that it denies others the conditions for well-being that it claims for itself. Examples of such identities can include self-proclaimed racist identities as well as cultural identities whose tenets conflict with claims for, say, gender equality.[3] Given this view, Mad identity is not morally objectionable,

---

[2] This does not occur for everyone of course, as some people cherish the diagnosis they receive, even more they seek a diagnosis and consider the moment they receive one to be a moment of validation (in recent times this can be seen with adult Attention Deficit Hyperactivity Disorder (ADHD) diagnoses).

[3] I have discussed these examples in section 5.3.2, and I refer the reader to that section.

or it would be only to the extent that it is constituted by beliefs that commit the same sort of error committed by self-proclaimed racist identities. A brief look at the Mad narratives discussed in section 9.3.3 shows that this error has not been committed. The narratives do not aim to reserve for themselves the conditions for well-being that they deny others, rather the aim is to extend those conditions to more people. Mad identity, thereby, is neither trivial nor (necessarily) morally objectionable; might it be irrational?

10.3.2 **Irrational identities**

In Chapter 7 I raised and examined the distinction between failed and controversial identities. I began by pointing out that every demand for recognition—all gaps in social validation—involves the perception by each side that the other is committing a mistake. Given this, I formulated the question that we had to address as follows: How do we sort out those mistakes that can be addressed within the scope of recognition (controversial identities) from those that cannot (failed identities)? The implication was that a failed identity involves a mistake that cannot be corrected by revising the category with which a person identifies, while a controversial identity involves a mistake that can, in principle, be corrected in that way. The issue I am concerned with here is no longer the identity claim as such but the validity of the collective category itself; the question is no longer "what kind of mistake is the person identifying as x implicated in?" but "is x a valid category?". This question features as an element of adjudication for the reason that some social identities can be irrational in such a way that they cannot be regarded as meriting a positive social or a political response. As Appiah (2005, p. 181) writes:

> Insofar as identities can be characterised as having both normative and factual aspects, both can offend against reason: an identity's basic norms might be in conflict with one another; its constitutive factual claims might be in conflict with the truth.

For example, consider members of the Flat Earth Society if they were to identify as Flat-Earthers and demand recognition of the validity of their identity. They may successfully demonstrate that society's refusal to recognize them as successful agents incurs on them a range of social harms such as disqualification. Yet it is clear that their identity does not merit further consideration and this for the reason that it is false: the Earth is not flat. A similar predicament befalls some Creationists; Young-Earth Creationists, for example, believe that Earth is about ten thousand years old and was created over a period of six days, a belief that stands against all scientific evidence. It is not unreasonable to suggest that neither the Flat-Earthers nor the Young-Earth Creationists ought to have their identity claims taken seriously, as the facts that constitute their identities do not measure up to what we know to be true, given the best evidence we now possess. To put it bluntly, whatever else might be at stake between us and the Flat-Earthers or Young-Earth Creationists, the shape of the Earth, its age, and the emergence and development of life on it are not.

Who does "us" refer to in this context? To those who regard *scientific rationality* as an important value to uphold in society. By scientific rationality I mean an epistemological and methodological framework that prioritizes procedural principles of knowledge acquisition (such as empirical observation, atomization of evidence, and nonmetaphysical, nondogmatic reasoning), and eschews substantive convictions about the world derived from a sacred, Divine, or otherwise infallible, authority (see Gellner 1992, pp. 80–4). In rejecting the demands of Flat-Earthers and Young-Earth Creationists, we are prioritizing the value of scientific rationality over the value of an individual's attachment to a particular identity. We are saying: we know that it matters to you that your view of the world is accepted by us, but to accept it is to undermine what we consider, in this instance, to be a more important value. Note that such a response preserves the value of free-speech—Flat-Earthers and Young-Earth Creationists are free to espouse their views. Note also that refusing to accord these identities a positive response is a separate issue from taking an active stand against them (an example of the latter would be government intervention to ban the teaching of creationism in schools).[4] What we are trying to determine here is not who should receive a negative response but who is a legitimate candidate for a positive one. Owing to the irrationality of their constituting claims, Flat-Earthers and Young-Earth Creationists are not.

At this point in the argument someone could object to the premise of assessing the rationality of identities. They could object on two grounds: they could say that there is no stance from where we can make such assessments; or they could say that even if such a stance exists and it is possible to determine the rationality of an identity, such a determination is always trumped by the demand for recognition and by individuals' attachment to their identities. Both positions could further argue that as long as an identity is neither trivial nor morally objectionable, it ought to be considered for a positive response. We can recognize in the first position a commitment to cognitive relativism, and in the second position we can recognize an extreme form of liberal tolerance. Both positions are problematic, as I argue in what follows.

Cognitive relativism begins with the idea that all knowledge claims are relative to a particular perspective, where perspective includes things like our conceptual schemes and perceptual realities (Claim 1).[5] That, in itself, is not an alarming claim, for it merely indicates that knowledge is always from a standpoint, leaving the possibility that a particular standpoint has a justifiable claim to the truth. For example, the concepts of space and time, as Kant had argued, are the conditions of possibility of all experience. This does not mean that one can no longer pursue objective truths, it means that one can only do so through a conceptual apparatus. But relativists intend a much stronger claim, the idea that owing to the plurality of conceptual schemes, no standpoint can assert a privileged status vis-a-vis others: there is no transcendental point of view that can subsume all others (Claim 2). From this claim, things tend to escalate rather quickly. Some take it to imply that we might as well give up on

---

[4] For an example of what an active stance would look like in such cases and the problems this raises, see Appiah (2005, pp. 182–9) for an ingenious thought experiment based in the mythical Republic of Cartesia. The regime in Cartesia encourages the creed of hard rationalism and actively seeks to transform *any* deviations from rationality among its citizens.

[5] There are numerous accounts of, and arguments for and against, cognitive relativism, for example, Hollis and Lukes (1982), Gellner (1987, 1992), Nagel (1997), Rorty (1998), Boghosian (2006), and Lukes (2008).

"truth" as the aim of inquiry and focus instead on pragmatic concerns such as the relative utility of our descriptions of the world; others go further by denying objectivity altogether (not merely pragmatically but ontologically), replacing it with a variety of conceptual schemes that construct different realities. If we add to this latter claim the idea that different conceptual schemes are incommensurable, we arrive at the radical end of the relativist journey: not only is knowledge bound by perspective, there is also no possibility whatsoever of making judgments across perspectives: your claims are as valid as mine, or neither of our claims are valid—which amounts to the same thing—since by fully relativizing the criteria for validity we lose the notion of universal validity itself.[6]

I leave aside the radical view, as it is unlikely that many philosophers or social scientists take seriously the incommensurability thesis. What is more relevant to my concerns here is Claim 2, the idea that there is no privileged point of view. Claim 2 is relevant because the whole point of venturing into this debate is to defend the notion that one can assess the rationality of identities in cases where they are constituted by claims of a *factual* nature; that there is a justifiable stance from where we can make such assessments. Claim 2 is correct in asserting that there is no transcendental point of view, but wrong in asserting that there is no privileged point of view. But given that there is no transcendental point of view, there is no noncircular way of establishing privilege; as Ernest Gellner (1982, p. 188) puts it: "Other visions validate themselves by their own rules, and will not play according to ours. Hence any move which eliminates them also breaks their rules, and is consequently question begging." That being said, it is possible to argue for the priority of the scientific worldview in "partially non-question begging ways" (Gellner 1982). Toward this Gellner (1987, p. 90) proposes two converging arguments, an epistemological and a sociological:

> The epistemological . . . Initially anything may be true. We ask: how can we pick out the correct option of belief, seeing that we have no prior indication of what it may be? The answer is contained in the epistemological tradition which has accompanied the rise of modern science . . . The answer is, in rough outline: eliminate all self-maintaining circular belief systems. As the main device of self-maintaining systems is the package-deal principle, which brings about the self-maintaining circle of ideas, break up information into as many parts as possible, and scrutinize each item separately. This breaks up the circle and destroys self-maintenance. At the same time, assume nevertheless the regularity of nature, the systematic nature of the world, not because it is demonstrable, but because anything which eludes such a principle also eludes real knowledge.

---

[6] One problem with the radical form of cognitive relativism is that it refutes itself. This is a common objection and one that, in my view, effectively undermines that position. Gellner (1992, p. 49–50) describes it like this (you can replace "culture" with "form of life" or "world-view" and the argument remains the same): "If standards are inherently and inescapably expressions of something called culture, and can be nothing else, then no culture can be subjected to a standard, because (*ex hypothesi*) there cannot be a transcultural standard which would stand in judgement over it. No argument could be simpler or more conclusive". Or, if relativism is true, "why is your argument for relativism not itself relative?" (Lukes 2008, p. 13).

Communities that have consistently applied this kind of epistemology, have developed a scientific practice that produced enormous "cognitive wealth," the implementation of which has led to a "very powerful technology" adopted and valued by many communities around the world (Gellner 1987, p. 91). Steven Lukes (2008, pp. 13–14) expresses this point:

> No one *really* doubts that science yields objective knowledge that enables us to predict and control our environment and that there has been massive scientific and technological progress, and no one really supposes that judgements of the cognitive superiority of later over earlier phases of scientific or of scientific over prescientific modes of thought are merely prejudices relative to "our" local conceptual or explanatory scheme. People across the world live many-layered lives that can combine magic, religion and science in countless ways, but no longer in ways that preclude acceptance of the cumulating cognitive power of science. When people are ill, they can believe in miracles, prayer and surgery. Creationists and religious fundamentalists take flu vaccines whose development presupposes the truth of Darwinism, fly in aeroplanes, and surf the Web on computers. Members of tribes who consult witch doctors seek cures in local hospitals when they can; and although countless people in modern societies hold innumerable weird and apparently irrational beliefs, they do so against the massive background of science-compatible common sense. Those who most loudly proclaim their anti-modernism never reject the whole package. Anti-modernism is a modernist stance; there is no route back from modernity.

Together, the epistemological and the sociological arguments challenge Claim 2, and support the idea that scientific rationality does have a privileged position in relation to other standpoints in so far as factual claims about the world are concerned.

Moving on to the position of the extremely tolerant liberals, another problem presents itself. In passing a positive judgment despite being aware that the identity is irrational, their judgment manages to be both invalid and condescending.[7] It is invalid because in repudiating relevant criteria for assessment, it ceases to be a judgment. Note that the Flat-Earthers demand that we recognize the validity of their identity (i.e., the truth of the claims that make up their identity). The validity of our judgment, therefore, rests precisely on being informed by a determination of the truth of their claims. The extremely tolerant liberal's judgment is also condescending for the reason that it is a lie. In demanding recognition, people want to have their identities genuinely affirmed as valid and valuable, and not to be at the end of a socially orchestrated lie. There is no doubt that some people could be satisfied with an insincere yet positive judgment. Writ large, however, a society in which people constantly lie to each other by offering positive views of their respective ways-of-life or identities is very far from instantiating the ideal of recognition that we are aiming for; in fact, such a society, in being partly constituted by an essential contradiction between people's actual views and their advertised judgments is borderline dystopian.

We can now respond to those objecting to the premise of judging the rationality of identities as follows: contra cognitive relativism, it is possible to argue for the priority of one standpoint over others, a standpoint from where we can judge the rationality of identities. Equally important, we have to endorse the criteria that inform

---

[7] This argument has appeared at several points in the book; see sections 5.3.3 and 5.5.

our judgments; not to do so leaves us with invalid and condescending judgments, which is the predicament of the extremely tolerant liberal. If there is no escaping judgment—if there is no escaping that we stand somewhere in adjudicating demands for recognition—is it always appropriate to take the stance of scientific rationality?

Scientific rationality is the stance of the Enlightenment and can be contrasted with other stances such as religious fundamentalism and cultural traditionalism. Naturally, if one were to adopt, say, a religious fundamentalist stance, one is likely to come to a different view on all the questions we might ask about the rationality and moral acceptability of identities (assuming one comes as far as thinking in terms of identity and recognition). Aside from the arguments for scientific rationality presented earlier, I will continue to operate with it as a stance for the following reasons: first, scientific rationality (or something close to it) is the stance, I assume, of many of the people who are reading this book; second, it is the stance of the book itself, immersed as it is in the contemporary philosophical tradition; third, the confrontation between madness and society is mediated via psychiatry which, in this confrontation, stands in for scientific rationality: the possibility of resolving this conflict therefore requires that we deal with the confrontation in the terms in which it occurs. However, to adopt the stance of scientific rationality does not mean that it is always an appropriate stance for assessing identities; some cases might fall outside its purview. How can this come about?

Perhaps we were able to pass judgment on the rationality of Flat-Earth and Young-Earth Creationist identities because they are engaged in the same "game" that we are engaged in, it just happens that they are not very good at it. The game in question is one where participants make observations, formulate hypotheses, gather data to test hypotheses, and eventually develop theories. Of course, individually, few of us adopt such a rigorous method in forming our beliefs, but we generally accept that something like this method is our best bet for getting things right about the nature of the world.[8] And if through further experimentation and theorization it turns out that a well-established fact is not true, then we change our views accordingly. Other times, with other identities, it is not at all obvious that that is the game being played; it is not obvious that people are engaging with the world in order to get things right in the sense advocated by scientific rationality. They are not aiming to get things wrong either, but are playing a different sort of game. There are many ways of engaging with the world, and if we suspect that that is the case, then scientific rationality is not an appropriate framework for assessing the constituting claims of those identities. What other modes of engagement with the world are there? I briefly explore this by looking at the distinction between doctrine and practice, a distinction that applies to belief systems in general including the monotheistic religions. Let us begin with a case where doctrine is emphasized over practice (or ritual).

---

[8] Most of the time we acquire our knowledge from designated experts such as scientists and researchers who have the requisite knowledge and training to study natural and social phenomena. In some contexts today, the idea of the "expert" is under threat in the midst of the "horizontality" of information production and distribution that has been made possible by social media outlets, and the derision of hitherto trusted sources of information now routinely described as "fake news."

Referring to religious fundamentalism, Gellner (1992, p. 2) writes:

> The underlying idea is that a given faith is to be upheld firmly in its full and literal form, free of compromise, softening, re-interpretation or diminution. It presupposes that the core of religion is *doctrine*, rather than ritual, and also that this doctrine can be fixed with precision and finality.

Religious doctrine includes fundamental ideas about our nature, the nature of the world and the cosmos, and the manner in which we should live and treat each other. In following to the letter the doctrines of one's faith, believers are trying to get it right, where getting it right means knowing with exactness what God intended for us. In the case of Islam, the tradition I know most about, the Divine intent can be discerned from the Qur'an (considered to be the word of God) and the Traditions (the sayings) attributed to the Prophet (see Rashed 2015b).[9] The process of getting it right, therefore, becomes an interpretive one, raising questions such as: how do we understand this verse; what does God mean by the words "dust" and "clot" in describing human creation; who did the Prophet intend by this Tradition; does this Tradition follow a trusted lineage of retellers?

We can see that "getting it right" for the religious fundamentalist and for the scientific rationalist mean different things—interpreting the Divine intent, and producing true explanations of the nature of the world, respectively. But then we have a problem, for religious doctrine often involves claims whose truth—in the sense of their relation to reality—can, in principle, be established. Yet in being an interpretive enterprise, religious fundamentalism cannot claim access to the truth in this sense. The religious fundamentalist can immediately respond by pointing out that the Divine word corresponds to the truth; it *is* the truth. If we press the religious fundamentalist to tell us why this is so, we might be told that the truth of God's pronouncements in the Qur'an is guaranteed by God's pronouncement (also in the Qur'an) that His word is the truth and will be protected for all time from distortion.[10] Such a circular argument, of course, is unsatisfactory, and simply points to the fact that matters of evidence and logic have been reduced to matters of faith. If we press the religious fundamentalist further we might encounter what has become a common response: the attempt to justify the truth of the word of God by demonstrating that the Qur'an had anticipated modern scientific findings, and had done so over 1,400 years ago. This is known as the "scientific miracle of the Qur'an", where scholars interpret certain ambiguous, almost poetic verses to suggest discoveries such as the relativity of time, the process of conception, brain functions, the composition of the Sun, and many others. The irony in such an attempt is that it elevates scientific truths to the status of arbiter of the truth of the word of God. But the more serious problem is that science is a self-correcting progressive enterprise—what we know today to be true may turn out tomorrow to be false. The Qur'an, on the other hand, is fixed; every scientific claim in the Qur'an (assuming there are any that point to current scientific discoveries) is going to be refuted the moment

---

[9] The analysis in the text can equally be applied to Christianity and Judaism.

[10] I have heard several religious scholars give this sort of argument.

our science develops. You cannot use a continually changing body of knowledge to validate the eternally fixed word of God.

Neither the faith-based response nor the "scientific miracle of the Qur'an" response can tie the Divine word to the truth. From the stance of scientific rationality, all the religious fundamentalist can do is provide interpretations of the "Divine" intent as the latter can be discerned in the writings of his or her tradition. Given this, when we are presented with identities constituted by doctrinal claims whose truth can, in principle, be established (and which therefore stand or fall subject to an investigation of their veracity), we cannot extend a positive response to these identities; scientific rationality is within its means to pass judgment.

But not all religion is purely doctrinal in this sense or, more precisely, its doctrines are not intended as strictly factual claims about the world. Appiah (2005, p. 188) makes the following point:

> Gore Vidal likes to talk about ancient mystery sects whose rites have passed down so many generations that their priests utter incantations in language they no longer understand. The observation is satirical, but there's a good point buried here. Where religious observance involves the affirmation of creeds, what may ultimately matter isn't the epistemic content of the sentences ("I believe in One God, the Father Almighty . . . ") but the practice of uttering them. By Protestant habit, we're inclined to describe the devout as believers, rather than practitioners; yet the emphasis is likely misplaced.

This is a reasonable point; for many people, religion is a practical affair: they attend the mosque for Friday prayers with their family members, they recite verses from the Qur'an and repeat invocations behind the Imam, and they socialize with their friends after the prayer, and during all of this, "doctrine" is the last thing on their minds. They might even get overwhelmed with spiritual feelings of connectedness to the Divine. In the course of their ritual performance, they are likely to recite verses the content of which involves far-fetched claims about the world. It would be misguided to press them on the truth of those claims (in an empirical or logical sense), as it would be to approach, to use Taylor's (1994a, p. 67) example, "a raga with the presumptions of value implicit in the well-tempered clavier"; in both cases we would be applying the wrong measure of judgment, it would be "to forever miss the point".[11]

And then there is the possibility that the "truths" in question are metaphorical truths, symbolic expressions of human experience, its range and its moral heights and depths. Charles Taylor (2007, 1982) often talks about the expressive dimension of our experience, a dimension that has been largely expunged from scientific research and its technological application. Human civilizations have always developed rich languages of expression, religious languages being a prominent example. The rarefied language

---

[11] Another common error is to infer from people's behavior a set of beliefs to which they supposedly subscribe. We cannot take for granted individuals' conscious subscription to a body of beliefs on the basis of the assumption that their practices seem to be motivated by such beliefs. The practices might be so deeply habitual and unreflective that the motivations for performing them are not always immediately accessible. A person might find it comforting to carry an amulet for protection without this implying that they believe in a supernatural being that offers them protection by virtue of wearing this amulet.

of scientific rationality and its attendant procedural asceticism are our best bet to get things right about the world, but they are often inadequate as a means to express our psychological, emotional, and moral complexity.

To judge the practical (ritualistic) and expressive dimensions of identities in light of the standards of scientific rationality is to trespass upon these identities. Our judgments are misplaced and have limited value. My contention is that every time we suspect that we do not possess the right kind of language to understand other identities, or that there is an experience or mode of engagement that overdetermines the language in which people can express their identities, we have a genuine problem of shared understanding; we are not within our means to pass judgments of irrationality on the narratives that constitute these identities. Now I am not suggesting that the distinctions between doctrine and practice, or between understanding the world and expressing ourselves, are easy to make. And neither am I suggesting that a particular case falls neatly on side or the other of these distinctions. But if we are going to adopt the stance of scientific rationality—given that we have to adopt *some* stance as I have argued earlier—then these are the issues we need to think about: (1) Is the narrative best apprehended in its factual or expressive dimension? (2) Are there experiences that overdetermine the kind of narrative that can adequately express them?

How do Mad narratives fare in relation to these two questions? Consider the first question in relation to narratives of spiritual transformation, in this instance one based on a radical ecological perspective (section 9.3.3). A key idea in this narrative is the fundamental connectedness between mental well-being and the overall well-being of life on Earth. From the standpoint of scientific rationality, one could take issue with the factual accuracy of this claim, assuming it is possible to define it more clearly and hence be able to test it. In my view, to do so is to risk missing the point of such narratives; it is to employ the wrong measure of judgment. On the one hand, a radical ecological narrative is intended to spur us to action to look after the planet's ecosystem (and in this respect it has to make some factual claims); on the other hand, in so far as it is a narrative of *spiritual transformation*, it amounts to an individual's calibration of his or her relationship with the environment (and in this respect is best understood in its expressive dimension).

Consider the first question, again, but now in relation to a version of the narrative of "healing voices," or some related narrative pertaining to "thought insertion" that allows for external authorship of mental states. This means that it is possible for external agents (whom no one else can perceive) to speak to a person and author his thoughts. From the stance of scientific rationality, these claims are unusual, if not bizarre; they presuppose cultural psychological assumptions pertaining to the boundaries of self and to the kind of beings there are in the world that are quite alien to the scientific standpoint. Understandably, the scientific rationalist might reject these assumptions as they are incompatible with her worldview on both epistemological and ontological grounds (she cannot know about these beings nor can she justifiably presuppose their existence). Even though it is understandable for her to take that position, when it comes to passing judgment on those claims the issue is not as straightforward as it might seem.

The complication here concerns the second question mentioned earlier: are there experiences that overdetermine the kind of narrative that can adequately express them? In the case of Mad narratives, the answer is yes. Here are some examples: With the narrative of "dangerous gifts" these experiences include unique thought processes and extreme emotional states; with the narrative of "healing voices" the experiences consist, primarily, in hearing voices that are external to one's mind; in the case of narratives that allow for external authorship of mental states, the experiences include thought insertion; in the case of "spiritual transformation" the experiences consist in breakdown of the habitual experience of self and world, and disruptions to the continuity of self. To say that the experiences overdetermine the interpretive-framework is to say that the gap between this framework and the framework offered by those who might not be familiar with those experiences cannot be overcome simply by insisting on the irrationality of the former (the Mad narratives) and the coherence of the latter (the scientific rationalist's narrative): there is a genuine deficit in mutual understanding that needs to be explored. In such cases, and in cases where a narrative is best apprehended in its expressive dimension, scientific rationality is not in a position to pass judgment on the constituting claims of these identities. It is precisely those identities where they are associated with a demand for recognition, and where they are neither trivial nor morally objectionable, that ought to be considered further by asking: What should be done in response to these demands?

10.4 **Responding to misrecognition**

What is it that should be done in response to Mad activism's demand for recognition? To come as far as asking this question is to have already established that: (1) The demand for recognition of Mad identity possesses normative force; and (2) Mad identity is not trivial, morally objectionable, or irrational. We can now examine what responding to misrecognition requires, guided by the account detailed in Chapter 5, sections 5.3 to 5.5, and summarized earlier in section 10.2.

10.4.1 **What is the intended outcome?**

The demand for recognition is for society to acknowledge the validity and value of a range of counternarratives of psychological diversity: Mad narratives. It is for a narrative such as "dangerous gifts" to be seen as a valid way of understanding the thought processes and experiences referred to as "bipolar disorder." Further, it is for those thought processes and experiences to be seen as potentially valuable, an evaluation consistent with the manner in which they are portrayed by the Mad narrative in question. The ideal outcome, therefore, is for social understandings of madness to overlap with a range of Mad narratives. It is for the validity and value of Mad narratives to be *freely* and *genuinely* registered by others; as I have argued at several points in this book, recognition cannot be forced and its value is undercut when it is disingenuous (see sections 5.3.3 and 5.5). The affirmation that is demanded cannot be offered unconditionally; it can only be offered through a process of actual engagement, understanding, and evaluation of the narratives in question. The vehicle for such engagement is "conversation" in a broad sense.

10.4.2 Through what vehicle can this outcome be realized?

A conversation begins with participants; in our case, who is conversing with who? There are many people who can be involved in these conversations including: activists who are advancing counternarratives and demanding recognition; service users and patients; mental health professionals of various backgrounds; academics and researchers; members of the public not directly involved in mental health. Activists demanding recognition are the focal point of such conversations, since they are the ones issuing a direct challenge to dominant narratives. At the risk of oversimplifying things, we can say that we have a range of Mad narratives on the one hand, and a range of psychiatric and psychological diagnostic categories, constructs, and formulations on the other. For example, a person considers his voices to bring useful information that can be utilized for personal "growth" (the "healing voices" narrative), while psychiatric and psychological narratives may regard voices as misattributed inner speech with no intrinsic value (auditory verbal hallucinations). Another regards the intense disruptions and changes to her experience of self, of others, and of the world around her to be part of a process of spiritual transformation, while psychiatric and psychological narratives may regard them, for example, as a schizophrenic or psychotic episode—in general, an illness that ought to be treated, not a journey through which the person ought to be guided and assisted.

This confrontation constitutes the dramatic moment of the encounter, and highlights the gaps in social validation that we need to overcome. This is the gap between my understanding of myself through a particular Mad narrative, and other people's understanding of me through a particular psychiatric or psychological narrative. From the perspective of those demanding recognition, psychiatric and psychological narratives in such an encounter constitute misrecognition of their identities. And the aim of the conversations is to address this through serious attempts to engage with and to understand Mad narratives.[12] But not any kind of conversation will do; what we need are conversations that can lead to an outcome of reconciliation. As we know, some conversations are conducted with no desire on either side to change or to understand the other. We therefore need to specify the right attitude that should inform these conversations.

10.4.3 What attitude should inform these conversations?

Responding to misrecognition requires that we approach our conversations with others with an attitude of reconciliation. I described this attitude at length in section 5.4. It involves acknowledging, from the start, that other people's ability to find themselves validated in the social world matters as much as my own. This means that it is

---

[12] Conversations can be direct or indirect; you can sit with people in the same room and get to know them, or you can get to know them through their writings and their attempts to represent themselves. This raises questions of representation—who gets to speak on behalf of who—but these questions arise for any social and political activity that appeals to a notion of group identity (see section 4.2.4).

important for the person over there, just as it is important for me, to find a place in the social world for her identity and projects, and to receive affirmation of their validity. With this attitude in place one can, at least, begin to listen to the other and engage in conversations with the possibility of reconciliation on the agenda. It can only be a *possibility* since, as I have pointed out earlier, recognition has to be freely and genuinely offered subject to engagement, understanding, and evaluation of the narratives in question.

But why should we approach others with an attitude of reconciliation? In section 5.4.2 I argued that this is not a question we would ask of our closest friends and partners. In the best of cases, friendships and partnerships are defined by an unconditional and mutual attitude of reconciliation. Extending this attitude to others requires that we expand the scope of our concern to include those who are not our friends or partners. There are numerous obstacles that stand in the way of such an accomplishment such as the lack of an emotional connection, motivational and social-psychological issues (e.g., apathy, denial, the bystander effect), and economic and political problems that limit our concern to those with whom we normally identify. Another key obstacle is when we portray others as fundamentally unlike us, for example, as incapable of suffering in the same way or to the extent that we do, or that they lack some fundamental human value or capacity. Invariably, such assumptions are prejudices based on imagined conceptions. While reversing these conceptions and humanizing others can go some way toward expanding our range of concern, it is unlikely that it will be sufficient on its own due to the other obstacles just indicated.[13] But it is a start, and it goes some way toward addressing misrecognition.

10.4.4 What kind of activities can facilitate reconciliation?

An attitude of reconciliation can be facilitated by reversing popular prejudices concerning others, the kind of prejudices that render them unworthy of our concern (in the sense that their ability to find themselves at home in the social world does not matter). In the case of madness, there are a range of popular, negative prejudices that can contribute to this, including: mad people are especially violent; mad people are powerless and deserve only pity; mad people have only neurochemical and neurological changes—there is no point searching for meaning in their experiences; madness is a chronic degenerative condition. The upshot of such prejudices is that others are deemed too different to us, and on account of this we are less likely to approach them with an attitude of reconciliation. In this respect, the work of mental health charities to combat stigma is of exceptional importance (charities such as Mind and Rethink in the United Kingdom).

But fighting mental health prejudice still leaves us with the question of the positive view that should be promoted. In general, this view tends to be a version of the view that mental illness is like physical illness. For example, in 2017 the UK government launched a program of mental health reform that re-emphasized the objective

---

[13] See section 5.4.2 for details of this argument.

of achieving a "parity of esteem" between mental and physical illness.[14] Similarly, the recent campaign Heads Together—a coalition of eight charities under the patronage of the Royal Family—seeks to "change the conversation on mental health," and adopts the view that mental health is the same as physical health.[15] This popular analogy does not mean, of course, that mental and physical illnesses are similar kinds of problems (either phenomenologically or in terms of their causes). The analogy is intended, in part, to draw upon the positive aspects of ascriptions of physical illness; it is to say that, like physical illness, mental illness is not something to be ashamed of, it is not the person's fault, it is not a sign of weakness, and it can be treated.[16] That, of course, is the sort of medical view that Mad activism seeks to resist by introducing counternarratives of psychological, emotional, and experiential diversity. Though we are, perhaps, some distance from achieving this, it would be welcome to see campaigns of the kind just mentioned advance, in addition to the medical view, a plurality of alternative narratives of madness. Doing so can increase the public's exposure to these narratives and can play a role in facilitating reconciliation. A notable, recent example is the documentary *Why Did I Go Mad?* aired in 2017 on the BBC Horizon series. It advanced ideas close to the "healing voices" narrative described in section 9.3.3. The reach of the BBC, and of similar major broadcasting corporations, makes them ideal for publicizing alternative narratives of madness.

We have now addressed the two main questions identified in section 10.1. In the concluding section of this chapter, I shall briefly consider some anticipated benefits of a successful process of reconciliation.

10.5 **Mad narratives and the cultural repertoire**

An anticipated benefit of a successful process of reconciliation with Mad narratives is a broadening of our cultural repertoire as it pertains to madness beyond medical and psychological theories. What is the "cultural repertoire" and what are the concrete benefits of genuinely incorporating Mad narratives within it?

The notion of a "cultural repertoire" was introduced by Ann Swidler (1986, p. 273) who viewed culture as a "'tool kit' of symbols, stories, rituals, and world-views, which people may use in varying configurations to solve different kinds of problems." This notion challenged the idea of culture as a monolithic entity that overdetermines individual agency and experience, an idea that was prevalent in early anthropological studies (and can still be seen today in some public discourse in the form of the supposed uniformity of the traits and motivations of individuals by virtue of their "cultural" belonging) (see Rashed 2013b). Medical anthropological studies of madness that operated with the notion of culture as a "resource" or a "tool kit" were able to show

---

[14] See the following report: The Government's response to the Five Year Forward View for Mental Health. January 2017. Online: https://www.gov.uk/government/publications/five-year-forward-view-for-mental-health-government-response

[15] Online: https://www.headstogether.org.uk/

[16] See section 2.2.4 for more on this idea.

that individuals are actively and creatively involved in making sense of their experiences (see section 9.5). Naturally, this process occurs under a range of constraints that include the nature and the intensity of the experiences, the response of the designated experts, the input of family members, the capacity for individual creativity, and social positioning and power (see Rashed 2012). Further, while there certainly is scope for the conscious and creative "use" of the cultural repertoire, we must note that fundamental aspects of our thinking, behaving, and embodied experience are culturally inscribed yet are not ordinarily available for us to transform or reject; neither cultural determinism nor individual agency have full reign.

All that being the case, a key limitation on people's ability to make sense of their experiences is an impoverished cultural repertoire. It is, for example, to find oneself attracted to members of the same sex in a society where such attraction can only be one of two things: a sin or a crime. And in the case of madness, it is to be in a society where a range of experiences, emotional expressions, and psychological states are invariably understood as mental disorder, mental illness, or psychological dysfunction, to name some key notions. In this sense, we can understand Gay activism and Mad activism as broadening our cultural repertoire as it pertains to sexuality and madness, respectively. In the case of madness, Mad activism seeks to introduce a range of Mad narratives that are more faithful to people's experiences and can help them make sense of what they are going through (see section 9.3.3). To the extent that Mad activism is successful, these narratives become part of the cultural repertoire; that is, they are socially understood, valued, and accepted. But success here, as I have argued in Chapter 5 and in this chapter, is the outcome of a process of reconciliation: that outcome cannot be anticipated or forced. We cannot anticipate that people are going to *understand, value,* or *accept* a set of ideas (and we cannot, obviously, force them to); what we can do is to set things on the right track and encourage people to approach each other with an attitude of reconciliation, as I have argued in section 10.4.

Nevertheless, in the spirit of positive anticipation, I shall conclude my investigation of Mad activism's demand for recognition by outlining some possible benefits of broadening our cultural repertoire to include Mad narratives. Mad narratives, I contend, can become a cultural form of societal adjustment—a "cultural adjustment"— and hence a resource that can bring benefits for many people in society beyond the activists who played a key role in constructing and popularizing these narratives. An analogy with physical adjustments can illuminate this point (see Table 10.1). For physical adjustments—I will use the example of ramps that provide wheelchair access to buildings—we can conceive of immediate and delayed beneficiaries, as well as an overall social benefit. Immediate beneficiaries, typically, are people who use wheelchairs; they are the intended beneficiaries of the adjustment. Unintended, immediate beneficiaries are people with mobility difficulties who already find it difficult to navigate stairs, and parents with prams who otherwise have to face the cumbersome task of carrying the pram up a flight of stairs. Delayed beneficiaries are people who are well today but may experience mobility difficulties in the future, and people who are bed-bound today but are expected to use a wheelchair soon. In terms of overall social benefit, physical adjustments such as wheelchair ramps sensitize the public to people's

Table 10.1 Physical adjustments and cultural adjustments

Domain	Physical adjustments	Cultural adjustments
Example	Wheelchair ramps	Mad narratives
Immediate beneficiaries	(a) Intended: wheelchair users. (b) Unintended: people with mobility difficulties who do not use wheelchairs; parents with prams.	People experiencing phenomena of madness and actively searching for ways to make sense of their experiences (see section 9.5).
Delayed beneficiaries	People who are bed-bound today but will use a wheelchair in the future. People who are healthy today but may become frail in the future.	People experiencing severe thought disorder and cognitive difficulties in the present but who may be in a therapeutic position to make use of Mad narratives in the future. People who are not experiencing phenomena of madness today but may do so in the future.
Overall social benefit	Increased awareness of and sensitivity toward the needs of people with mobility difficulties. Enabling people with mobility difficulties to take part in employment.	Increased awareness of the different meanings of madness. Increased intelligibility and acceptance of phenomena of madness and of psychological/ experiential difference more broadly (see section 2.2.5).
Nonbeneficiaries[1]	People with mobility difficulties who do not wish to use a wheelchair, opting for prostheses or medical correction. People who will never experience mobility difficulties.	People who opt for an exclusively medical, diagnostic understanding of their experiences. People who will never experience the relevant mental health phenomena.

[1] In some sense, there is no such thing as a nonbeneficiary. As citizens in a community and as members of society, our well-being is connected to the well-being of others, though this is not always directly evident. That being said, we can still consider who would be a nonbeneficiary in the most immediate sense of the term; that is, people who will never personally make use of a wheelchair ramp or a Mad narrative.

different needs and abilities. They also enable people with mobility difficulties to take a more substantial part in public life, including employment.

The same typology of benefits can be discerned in relation to Mad narratives, now that we conceive of them as cultural adjustments. Immediate beneficiaries are people experiencing phenomena such as passivity experiences, voices, extreme emotional states, and disruptions to the unity and continuity of self, and who are actively searching for ways to make sense of their experiences. A rich cultural repertoire of narratives pertaining to these experiences can help people find a sense of meaning, purpose, agency, and unity and continuity of self. Crucially, the anticipated social acceptability of these narratives means that in developing a personalized understanding of her experiences in light of a Mad narrative, the person would not be left with an idiosyncratic sub-jective narrative but with one that is more likely to be socially sanctioned. Delayed beneficiaries are people who are experiencing severe cognitive difficulties at present, and who by virtue of this cannot make use of Mad narratives now, but who may be able to do so in the future, perhaps in a therapeutic context. Of course, anyone at some point in their life can experience phenomena of madness, and in this respect everyone is in some sense a delayed beneficiary. Overall social benefit is more marked here than it is with physical adjustments. Diversifying the social meanings of madness beyond illness and pathology can improve acceptance of unusual experiences and of psychological and behavioral difference more broadly. Despite the obvious differences between physical and cultural adjustments, we can see that in both cases—exemplified by wheelchair ramps and Mad narratives—the adjustments can have benefits that go beyond the immediate, intended beneficiaries.

If we can imagine a future where a range of Mad narratives have become an estab-lished part of the cultural repertoire, a future in which the benefits I outlined here earlier are evident, we must ensure that it is a future where one particular narrative has not become a *master* narrative. I began this book by pointing to the dominance in contemporary culture of the view that madness is a disorder (or a dysfunction or an illness) of the mind. Mad activism rose against the dominance and inadequacies of this view and sought to populate our culture with alternative narratives of madness. Creating a rich cultural repertoire in which a diversity of people with a diversity of experiences can find themselves is an important goal. Once achieved, however, this goal would be compromised at the point where one narrative claims dominance and undermines all others. And while this is a social process that we cannot fully anticipate or control, it is a process of which we must remain aware.

10.6 **Conclusion**

This chapter addressed the following questions: (1) Does the demand for recogni-tion of Mad identity possess normative force? (2) How should society respond to the demand for recognition of Mad identity? With regard to the first question I argued that a demand for recognition possesses normative force if it can satisfy two require-ments: first, demonstrate the presence of social harms owing to misrecognition; sec-ond, there are no other reasons that deflate the demand of normative force (i.e., the identity for which recognition is demanded is not trivial, morally objectionable, or irrational). As I have argued at length in section 10.3, Mad identity can satisfy these two requirements.

In answering the second question, I developed a framework for responding to mis-recognition. This framework consists in several interlocking requirements. The core of the response are the conversations that need to occur between, on the one hand, activists and others advancing counternarratives of madness and, on the other, propo-nents of medical and psychological narratives of madness. If these conversations are to have a chance of succeeding they need to be informed by an attitude of reconcilia-tion. This attitude, in turn, can be facilitated through campaigns that seek to reverse negative prejudices pertaining to madness, and to advance alternative narratives of madness beyond the analogy with physical health. Achieving an outcome of reconciliation cannot be anticipated or forced. Conversations with madness, and the social changes that need to occur, have to take their course. The intention behind constructing a framework for responding to misrecognition, as attempted in this chapter, was to chart a possible path that can be taken.

Chapter 11

Conclusion: Pathways to reconciliation

11.1 Reconciling skeptics and supporters

In the Introduction to this book, I noted two responses that this project could meet even before it starts: skeptical and supportive. Skeptics unconditionally reject the claims and demands of Mad activism while supporters unconditionally accept them. Both do not see the point of examining those claims and demands for they consider them to be fundamentally incoherent and/or irrelevant (the skeptic's position) or fundamentally correct (the supporter's position) (see Introduction). It is fitting, therefore, to conclude this book by responding to the skeptics and the supporters given what we have acquired over the past chapters in terms of an analysis of the claims and demands of Mad activism. In offering this response, there may also be a prospect of reconciling skeptics and supporters in their mutually exclusive positions.

The two fundamental points on which the prospect of reconciliation rests are: (1) whether or not madness can be grounds for identity (a question of possibility); and (2) the relevance of Mad activism beyond activists themselves (a question of scope).

11.1.1 The possibility-objection

The possibility-objection, as it has been formulated and discussed in Part III, goes like this: if madness cannot be grounds for identity, then the notion of Mad identity is incoherent—it claims a basis in phenomena that undermine its very possibility. And if that is the case, then skeptics could be justified in their unconditional rejection of the central claim of Mad activism. On the other hand, if madness can be grounds for identity, then the skeptics would need to reconsider their position, and a meeting point with the supporters could be in view. The importance of this issue led to its consideration over the course of three chapters (7 to 9). The problem is that certain mental health phenomena appear to undermine key requirements that must be met in order for an identity claim to be the kind of claim that can be considered within the scope of recognition. We have seen that an identity claim must be a controversial and not a failed claim, must be an expression of a unified mental life, and must persist over a sufficient period of time. These requirements are jeopardized by, respectively, delusions, passivity phenomena, and the discontinuities of self often seen in the conditions of schizophrenia and bipolar disorder. If madness (represented here by the aforementioned phenomena) is to be grounds for identity, then it has to be shown that these phenomena do not necessarily undermine these requirements, or that they only *appear* to do so, or that they *actually* do so but there is a way of overcoming this. Each of the phenomena examined in Chapters 7 and 8 have their own distinctive fate:

- *Delusions and the requirement that an identity claim is a controversial and not a failed claim*: Delusions, where they to enter into a person's self-understanding, do not necessarily result in a failed claim; some delusional identities are controversial identities in the sense that the claim is not mistaken on its own terms but is presenting a radical view of the category with which the person is identifying.

- *Passivity phenomena and disunity of self*: The judgment that passivity phenomena undermine unity of self presupposes certain cultural psychological assumptions about self and world, assumptions pertaining to the possibility of external authorship of mental states. In contexts where such authorship is deemed possible, then passivity phenomena can constitute an enrichment and not a disunity of self. In contexts where it is not deemed possible, there remains a possibility for overcoming judgments of disunity by creating new contexts of judgment through activism.

- *Schizophrenia, bipolar disorder, and discontinuity of self*: These conditions can manifest in discontinuity of self of a longitudinal and a cyclical nature, respectively. Narratives discontinuities of this sort can be overcome through unifying narratives that retain social intelligibility.

With the aforementioned conclusions at hand, we can ask again: Can madness be grounds for identity? In many cases, madness can only be grounds for identity once it is ordered in some way. The task of ordering madness is a dual achievement: the resolution of impairments to identity formation *and* the preservation of something of the phenomenology of madness. Mad narratives—the narratives of psychological, emotional, and experiential diversity advanced by activists—can, in principle, provide the required unity and continuity of self while remaining faithful to the phenomenology of madness (see sections 9.2.2 and 9.3). In conclusion, madness can be grounds for identity: the possibility-objection cannot be upheld.

Establishing the possibility for madness to be grounds for identity does not mean that it always can be in practice. Skeptics therefore can concede the point that madness can be grounds for identity while raising another objection: they can concede that Mad identity is not an incoherent notion but that it does not apply to them or to the people they see in the clinic.

11.1.2 **The scope-objection**

The scope-objection accepts the coherence of Mad activism but limits the latter's relevance to the activists themselves, to those people who have lived-experience of mental health phenomena, and who are already demanding recognition and constructing counternarratives of psychological diversity. Skeptics who have clinical roles can point out—and indeed they are correct to do so—that some of the people they see on acute wards and rehabilitation units may have, for example, severe disturbances of the thinking process, significant cognitive difficulties, and a fragmented sense of self such that the claims and demands of Mad activism do not apply to them. Those individuals—the skeptics can continue—require treatment and care, not political recognition for a self-understanding they do not appear able to express. Similarly, skeptics who are service users and adopt a medical understanding of their experiences might not regard Mad activism to be speaking to them. If Mad activism is not to fall into irrelevance, it has to demonstrate the extended benefit it can bring to various groups of people and to society in general.

The wider benefits of Mad activism can be encapsulated in the notion, outlined in Chapter 10, that Mad narratives are *cultural adjustments*: a broadening of our cultural repertoire as it pertains to madness beyond medical and psychological theories; a resource of ideas about madness that are available for individuals to utilize to make sense of their experiences. Though obviously different in key ways, I drew an analogy with physical adjustments to parse out the range of benefits (Table 10.1). We have seen that Mad narratives have benefits that go beyond the groups of activists advancing these notions. The scope-objection advanced by the skeptics is too severe in its limitation of the benefits of Mad activism.

In conclusion, the possibility-objection and the scope-objection advanced by skeptics are inaccurate: as I have argued in this book, madness *can* be grounds for identity, and the benefits of Mad activism can have wide relevance. In demonstrating this, we have generated a possibility for reconciling skeptics and supporters, with supporters able to qualify and defend those claims and demands and not merely to unconditionally accept them.

11.2 **Reconciling madness and society**

Reconciling skeptics and supporters is only part of the issue; the broader challenge is to reconcile madness with society. The process of reconciliation was examined by asking the following question: Does the demand for recognition of Mad identity possess normative force and, if it does, how should society respond to it? Given the philosophical and political account of recognition detailed in Part II, and in light of the criteria for adjudication outlined in Part IV, a demand for recognition possesses normative force if it can satisfy the following two steps: (1) Demonstrate that individuals are experiencing the social harms of disqualification and/or identity impairment owing to social relations that fail to recognize them as successful agents. (2) There are no reasons that deflate the demand of normative force (i.e., the demand is not trivial, morally objectionable, or irrational). The demand for recognition of Mad identity satisfies the first step: social disqualification is the hallmark of the distinctive form of misrecognition experienced by those considered to be "mentally ill" or to have a "mental disorder." The demand also satisfies the second step in that the narratives that make up Mad identity are neither trivial nor morally objectionable. The question of irrationality, however, is more complex.

We have seen that some identities are constituted by false claims, a clear example being an identity based on membership of the Flat Earth Society. Such identities, though they may not be trivial nor morally objectionable, are irrational in a way that it would be counterintuitive to suggest that we ought to somehow expend an effort to reconcile with its holders (where such reconciliation requires that the correct shape of the Earth is at stake between us). In this case, we are prioritizing the value of scientific rationality over the value of an individual's attachment to a particular identity.

A legitimate question to ask is whether scientific rationality ought to be prioritized in such cases. In the example of the Flat Earth Society I am confident that it ought to be, for otherwise we would be peddling in what we know—given the best evidence we now possess—to be falsehoods. In other cases, however, our confidence must be tempered, for it might be that scientific rationality is not an appropriate framework for approaching the identity in question. Some claims, though they appear to concern factual matters, are better apprehended in their performative and expressive aspects. In some cases, we might not possess at the outset the appropriate vocabulary to understand the beliefs and practices we are encountering. In other cases, the claims of the identity in question are interpretations of experience and hence are not directly touched by the criteria of factual accuracy. In all these cases, we must suspend our judgments of irrationality, for there appears to be a deficit in mutual understanding that precludes such judgments. As I argue in Chapter 10, this is exactly what we need to do in relation to Mad narratives such as "dangerous gifts," "spiritual emergence," and "healing voices". These narratives are best apprehended as interpretive, meaning-giving frameworks (rather than factual claims to be tested empirically). Further, they are constructed to make sense of experiences with which the person passing the ill-advised judgment of irrationality might not be familiar. On the question of irrationality, Mad narratives do not deflate the demand for recognition of its normative force.

Having satisfied the two aforementioned steps, the demand for recognition of Mad identity is a justified demand. Political reform and interpersonal reconciliation are two possible responses to justified demands for recognition (see Chapter 5). Political reform can involve coercive and/or incentivizing institutional activities aimed at addressing misrecognition. In the case of Mad activism this could involve, for example, the treatment of certain psychiatric terms in the same way that racial slurs are regarded today. However, coercion and incentive are not adequate responses to misrecognition given the requirement that recognition is freely and genuinely offered. As we know from the state of race and interfaith relations in many communities, banning certain terms or criminalizing their use might not lead to genuine and mutual recognition. In fact, such political actions are perceived by some as an infringement on free speech and may have the opposite effect by breeding resentment. Where political action can be helpful is when it creates favorable conditions for people to meet, for instance, by promoting humanizing narratives concerning misrecognized groups in society, or by the extension of hitherto denied legal and civil rights. Favorable conditions of this sort can encourage what is ultimately the required response to demands for recognition: the achievement of interpersonal reconciliation.

Reconciliation involves accommodation between individuals in the life contexts in which they interact, mediated via the narratives that inform these interactions. Reconciliation is both an attitude and an outcome. As an attitude it involves approaching others with the acknowledgment that their ability to find their identity validated in the social world matters as much as my own. As an outcome it is to achieve reconciliation in the sense that the narratives that make up their identity are actually validated. In the case of Mad activism, it is for counternarratives such as "spiritual emergence" and "dangerous gifts" to be accepted as valid narratives and in this way to become components of our cultural repertoire as it pertains to madness. But whereas that is the ideal to aim for, it cannot be forced as that would undercut the value of such acceptance and undermine the genuine social change in beliefs that is demanded. What needs to happen is for people to interact where such interactions are informed by an attitude of reconciliation. These interactions, where they involve activists and mental health professionals or members of the public, tend to begin with a confrontation of two sets of opposing narratives: a range of Mad narratives on the one hand, and a range of psychiatric/psychological narratives on the other. With the right attitude in place, what should happen next is a conversation where the narratives of Mad identity would no longer be dismissed as "incoherent" or "irrational." Instead, there would be genuine attempts to understand these narratives and to register their value.

Interrogating the concepts and methods of understanding that must inform these conversations if they are to be successful at achieving reconciliation is a further project to be considered. What I hope to have achieved in this book is to have cleared the ground for such a project by showing that madness can be grounds for identity, that Mad activism has relevance beyond the group of activists themselves, and that Mad narratives cannot be immediately dismissed as irrational. The demand for recognition of Mad identity possesses normative force: conversations with madness are ones that society ought to have.

References

Al-Ghazali, M. (2010). *The Alchemy of Happiness*. C. Field (Trans.). New York: Cosimo Publishers.

American Psychiatric Association (1994). *Diagnostic and Statistical Manual of Mental Disorders*, 4th edition. New York: American Psychiatric Association.

American Psychiatric Association (2000). *Diagnostic and Statistical Manual of Mental Disorders IV-TR*. [Revised 4th edition]. New York: American Psychiatric Association.

Amundson, R. (1992). Disability, Handicap, and the Environment. *Journal of Social Philosophy*, 23(1), 105–19.

Amundson, R. (2000). Against Normal Function. *Studies in History and Philosophy of Biological and Biomedical Science*, 31(1), 33–53.

Amundson, R., and Tresky, S. (2007). On a Bioethical Challenge to Disability Rights. *Journal of Medicine and Philosophy*, 32(6), 541–61.

Anderson, J., and Honneth, A. (2005). Autonomy, Vulnerability, Recognition, and Justice. In: J. Christman and J. Anderson (eds.). *Autonomy & Challenges to Liberalism*. Cambridge: Cambridge University Press, pp. 127–49.

Anscombe, E. (1958). Modern Moral Philosophy. *Philosophy*, 33(124), 1–16.

Appiah, A. (1994a). Race, Culture, Identity: Misunderstood Connections. *The Tanner Lecture on Human Values*. Delivered at University of California, San Diego. Online: http://tannerlectures.utah.edu/_documents/a-to-z/a/Appiah96.pdf

Appiah, K. (1994b). Identity, Authenticity, Survival: Multicultural Societies and Social Reproduction. In: A. Gutmann (ed.). *Multiculturalism: Examining the Politics of Recognition*. New Jersey: Princeton University Press, pp. 149–63.

Appiah, K. (2005). *The Ethics of Identity*. New Jersey: Princeton University Press.

Ayer, A. J. (1946). *Language, Truth and Logic*, 2nd edition. London: Victor Gollancz.

Barker, P., Campbell, P., and Davidson, B. C. (eds.) (1999). *From the Ashes of Experience: Reflections on Madness, Survival, and Growth*. London: Whurr Publishers.

Bayne, T. (2013). The Disunity of Consciousness in Psychiatric Disorders. In: K. W. M. Fulford, M. Davies, R. Gipps, G. Graham, J. Sadler, G. Stanghellini, and T. Thornton (eds.). *The Oxford Handbook of Philosophy and Psychiatry*. Oxford: Oxford University Press, pp. 673–88.

Bell, D. (2005). A Communitarian Critique of Liberalism. *Analyse & Kritik*, 27, 215–38.

Beresford, P. (2000). What Have Madness and Psychiatric System Survivors Got to Do with Disability and Disability Studies? *Disability and Society*, 15(1), 167–72.

Beresford, P. (2005). Social Approaches to Madness and Distress: User Perspectives and User Knowledge. In: J. Tew (ed.). *Social Perspectives in Mental Health: Developing Social Models to Understand and Work with Mental Distress*. London: Jessica Kingsley Publishers, pp. 32–52.

Beresford, P., Nettle, M., and Perring, R. (2010). Towards a Social Model of Madness and Distress: Exploring What Service Users Say. Joseph Rowntree Foundation. Online: https://www.jrf.org.uk/sites/default/files/jrf/migrated/files/mental-health-service-models-full.pdf

Boghosian, P. (2006). *Fear of Knowledge: Against Relativism and Constructivism*. Oxford: Clarendon Press.

Bolton, D. (2007). The Usefulness of Wakefield's Definition for the Diagnostic Manuals. *World Psychiatry*, **6**, 164–65.

Bolton, D. (2008). *What is Mental Disorder? An Essay in Philosophy, Science and Values*. Oxford: Oxford University Press.

Bolton, D. (2013). What Is Mental Illness. In: K. W. M. Fulford, M. Davies, R. Gipps, G. Graham, J. Sadler, G. Stanghellini, and T. Thornton (eds.). *The Oxford Handbook of Philosophy and Psychiatry*. Oxford: Oxford University Press, pp. 434–50.

Boorse, C. (1997). A Rebuttal on Health. In: J. Humber and R. Almeder (eds.). *What Is Disease?* Totowa, NJ: Humana Press, pp. 1–134.

Boorse, C. (2011). Concepts of Health and Disease. In: F. Gifford (ed.). *Philosophy of Medicine*. Amsterdam: Elsevier, pp. 13–64.

Bortolotti, L. (2009). *Delusions and Other Irrational Beliefs*. Oxford: Oxford University Press.

Bortolotti, L. (2013). Rationality and Sanity: The Role of Rationality Judgements in Understanding Psychiatric Disorders. In: K. W. M. Fulford, M. Davies, R. Gipps, G. Graham, J. Sadler, G. Stanghellini, and T. Thornton (eds.). *The Oxford Handbook of Philosophy and Psychiatry*. Oxford: Oxford University Press, pp. 480–96.

Bortolotti, L. (2015). *Irrationality*. Cambridge: Polity Press.

Bortolotti, L., and Broome, M. (2009). A Role for Ownership and Authorship in the Analysis of Thought Insertion. *Phenomenology and Cognitive Science*, **8**, 205–24.

Bortolotti, L., Cox, R., Broome, M., and Mameli, M. (2012). Rationality and Self-Knowledge in Delusion and Confabulation: Implications for Autonomy as Self-Governance. In: L. Radoilska (eds.). *Autonomy and Mental Disorder*. Oxford: Oxford University Press, pp. 100–22.

Bourguignon, E. (1989). Multiple Personality, Possession Trance, and the Psychic Unity of Mankind. *Ethos*, **17**, 371–84.

Bourguignon, E. (2005). Spirit Possession. In: C. Casey and R. Edgerton (eds.). *A Companion to Psychological Anthropology: Modernity and Psychocultural Change*. Oxford: Blackwell Publishing, pp. 374–88.

Bracken, P., and Thomas, P. (2005). *Postpsychiatry: Mental Health in a Postmodern World*. Oxford: Oxford University Press.

Bracken, P., and Thomas, P. (2013). Challenges to the Modernist Identity of Psychiatry: User Empowerment and Recovery. In: K. W. M. Fulford, M. Davies, R. Gipps, G. Graham, J. Sadler, G. Stanghellini, and T. Thornton (eds.). *The Oxford Handbook of Philosophy and Psychiatry*. Oxford: Oxford University Press, pp. 123–38.

Bratman, M. (2007). *Structures of Agency: Essays*. Oxford: Oxford University Press.

Brubaker, R. (2016). *Trans: Gender and Race in an Age of Unsettled Identities*. New Jersey: Princeton University Press.

Burstow, B. (2013). A Rose by Any Other Name. In: B. LeFrançois, R. Menzies, and G. Reaume (eds.). *Mad Matters: A Critical Reader in Canadian Mad Studies*. Toronto: Canadian Scholars' Press, pp. 79–90.

Campbell, P. (1992). A Survivor's View of Community Psychiatry. *Journal of Mental Health*, **1**(2), 117–22.

Campbell, P. (2009). The Service User/Survivor Movement. In: J. Reynolds, R. Muston, T. Heller, J. Leach, M. McCormick, J. Wallcraft, and M. Walsh (eds.). *Mental Health Still Matters*. Basingstoke: Palgrave Macmillan, pp. 46–52.

Campbell, P., and Roberts, A. (2009). Survivors' History. *A Life in the Day*, **13**(3), 33–9.

Caney, S. (1992). Liberalism and Communitarianism: A Misconceived Debate. *Political Studies*, **40**(2), 273–89.

Carr, S. (2005). 'The Sickness Label Infected Everything We Said': Lesbian and Gay Perspectives on Mental Distress. In: J. Tew (ed.). *Social Perspectives in Mental Health: Developing Social Models to Understand and Work with Mental Distress*. London: Jessica Kingsley Publishers, pp. 168–83.

Chamberlin, J. (1988). *On Our Own. Patient Controlled Alternatives to the Mental Health System*. London: MIND.

Chamberlin, J. (1990). The Ex-Patients' Movement: Where We've Been and Where We're Going. *The Journal of Mind and Behavior*, **11**(3), 323–36.

Chamberlin, J. (1995). Rehabilitating Ourselves: The Psychiatric Survivor Movement. *International Journal of Mental Health*, **24**(1), 39–46.

Clare (2011). Mad Culture, Mad Community, Mad Life. *Asylum: The Magazine for Democratic Psychiatry*, **18**(1), 15–17.

Clark, S. (2013). Personal Identity and Identity Disorders. In: K. Fulford, M. Davies, R. Gipps, G. Graham, J. Sadler, G. Stanghellini, and T. Thornton (eds.). *The Oxford Handbook of Philosophy and Psychiatry*. Oxford: Oxford University Press, pp. 911–28.

Clay, S. (1999). Madness and Reality. In: P. Barker, P. Campbell, and B. Davidson (eds.). *From the Ashes of Experience: Reflections on Madness, Survival, and Growth*. London: Whurr Publishers, pp. 16–36.

Cohen, E. (2007). *The Mind Possessed: The Cognition of Spirit Possession in an Afro-Brazilian Religious Tradition*. Oxford: Oxford University Press.

Cohen, E. (2008). What Is Spirit Possession? Defining, Comparing and Explaining Two Possession Forms. *Ethnos*, **73**(1), 101–26.

Cooper, D. (1967). *Psychiatry and Anti-Psychiatry*. London: Tavistock Publications.

Cooper, D. (1978). *The Language of Madness*. London: Allen Lane.

Cooper, R. (2013). Natural Kinds. In: K. W. M. Fulford, M. Davies, R. Gipps, G. Graham, J. Sadler, G. Stanghellini, and T. Thornton (eds.). *The Oxford Handbook of Philosophy and Psychiatry*. Oxford: Oxford University Press, pp. 950–65.

Costa, L. (2015). Mad Pride in Our Mad Culture. *Consumer/Survivor Information Resource Centre Bulletin*, No. 535. Online: http://www.csinfo.ca/bulletin/Bulletin_535.pdf

Craigie, J., and Bortolotti, L. (2015). Rationality, Diagnosis, and Patient Autonomy in Psychiatry. In: J. Sadler, C. W. van Staden, and K. W. M. Fulford (eds.). *The Oxford Handbook of Psychiatric Ethics*, Volume 1. Oxford: Oxford University Press, pp. 387–404.

Crisp, R. (2006). *Reasons and the Good*. Oxford: Oxford University Press.

Crisp, R. (2013). Commentary: Value-Based Practice by a Different Route. In: K. W. M. Fulford, M. Davies, R. Gipps, G. Graham, J. Sadler, G. Stanghellini, and T. Thornton (eds.). *The Oxford Handbook of Philosophy and Psychiatry*. Oxford: Oxford University Press, pp. 411–12.

Crossley, N. (2004). Not Being Mentally Ill: Social Movement, System Survivors, and the Oppositional Habitus. *Anthropology & Medicine*, **11**(2), 161–80.

Crossley, N. (2006). *Contesting Psychiatry: Social Movements in Mental Health*. London: Routledge.

Curtis, T., Dellar, R., Leslie, E. and Watson, B. (2000). (eds.). *Mad Pride: A Celebration of Mad Culture*. Truro: Chipmunka Publishing.

Dain, N. (1989). Critics and Dissenters: Reflections on "Anti-Psychiatry" in the United States. *Journal of the History of the Behavioural Sciences*, **25**, 3–25.

Davis, K. (1938). Mental Hygiene and the Class Structure. *Psychiatry*, **1**, 55–64.

deBie, A. (2013). And What Is Mad Pride? Opening Speech of the First Mad Pride Hamilton Event on July 27, 2013. *This Insane Life*, **1**, 7–8.

Desjarlais, R. (1996). Struggling Along. In: M. Jackson (ed.). *Things as They Are: New Directions in Phenomenological Anthropology*. Bloomington: Indiana University Press, pp. 70–93.

Diamond, S. (2014). Feminist Resistance Against the Medicalization of Humanity: Integrating Knowledge about Psychiatric Oppression and Marginalized People. In: B. Burstow, B. LeFrançois, and S. Diamond (eds.). *Psychiatry Disrupted: Theorizing Resistance and Crafting the (R)evolution*. Montreal: Mc-Gill-Queen's University Press, pp. 194–207.

Disley, L. (2015). *Hegel, Love and Forgiveness: Positive Recognition in German Idealism*. London: Pickering and Chatto.

Dolezal, R. (2017). *In Full Color: Finding My Place in a Black and White World*. Dallas, TX: Benbella Books.

DuBrul, S. (2014). The Icarus Project: A Counter Narrative for Psychic Diversity. *Journal of Medical Humanities*, **35**, 257–71.

Dübgen, F. (2012). Africa Humiliated? Misrecognition in Development Aid. *Res Publica*, **18**, 65–77.

Dworkin, R. (1978). Liberalism. In: S. Hampshire (ed.). *Public and Private Morality*. Cambridge: Cambridge University Press, pp. 113–43.

DWP. (2009). *Realising Ambitions: Better Employment Support for People with a Mental Health Condition*. Department for Work and Pensions: The Stationery Office Limited.

Edwards, R. (1981). Mental Health as Rational Autonomy. *Journal of Medicine and Philosophy*, **6**, 309–22.

Fabrega, H. (1989). On the Significance of an Anthropological Approach to Schizophrenia. *Psychiatry*, **52**, 45–64.

Fabris, E. (2013). Mad Success: What Could go Wrong When Psychiatry Employs Us as "Peers"? In: B. LeFrançois, R. Menzies, and G. Reaume (eds.). *Mad Matters: A Critical Reader in Canadian Mad Studies*. Toronto: Canadian Scholars' Press, pp. 130–40.

Farber, S. (2012). *The Spiritual Gift of Madness: The Failure of Psychiatry and the Rise of the Mad Pride Movement*. Toronto: Inner Traditions.

Findlay, J. (1962). *The Philosophy of Hegel: An Introduction and Re-examination*. New York: Collier.

Finkler, L. (1997). Psychiatric Survivor Pride Day: Community Organising with Psychiatric Survivors. *Osgoode Hall Law Journal*, **35**(3/4), 763–72.

Fletcher, E. (2017). Uncivilizing "Mental Illness": Contextualizing Diverse Mental States and Posthuman Emotional Ecologies within The Icarus Project. *Journal of Medical Humanities*, pp. 1–15, doi: 10.1007/s10912-017-9476-y.

Foster, J. (1985). *Ayer*. London: Routledge.

Foucault, M. (2001). *Madness and Civilization: A History of Insanity in the Age of Reason*. London: Routledge.

Frankfurt, H. (1971). Freedom of the Will and the Concept of the Person. *Journal of Philosophy*, **67**(1), 5–20.

Fraser, N. (2001). Recognition without Ethics? *Theory, Culture & Society*, **18**(2–3), 21–42.

Fraser, N., and **Honneth, A.** (2003). *Redistribution or Recognition? A Political-Philosophical Exchange.* London: Verso.

Fraser, N. (2008). *Adding Insult to Injury: Nancy Fraser Debates Her Critics: Debating Redistribution, Recognition and Representation.* London: Verso.

Fraser, N. (2010). Rethinking Recognition. In: H. Schmidt am Busch, and C. Zurn (eds.). *The Philosophy of Recognition: Historical and Contemporary Perspectives.* Lanham: Lexington Books, pp. 211–22.

Fricker, M. (2007). *Epistemic Injustice: Power and the Ethics of Knowing.* Oxford: Oxford University Press.

Gaita, R. (2000). *A Common Humanity: Thinking About Love and Truth and Justice.* New York: Routledge.

Gans, C. (1998). Nationalism and Immigration. *Ethical Theory and Moral Practice,* **1**(2), 159–80.

Geekie, J., and **Read, J.** (2009). *Making Sense of Madness: Contesting the Meaning of Schizophrenia.* London: Routledge.

Gellner, E. (1982). Relativism and Universals. In: M. Hollis and S. Lukes (eds.). *Rationality and Relativism.* Massachusetts: MIT Press, pp. 181–200.

Gellner, E. (1987). *Relativism and the Social Sciences.* Cambridge: Cambridge University Press.

Gellner, E. (1992). *Postmodernism, Reason, and Religion.* London: Routledge.

Gilleen, J. and **David, A. S.** (2005). The Cognitive Neuropsychiatry of Delusions: From Psychopathology to Neuropsychology and Back Again. *Psychological Medicine,* **35**(1), 5–12.

Gillett, G. (2012). How Do I Learn to Be Me Again? Autonomy, Life Skills, and Identity. In: L. Radoilska (ed.). *Autonomy and Mental Disorder.* Oxford: Oxford University Press, pp. 233–51.

Glover, J. (2003). Towards Humanism in Psychiatry. *The Tanner Lectures on Human Values.* Delivered at the University of Princeton. Online: https://tannerlectures.utah.edu/_documents/a-to-z/g/glover_2003.pdf

Goering, S. (2009). "Mental Illness" and Justice as Recognition. *Philosophy and Public Policy Quarterly,* **29**(1/2), 14–18.

Gorman, R. (2013). Thinking Through Race, Class, and Mad Identity Politics. In: B. LeFrançois, R. Menzies, and G. Reaume (eds.). *Mad Matters: A Critical Reader in Canadian Mad Studies.* Toronto: Canadian Scholars' Press, pp. 269–80.

Graby, S. (2015). Neurodiversity: Bridging the Gap Between the Disabled People's Movement and the Mental Health System Survivors' Movement. In: H. Spandler, J. Anderson, and B. Sapey (eds.). *Madness, Distress and the Politics of Disablement.* Bristol: Policy Press, pp. 231–44.

Graham, G. (2010). *The Disordered Mind: An Introduction to Philosophy of Mind and Mental Illness.* London: Routledge.

Graham, G. (2015). Identity and Agency: Conceptual Lessons for the Psychiatric Ethics of Patient Care. In: J. Sadler, C. W. van Staden, and K. W. M. Fulford (eds.). *The Oxford Handbook of Psychiatric Ethics, Volume 1.* Oxford: Oxford University Press, pp. 372–86.

Graham, G., and **Stephens, G.** (1994). *Philosophical Psychopathology.* Cambridge, MA: MIT Press.

Gunn, R. (2016). On Thought Insertion. *Review of Philosophy and Psychology,* **7**, 559–75.

Hamilton, C. (2005). *Broken Open.* Milsons Point: Transworld Publishers.

Harris, H. (1997). *Hegel's Ladder. I: The Pilgrimage of Reason.* Indianapolis: Hackett Publishing Company.

Haslam, N. (2000). Psychiatric Categories as Natural Kinds: Essentialist Thinking About Mental Disorders. *Social Research,* **67**, 1031–47.

Haslam, N. (2002). Kinds of Kinds: A Conceptual Taxonomy of Psychiatric Categories. *Philosophy, Psychiatry and Psychology,* **9**, 203–17.

Hegel, G. W. F. (1892). *The Logic of Hegel: Part One of the Encyclopaedia of the Philosophical Sciences.* Oxford: Clarendon Press.

Hegel, G. W. F. (1969). *Hegel's Science of Logic.* New York: Routledge.

Hegel, G. W. F. (1971). *Philosophy of Mind: Part Three of the Encyclopaedia of the Philosophical Sciences.* Oxford: Clarendon Press.

Hegel, G. W. F. (1977). *Phenomenology of Spirit.* Oxford: Oxford University Press.

Hegel, G. W. F. (1983). *Hegel and the Human Spirit: A Translation of the Jena Lectures on the Philosophy of Spirit.* Detroit: Wayne State University Press.

Hegel, G. W. F. (1991). *Elements of the Philosophy of Right.* Cambridge: Cambridge University Press.

Heron, R., and Greenberg, N. (2013). Mental Health and Psychiatric Disorders. In: K. Palmer, I. Brown, and J. Hobson (eds.). *Fitness for Work: Medical Aspects.* Oxford: Oxford University Press, pp. 132–54.

Hervey, N. (1986). Advocacy or Folly: The Alleged Lunatics' Friend Society, 1845–63. *Medical History,* **30**, 245–75.

Heyes, C. (2000). *Line Drawings: Defining Women Through Feminist Practice.* Ithaca, NY: Cornell University Press.

Hollis, M., and Lukes, S. (eds.) (1982). *Rationality and Relativism.* Massachusetts: MIT Press.

Holmes, G. (2013). Toxic Mental Environments and Other Psychology in the Real World Groups. In: S. Coles, S. Keenan, and B. Diamond (eds.). *Madness Contested: Power and Practice.* Herefordshire: PCCS Books, pp. 247–66.

Honneth, A. (1996). *The Struggle for Recognition: The Moral Grammar of Social Conflicts.* Cambridge, MA: MIT Press.

Honneth, A. (1997). Recognition and Moral Obligation. *Social Research,* **64**(1), 16–35.

Honneth, A. (2001a). Invisibility: On the Epistemology of "Recognition". *Proceedings of the Aristotelian Society, Supplementary Volumes,* **75**, 111–26.

Honneth, A. (2001b). Recognition or Redistribution? Changing Perspectives on the Moral Order of Society. *Theory, Culture & Society,* **18**(2–3), 43–55.

Honneth, A. (2002). Grounding Recognition: A Rejoinder to Critical Questions. *Inquiry,* **45**(4), 499–519.

Honneth, A. (2007). *Disrespect: The Normative Foundations of Critical Theory.* Cambridge: Polity Press.

Honneth, A. (2012). *The I in We: Studies in the Theory of Recognition.* Cambridge: Polity Press.

Horwitz, A., and Wakefield, J. (2007). *The Loss of Sadness: How Psychiatry Transformed Normal Sorrow into Depressive Disorder.* Oxford: Oxford University Press.

Houlgate, S. (2003). G. W. F. Hegel: The Phenomenology of Spirit. In: R. Solomon and D. Sherman (eds.). *The Blackwell Guide to Continental Philosophy.* Oxford: Wiley-Blackwell, pp. 8–29.

Houlgate, S. (2005). *An Introduction to Hegel: Freedom, Truth and History.* Oxford: Blackwell Publishing.

Houlgate, S. (2013). *Hegel's Phenomenology of Spirit*. London: Bloomsbury.

Hoy, D. (2009). The Ethics of Freedom: Hegel on Reason as Law-Giving and Law-Testing. In: K. Westphal (ed.). *The Blackwell Guide to Hegel's Phenomenology of Spirit*. Oxford: Wiley-Blackwell, pp. 153–71.

Ikaheimo, H. (2002). On the Genus and Species of Recognition. *Inquiry*, **45**(4), 447–62.

Ikaheimo, H. (2007). Recognising Persons. *Journal of Consciousness Studies*, **14**(5–6), 224–47.

Ikaheimo, H. (2009). A Vital Human Need: Recognition as Inclusion in Personhood. *European Journal of Political Theory*, **8**(1), 31–45.

Ikaheimo, H. (2011). Holism and Normative Essentialism in Hegel's Social Ontology. In: H. Ikaheimo and A. Laitinen (eds.). *Recognition and Social Ontology*. Leiden: Brill, pp. 145–209.

Ikaheimo, H. (2012). Globalising Love: On the Nature and Scope of Love as a Form of Recognition. *Res Publica*, **18**, 11–24.

Jackson, M. (1996). *Things as They Are: New Directions in Phenomenological Anthropology*. Bloomington: Indiana University Press.

Jackson, M. (2007). The Clinician's Illusion and Benign Psychosis. In: M. Chung M, KWM Fulford, and G. Graham (eds.) *Reconceiving Schizophrenia*. Oxford: Oxford University Press, pp. 235–54.

Jackson, M., and **Fulford, K.** (1997). Spiritual Experience and Psychopathology. *Philosophy, Psychiatry, and Psychology*, **4**(1), 41–65.

Jaspers, K. (1963). *General Psychopathology*, 7th edition. Trans. J. Hoenig and M. W. Hamilton. Manchester: University of Manchester Press.

Jenkins J, and **Barrett, R.** (2004). Introduction. In: J. Jenkins and R. Barrett (eds.) *Schizophrenia, Culture and Subjectivity*. Cambridge: Cambridge University Press, pp. 1–28.

Jones, N., and **Kelly, T.** (2015). Inconvenient Complications: On the Heterogeneities of Madness and Their Relationship to Disability. In: H. Spandler, J. Anderson, and B. Sapey (eds.). *Madness, Distress and the Politics of Disablement*. Bristol: Policy Press, pp. 43–56.

Jost, A. (2009). Mad Pride and the Medical Model. *Hastings Center Report*, **39**(4), c3.

Jung, C. (1970a). *Civilization in Transition. Collected Works of Carl Jung*, Volume 10. London: Routledge and Kegan Paul.

Jung, C. (1970b). *Aion. Collected Works of Carl Jung*, Volume 9ii. London: Routledge and Kegan Paul.

Kant, I. (1952 [1781]). *Critique of Pure Reason*. London: Macmillan.

Kant, I. (1998). *Groundwork of the Metaphysics of Morals*. Cambridge: Cambridge University Press.

Keating, F. (2015). Linking "Race", Mental Health and a Social Model of Disability: What Are the Possibilities? In: H. Spandler, J. Anderson, and B. Sapey (eds.). *Madness, Distress and the Politics of Disablement*. Bristol: Policy Press, pp. 127–38.

Keil, G., **Keuck, L.**, and **Hauswald, R.** (2017). Vagueness in Psychiatry: An Overview. In: G. Keil, L. Keuck, and R. Hauswald (eds.). *Vagueness in Psychiatry*. Oxford: Oxford University Press, pp. 3–23.

Kennett, J. (2009). Mental Disorder, Moral Agency, and the Self. In: B. Steinbock (eds.). *The Oxford Handbook of Bioethics*. Oxford: Oxford University Press, pp. 91–113.

Kennett, J., and **Matthews, S.** (2003). The Unity and Disunity of Agency. *Philosophy, Psychiatry, and Psychology*, **10**(4), 305–12.

Kingma, E. (2007). What Is It to Be Healthy? *Analysis*, **67**, 128–33.

Kingma, E. (2013). Naturalist Accounts of Mental Disorder. In: K. W. M. Fulford, M. Davies, R. Gipps, G. Graham, J. Sadler, G. Stanghellini, and T. Thornton (eds.). *The Oxford Handbook of Philosophy and Psychiatry*. Oxford: Oxford University Press, pp. 363–84.

Korsgaard, C. (1989). Personal Identity and the Unity of Agency: A Kantian Response to Parfit. *Philosophy and Public Affairs*, **18**(2), 101–32.

Korsgaard, C. (1996). *The Sources of Normativity*. Cambridge: Cambridge University Press.

Kraepelin, E. (1909). *Psychiatrie*, 8th edition. Leipzig, Austria: Barth.

Kukathas, C. (1992). Are There Any Cultural Rights? *Political Theory*, **20**(1), 105–39.

Kymlicka, W. (1991). *Liberalism, Community, and Culture*. Oxford: Oxford University Press.

Kymlicka, W. (1995). *Multicultural Citizenship: A Liberal Theory of Minority Rights*. Oxford: Oxford University Press.

Kymlicka, W. (2001). *Politics in the Vernacular: Nationalism, Multiculturalism, and Citizenship*. Oxford: Oxford University Press.

Kymlicka, W. (2010). The Rise and Fall of Multiculturalism? New Debates on Inclusion and Accommodation in Diverse Societies. *International Social Science Journal*, **61**(199), 97–112.

Laing, R. D. (1965). *The Divided Self: An Existential Study in Sanity and Madness*. London: Penguin Books.

Laing, R. D. (1967). *The Politics of Experience and the Bird of Paradise*. London: Penguin Books.

Laitinen, A. (2002). Interpersonal Recognition: A Response to Value or a Precondition of Personhood? *Inquiry*, **45**, 463–78.

Larsen, J. (2004). Finding Meaning in First Episode Psychosis: Experience, Agency and the Cultural Repertoire. *Medical Anthropology Quarterly*, **18**(4), 447–71.

Lauer, Q. (1993). *A Reading of Hegel's Phenomenology of Spirit*. New York: Fordham University Press.

Liegghio, M. (2013). A Denial of Being: Psychiatrization as Epistemic Violence. In: B. LeFrançois, R. Menzies, and G. Reaume (eds.). *Mad Matters: A Critical Reader in Canadian Mad Studies*. Toronto: Canadian Scholars' Press, pp. 122–9.

Littlewood, R. (1993). *Pathology and Identity: The Work of Mother Earth in Trinidad*. Cambridge: Cambridge University Press.

Littlewood, R. (1997). Commentary on "Spiritual Experience and Psychopathology." *Philosophy, Psychiatry, & Psychology*, **4**(1), 67–73.

Littlewood, R. (2004). Multiple Personality Disorder: A Clinical and Cultural Account. *Psychiatry*, **3**(8), 11–13.

Littlewood, R., and Douyon, C. (1997). Clinical Findings in Three Cases of Zombification. *The Lancet*, **350**, 1094–6.

Littlewood, R., and Lipsedge, M. (2004). *Aliens & Alienists: Ethnic Minorities & Psychiatry*. New York: Brunner-Routledge.

Longden, E. (2013). TED Talk: *The Voices in my Head*. Online: https://www.ted.com/talks/eleanor_longden_the_voices_in_my_head/up-next

Longden, E., Corstens, D., and Dillon, J. (2013). Recovery, Discovery, and Revolution: The Work of Intervoice and the Hearing Voices Movements. In: S. Coles, S. Keenan, and B. Diamond (eds.). *Madness Contested: Power and Practice*. Herefordshire: PCCS Books, pp. 161–80.

Lukes, S. (2008). *Moral Relativism*. London: Profile Books.

MacIntyre, A. (1984). *After Virtue: A Study in Moral Theory.* Notre Dame: University of Notre Dame Press.

Margalit, A. (2001). Recognizing the Brother and the Other. *Proceedings of the Aristotelian Society, Supplementary Volumes,* **75**, 127–39.

Margalit, A., and Halbertal, M. (1994). Liberalism and the Right to Culture. *Social Research,* **61**(3), 491–510.

Markell, P. (2003). *Bound by Recognition.* New Jersey: Princeton University Press.

Mead, G. (1967). *Mind, Self, and Society: From the Standpoint of a Social Behaviorist.* Illinois: University of Chicago Press.

Mende, J. (2016). *A Human Right to Culture and Identity: The Ambivalence of Group Rights.* London: Rowman and Littlefield.

Menzies, R., LeFrançois, B., and Reaume, G. (2013). Introducing Mad Studies. In: B. LeFrançois, R. Menzies, and G. Reaume (eds.). *Mad Matters: A Critical Reader in Canadian Mad Studies.* Toronto: Canadian Scholars' Press, pp. 1–22.

McBride, C. (2013). *Recognition.* Cambridge: Polity Press.

McKay, R., and Cipolotti, L. (2007). Attributional Style in a Case of Cotard Delusion. *Consciousness and Cognition,* **16**(2), 349–59.

McLean, A. (1995). Empowerment and the Psychiatric Consumer/ Ex-patient Movement in the United States: Contradictions, Crisis and Change. *Social Science and Medicine,* **40**(8), 1053–71.

McNay, L. (2008). *Against Recognition.* Cambridge: Polity Press.

McWade, B., Milton, D., and Beresford, P. (2015). Mad Studies and Neurodiversity: A Dialogue. *Disability and Society,* **30**(2), 305–9.

Midgley, M. (1991). *Can't We Make Moral Judgments?* Bristol: Bristol Press.

Morris, S. (2000). Heaven Is a Mad Place on Earth. In: T. Curtis, R. Dellar, E. Leslie, and B. Watson (eds.). *Mad Pride: A Celebration of Mad Culture.* Truro: Chipmunka Publishing, pp. 207–8.

Morrison, L. (2005). *Talking Back to Psychiatry: The Psychiatric Consumer/ Survivor/ Ex-Patient Movement.* London: Routledge.

Moynihan, P. J. (2016). Healing Voices. Online: http://healingvoicesmovie.com/

Mulvany, J. (2000). Disability, Impairment or Illness? The Relevance of the Social Model of Disability to the Study of Mental Disorder. *Sociology of Health and Illness,* **22**(5), 582–601.

Murdoch, I. (1999). Vision and Choice in Morality. In: P. Conradi (ed.). *Existentialists and Mystics: Writings on Philosophy and Literature.* London: Penguin, pp. 80–1.

Nagel, T. (1997). *The Last Word.* Oxford: Oxford University Press.

Neuhouser, F. (2009). Desire, Recognition, and the Relation between Bondsman and Lord. In: K. Westphal (ed.). *The Blackwell Guide to Hegel's Phenomenology of Spirit.* Oxford: Wiley-Blackwell, pp. 37–54.

Nordenfelt, L. (1997). The Importance of a Disability/Handicap Distinction. *The Journal of Medicine and Philosophy,* **22**, 607–22.

Novotny, K. (1998). "Taylor"-Made? Feminist Theory and the Politics of Identity. *Women and Politics,* **19**(3), 1–18.

Oliver, M. (1990). *The Politics of Disablement.* Basingstoke: Macmillan.

Oliver, M. (1996). *Understanding Disability.* Basingstoke: Macmillan.

Oliver, M. (2004). The Social Model in Action: If I had a Hammer. In: C. Barnes and G. Mercer (eds.). *Implementing the Social Model of Disability: Theory and Research*. Leeds: Disability Press, pp. 18–31.

Olson, E. (2003). Personal Identity. In: S. Stich and T. Warfield (eds.). *The Blackwell Guide to Philosophy of Mind*. Oxford: Blackwell Publishing, pp. 352–68.

Padden, C., and Humphries, T. (2005). *Inside Deaf Culture*. London: Harvard University Press.

Parfit, D. (1984). *Reasons and Persons*. Oxford: Oxford University Press.

Peddie, J. (2014). *Understanding Experience and Constructing Identity in Spiritually Transformative Accounts of Psychosis*. University of East London PhD Thesis. Online: http://roar.uel.ac.uk/4607/1/James%20Peddie.pdf

Peirce, C. (1958). *The Collected Papers of C. S. Peirce*, Volumes 1–8. Cambridge, MA: Harvard University Press.

Perring, C. (2009). "Madness" and "Brain Disorders": Stigma and Language. In: K. White (ed.). *Configuring Madness: Representation, Context and Meaning*. Oxford: Inter-Disciplinary Press, pp. 3–24.

Peterson, D. (1982). (ed.). *A Mad People's History of Madness*. Pennsylvania: University of Pittsburgh Press.

Phillips, J. (2003). Self-Narrative in Schizophrenia. In: T. Kircher and A. David (eds.). *The Self in NeuroScience and Psychiatry*. Cambridge: Cambridge University Press, pp. 319–35.

Pilgrim, D., and Tomasini, F. (2012). On Being Unreasonable in Modern Society: Are Mental Health Problems Special? *Disability and Society*, 27(5), 631–46.

Pinkard, T. (1994). *Hegel's Phenomenology: The Sociality of Reason*. Cambridge: Cambridge University Press.

Pinkard, T. (2002). *German Philosophy 1760–1860: The Legacy of Idealism*. Cambridge: Cambridge University Press.

Pippin, R. (1989). *Hegel's Idealism: The Satisfactions of Self-Consciousness*. Cambridge: Cambridge University Press.

Pippin, R. (2000). What Is the Question for Which Hegel's Theory of Recognition is the Answer? *European Journal of Philosophy*, 8(2), 155–72.

Pippin, R. (2008a). *Hegel's Practical Philosophy: Rational Agency as Ethical Life*. Cambridge: Cambridge University Press.

Pippin, R. (2008b). Recognition and Reconciliation: Actualised Agency in Hegel's Jena Phenomenology. In: B. Van Den Brink, and D. Owen (eds.). *Recognition and Power: Axel Honneth and the Tradition of Critical Social Theory*. Cambridge: Cambridge University Press, pp. 57–78.

Pippin, R. (2010). *Hegel on Self-Consciousness: Desire and Death in the Phenomenology of Spirit*. New Jersey: Princeton University Press.

Plumb, S. (2005). The Social/Trauma Model: Mapping the Mental Health Consequences of Childhood Sexual Abuse and Similar Experiences. In: J. Tew (ed.). *Social Perspectives in Mental Health: Developing Social Models to Understand and Work with Mental Distress*. London: Jessica Kingsley Publishers, pp. 112–28.

Polvora (2011). Diagnosis "Human". *Icarus Project Zine*. April 2011, 4–5. Online: http://www.theicarusproject.net/article/community-zines

Poole, J., and Ward, J. (2013). "Breaking Open the Bone": Storying, Sanism, and Mad Grief. In: B. LeFrançois, R. Menzies, and G. Reaume (eds.). *Mad Matters: A Critical Reader in Canadian Mad Studies*. Toronto: Canadian Scholars' Press, pp. 94–104.

Price, M. (2013). Defining Mental Disability. In: L. Davis (ed.). *The Disability Studies Reader.* New York: Taylor & Francis, pp. 298–307.

Quante, M. (2010). "The Pure Notion of Recognition": Reflections on the Grammar of the Relation of Recognition in Hegel's *Phenomenology of Spirit.* In: H. Schmidt am Busch and C. Zurn (eds.). *The Philosophy of Recognition: Historical and Contemporary Perspectives.* Lanham: Lexington Books, pp. 89–106.

Quinton, A. (1991). Ayer's Place in the History of Philosophy. In: Phillips Griffiths (ed.). *A. J. Ayer: Memorial Essays.* Cambridge: Cambridge University Press, pp. 31–48.

Radden, J. (1985). *Madness and Reason.* London: George, Allen, and Unwin.

Radden, J. (1996). *Divided Minds and Successive Selves: Ethical Issues in Disorders of Identity and Personality.* Cambridge, MA: MIT Press.

Radden, J. (1998). Pathologically Divided Minds, Synchronic Unity and Models of Self. *Journal of Consciousness Studies,* **5**(5–6), 658–72.

Radden, J. (2003). Learning from Disunity. *Philosophy, Psychiatry, and Psychology,* **10**(4), 357–9.

Radden, J. (2004). Identity: Personal Identity, Characterization Identity, and Mental Disorder. In: J. Radden (ed.). *The Philosophy of Psychiatry: A Companion.* Oxford: Oxford University Press, pp. 133–46.

Radden, J. (2011). *On Delusion.* London: Routledge.

Radden, J. (2012). Recognition Rights, Mental Health Consumers and Reconstructive Cultural Semantics. *Philosophy, Ethics and Humanities in Medicine,* **7**(6), 1–8.

Radden, J., and Sadler, J. (2010). *The Virtuous Psychiatrist: Character Ethics in Psychiatric Practice.* Oxford: Oxford University Press.

Rashed, M. A. (2010). Religious Experience and Psychiatry: Analysis of the Conflict and Proposal for a Way Forward. *Philosophy, Psychiatry & Psychology,* **17**(3), 185–204.

Rashed, M. A. (2012). *Subjectivity, Society, and the Experts: Discourses of Madness.* PhD Thesis, University College London.

Rashed, M. A. (2013a). Culture, Salience, and Psychiatric Diagnosis: Exploring the Concept of Cultural Congruence and Its Practical Application. *Philosophy, Ethics and Humanities in Medicine,* **8**(5), 1–12.

Rashed, M. A. (2013b). Talking Past Each Other: Conceptual Confusion in Culture and Psychopathology. *South African Journal of Psychiatry,* **19**(1), 12–15.

Rashed, M. A. (2013c). Psychiatric Judgements Across Cultural Contexts: Relativist, Clinical-Ethnographic, and Universalist-Scientific Perspectives. *Journal of Medicine and Philosophy,* **38**(2), 128–48.

Rashed, M. A. (2015a). A Critical Perspective on Second-order Empathy in Understanding Psychopathology: Phenomenology and Ethics. *Theoretical Medicine and Bioethics,* **36**, 97–116.

Rashed, M. A. (2015b). Islamic Perspectives on Psychiatric Ethics. In: J. Sadler, C. W. van Staden, and K. W. M. Fulford (eds.). *The Oxford Handbook of Psychiatric Ethics,* Volume 1. Oxford: Oxford University Press, pp. 495–519.

Rashed, M. A. (2018a). In Defence of Madness: The Problem of Disability. *Journal of Medicine and Philosophy.* doi: org/10.1093/jmp/jhy016.

Rashed, M. A. (2018b). More Things in Heaven and Earth: Spirit Possession, Mental Disorder, and Intentionality. *Journal of Medical Humanities.* doi: org/10.1007/s10912-018-9519-z.

Rawls, J. (1973). *A Theory of Justice.* Cambridge, MA: The Belknap Press.

Read, J., and Dillon, J. (eds.) (2013). *Models of Madness: Psychological, Social, and Biological Approaches to Psychosis.* London: Routledge.

Read, J., Haslam, N. Sayce, L. and Davies, E. (2006). Prejudice and Schizophrenia: A Review of the "Mental Illness is an Illness Like Any Other" Approach. *Acta Psychiatr Scand,* **114**, 303–18.

Reaume, G. (2008). A History of Psychiatric Survivor Pride Day During the 1990s. *Consumer/ Survivor Information Resource Centre Bulletin,* No. 374: 2–3. Online: http://www.csinfo.ca/bulletin/Bulletin_374.pdf

Reeves, D. (2015). Psycho-emotional Disablism in the Lives of People Experiencing Mental Distress. In: H. Spandler, J. Anderson, and B. Sapey (eds.). *Madness, Distress and the Politics of Disablement.* Bristol: Policy Press, pp. 99–112.

Reiss, B. (2004). Letters from Asylumia: The Opal and the Cultural Work of the Lunatic Asylum, 1851–1860. *American Literary History,* **16**(1), 1–28.

Rethink. (2012). *What's Reasonable at Work? A Guide to Rights at Work for People with a Mental Illness.* London: Rethink Mental Illness.

Reznek, L. (2010). *Delusions and the Madness of the Masses.* New York: Rowman and Littlefield.

Rice, C. (2013). Defending the Objective List Theory of Well-Being. *Ratio,* **XXVI**(2 June), 196–211.

Risjord, M. (2012). Models of Culture. In: H. Kincaid (ed.). *The Oxford Handbook of Philosophy of Social Sciences.* Oxford: Oxford University Press, pp. 387–408.

Roe, D., and Davidson, L. (2005). Self and Narrative in Schizophrenia: Time to Author a New Story. *Medical Humanities,* **31**, 89–94.

Rorty, R. (1998). *Truth and Progress: Philosophical Papers,* Volume **3**. Cambridge: Cambridge University Press.

Rorty, R. (1999). *Philosophy and Social Hope.* London: Penguin.

Rosenthal, K. P. (2010). *Crooked Beauty.* From *Mad Dance Mental Health Film Trilogy.* Online: https://vimeo.com/28315394

Rossi, A. (1962). Some Pre-World War II Antecedents of Community Mental Health Theory and Practice. *Mental Hygiene,* **46**, 78–98.

Sacks, O. (1989). *Seeing Voices: A Journey into the World of the Deaf.* Berkeley: University of California Press.

Sanati, A., and Kyratsous, M. (2015). Epistemic Injustice in Assessment of Delusions. *Journal of Evaluation in Clinical Practice,* **21**(3), 479–85.

Sandel, M. (1982). *Liberalism and the Limits of Justice.* Cambridge: Cambridge University Press.

Sass, L. (2003). Self-disturbance in Schizophrenia: Hyperreflexivity and Diminished Self-affection. In: T. Kircher and A. David (eds.). *The Self in Neuroscience and Psychiatry.* Cambridge, UK: Cambridge University Press, pp. 242–71.

Sass, L., and Parnas, J. (2007). Explaining Schizophrenia: The Relevance of Phenomenology. In: M. Chung, K. W. M. Fulford, and G. Graham (eds.). *Reconceiving Schizophrenia.* Oxford: Oxford University Press, pp. 63–96.

Sass, L., and Pienkos, E. (2013). Delusion: The Phenomenological Approach. In: K. W. M. Fulford, M. Davies, R. Gipps, G. Graham, J. Sadler, G. Stanghellini, and T. Thornton (eds.). *The Oxford Handbook of Philosophy and Psychiatry.* Oxford: Oxford University Press, pp. 632–57.

Schrader, S., Jones, N., and Shattell, M. (2013). Mad Pride: Reflections on Sociopolitical Identity and Mental Diversity in the Context of Culturally Competent Psychiatric Care. *Issues in Mental Health Nursing*, **34**, 62–4.

Sen, D. (2011). What Is Mad Culture? *Asylum: The Magazine for Democratic Psychiatry*, **18**(1), 5.

Shapiro, I. (2003). *The Moral Foundations of Politics*. New Haven: Yale University Press.

Siep, L. (2011). Mutual Recognition: Hegel and Beyond. In: H. Ikaheimo and A. Laitinen (eds.). *Recognition and Social Ontology*. Leiden: Brill, pp. 117–44.

Siep, L. (2014). *Hegel's Phenomenology of Spirit*. Cambridge: Cambridge University Press.

Silvers, A. (2010). An Essay on Modelling: The Social Model of Disability. In: D. Ralston and J. Ho (eds.). *Philosophical Reflections on Disability*. Dordrecht: Springer, pp. 19–36.

Sims, A. (2003). *Symptoms in the Mind*. Philadelphia: Elsevier.

Smiles, S. (2011). Indicator Species. *Icarus Project Zine*. April 2011, 8–9. Online: http://www.theicarusproject.net/article/community-zines

Solomon, R. (1983). *In the Spirit of Hegel: A Study of G. W.F. Hegel's Phenomenology of Spirit*. Oxford: Oxford University Press.

Spandler, H., and Anderson, J. (2015). Unreasonable Adjustments? Applying Disability Policy to Madness and Distress. In: H. Spandler, J. Anderson, and B. Sapey (eds.). *Madness, Distress and the Politics of Disablement*. Bristol: Policy Press, pp. 13–25.

Sparrow, R. (2005). Defending Deaf Culture: The Case of Cochlear Implants. *The Journal of Political Philosophy*, **13**(2), 135–52.

Stanghellini, G. (2004). *Disembodied Spirits and Deanimated Bodies: The Psychopathology of Common Sense*. Oxford: Oxford University Press.

Stern, R. (2002). *Hegel and the Phenomenology of Spirit*. London: Routledge.

Stern, R. (2009). *Hegelian Metaphysics*. Oxford: Oxford University Press.

Stone, A. (2004). Essentialism and Anti-Essentialism in Feminist Philosophy. *The Journal of Moral Philosophy*, **1**(2), 135–53.

Sullivan-Bissett, E., Bortolotti, L., Broome, M., and Mameli, M. (2017). Moral and Legal Implications of the Continuity Between Delusional and Non-Delusional Beliefs. In: G. Keil, L. Keuck, and R. Hauswald (eds.). *Vagueness in Psychiatry*. Oxford: Oxford University Press. doi: 10.1093/med/9780198722373.003.0010.

Sunderland, M. (2015). In Rachel Dolezal's Skin. *Broadly Online Magazine*. Online: https://broadly.vice.com/en_us/article/gvz79j/rachel-dolezal-profile-interview

Sutherland, S. (1991). Language, Newspeak and Logic. In: P. Griffiths (eds.). *A. J. Ayer: Memorial Essays*. Cambridge: Cambridge University Press, pp. 77–88.

Swidler, A. (1986). Culture in Actions: Symbols and Strategies. *American Sociological Review*, **51**(2), 273–86.

Szasz, T. (1960). The Myth of Mental Illness. *American Psychologist*, **15**, 113–18.

Tamir, Y. (1998). A Strange Alliance: Isaiah Berlin and the Liberalism of the Fringes. *Ethical Theory and Moral Practice*, **1**(2), 279–89.

Taylor, C. (1979). *Hegel and Modern Society*. Cambridge: Cambridge University Press.

Taylor, C. (1982). Rationality. In: M. Hollis and S. Lukes (eds.). *Rationality and Relativism*. Cambridge, MA: The MIT Press, pp. 87–105.

Taylor, C. (1985). *Human Agency and Language: Philosophical Papers I*. Cambridge: Cambridge University Press.

Taylor, C. (1989). *Sources of the Self: The Making of the Modern Identity.* Cambridge: Cambridge University Press.

Taylor, C. (1991). *The Ethics of Authenticity.* London: Harvard University Press.

Taylor, C. (1994a). The Politics of Recognition. In: A. Gutmann (ed.). *Multiculturalism: Examining the Politics of Recognition.* New Jersey: Princeton University Press, pp. 25–73.

Taylor, C. (1994b). Can Liberalism be Communitarian? *Critical Review,* **8**(2), 257–62.

Taylor, C. (2007). *A Secular Age.* Cambridge, MA: Belknap Press.

Tempelman, S. (1999). Constructions of Cultural Identity: Multiculturalism and Exclusion. *Political Studies,* **47**(1), 17–31.

Tenney, L. (2006). Who Fancies to Have a Revolution Here? The Opal Revisited (1851–1860). *Radical Psychology,* **5**. Online: http://www.radpsynet.org/journal/vol5/Tenney.html

Terzi, L. (2004). The Social Model of Disability: A Philosophical Critique. *Journal of Applied Philosophy,* **21**(2), 141–57.

Tew, J. (2005). Core Themes of Social Perspectives. In: J. Tew (ed.). *Social Perspectives in Mental Health: Developing Social Models to Understand and Work with Mental Distress.* London: Jessica Kingsley Publishers, pp. 13–31.

Tew, J. (2015). Towards a Socially Situated Model of Mental Distress. In: H. Spandler, J. Anderson, and B. Sapey (eds.). *Madness, Distress and the Politics of Disablement.* Bristol: Policy Press, pp. 69–82.

Thomas, C. (2004). Developing the Social Relational in the Social Model of Disability: A Theoretical Agenda. In: C. Barnes and G. Mercer (eds.). *Implementing the Social Model of Disability: Theory and Research.* Leeds: Disability Press, pp. 32–47.

Thomas, P. (2013). Soteria: Contexts, Practice, and Philosophy. In: S. Coles, S. Keenan, and B. Diamond (eds.). *Madness Contested: Power and Practice.* Herefordshire: PCCS Books, pp. 141–58.

Thomas, P. and Bracken, P. (2008). Power, Freedom, and Mental Health: A Postpsychiatry Perspective. In: C. Cohen and S. Timimi (eds.). *Liberatory Psychiatry: Philosophy, Politics, and Mental Health.* Cambridge: Cambridge University Press, pp. 35–53.

Thornicroft, G., Brohan, E., Kassam, A., and Lewis-Holmes, E. (2008). Reducing Stigma and Discrimination: Candidate Interventions. *International Journal of Mental Health Systems,* **2**(3), 1–7.

Triest, A. (2012). Mad? There's a Movement for That. *Shameless Magazine,* **21**, 20–1.

Tuvel, R. (2017). In Defense of Transracialism. *Hypatia,* **32**(2), 263–78.

Tylor, E. (1891). *Primitive Culture: Researches into the Development of Mythology, Philosophy, Religion, Language, Art, and Custom.* London: John Murray.

Wakefield, J. (1992). The Concept of Mental Disorder: On the Boundary Between Biological Facts and Social Values. *American Psychologist,* **47**(3), 373–88.

Wallcraft, J., Read, J., and Sweeney, A. (2003). *On Our Own Terms: Users and Survivors of Mental Health Services Working Together for Support and Change.* London: The Sainsbury Centre for Mental Health.

Wartenberg, T. (1993). Hegel's Idealism: The Logic of Conceptuality. In: F. Beiser (ed.). *The Cambridge Companion to Hegel.* Cambridge: Cambridge University Press, pp. 102–29.

Watson, B. (2000). Towards a Critical Madness. In: T. Curtis, R. Dellar, E. Leslie, and B. Watson (eds.). *Mad Pride: A Celebration of Mad Culture.* Truro: Chipmunka Publishing, pp. 105–24.

Wells, L. (2003). Discontinuity in Personal Narrative: Some Perspectives of Patients. *Philosophy, Psychiatry, and Psychology*, **10**(4), 297–303.

Westphal, K. (1989). *Hegel's Epistemological Realism: A Study of the Aim and Method of Hegel's Phenomenology of Spirit*. Dordrecht and Boston: Kluwer.

Williams, R. (1958). *Culture and Society: Coleridge to Orwell*. London: Chatto and Windus.

Williams, R. (1992). *Recognition: Fichte and Hegel on the Other*. New York: State University of New York Press.

Williams, R. (1997). *Hegel's Ethics of Recognition*. Berkeley: University of California Press.

Withers, A. (2014). Disability, Divisions, Definitions, and Disablism: When Resisting Psychiatry is Oppressive. In: B. Burstow, B. LeFrançois, and S. Diamond (eds.). *Psychiatry Disrupted: Theorizing Resistance and Crafting the (R)evolution*. Montreal: Mc-Gill-Queen's University Press, pp. 114–28.

Woods, A. (2013). The Voice-Hearer. *Journal of Mental Health*, **22**(3), 263–70.

Young, A., and Leafhead, K. (1996). Betwixt Life and Death: Case Studies of the Cotard Delusion. In: P. Halligan and J. Marshall (eds.). *Method in Madness: Case Studies in Cognitive Neuropsychiatry*. New York: Taylor and Francis, pp. 147–72.

Zachar, P. (2000). Psychiatric Disorders Are Not Natural Kinds. *Philosophy, Psychiatry and Psychology*, **7**, 167–82.

Zachar, P. (2015). Psychiatric Disorders: Natural Kinds Made by the World or Practical Kinds Made by Us? *World Psychiatry*, **14**(3), 288–90.

Zurn, C. (2000). Anthropology and Normativity: A Critique of Axel Honneth's "Formal Conception of Ethical Life". *Philosophy & Social Criticism*, **26**(1), 115–24.

Author Index